Civil War Camps

and

Soldier Health

INTERPRETING THE CIVIL WAR

Texts and Contexts

The **Interpreting the Civil War** series focuses on America's long Civil War era, from the rise of antebellum sectional tensions through Reconstruction.

These studies, which include both critical monographs and edited compilations, bring new social, political, economic, or cultural perspectives to our understanding of sectional tensions, the war years, Reconstruction, and memory. Studies reflect a broad, national perspective; the vantage point of local history; or the direct experiences of individuals through annotated primary source collections.

Civil War Camps and Soldier Health

Sanitation and Military Effectiveness in the Union Army

Earl J. Hess

The Kent State University Press

Kent, Ohio

ISBN 978-1-60635-505-3 (paperback)
ISBN 978-1-63101-583-0 (epub)

The manufacturer's authorized representative in the EU for product safety is Mare Nostrum Group B.V., Mauritskade 21D, 1091 GC Amsterdam, The Netherlands, email gpsr@mare-nostrum.co.uk.

Cataloging information for this title is available at the Library of Congress.

For Pratibha and Julie,
With Love

Contents

Introduction

Soon after the end of the Civil War, Charles Anderson, then governor of Ohio, wrote to Secretary of War Edwin M. Stanton about the complaints volunteer soldiers often had lodged about their living conditions in the army. Those complaints that related "to their food, exposures, diseases, & c." were "in fact unavoidable incidents to all military service," Anderson correctly noted. In fact, he identified the major challenges to soldier health and simultaneously relegated them to a category of ills that had to be accepted to some degree or other if one wanted to organize a large military force.[1]

A sizeable and important group of people in the Northern states would have agreed with Anderson that those camp ills were to be expected, but they would have strongly disagreed with him that they had to be accepted. The Civil War was a potential watershed in awareness of preventive healthcare in the army, the first conflict in American history in which serious attempts were launched to educate officers and men that camp diseases could be attacked by changing the camp environment. These attempts were made mostly through the US Sanitary Commission, a nongovernmental organization sanctioned by the Federal government as an advisory agency. Sanitary Commission workers moved throughout the Union army to inspect camps; evaluate the living conditions from a "sanitary," or health, perspective; and make recommendations to regimental commanders and surgeons about how to improve conditions. Their recommendations were not mandatory; the commission had no authority to enforce anything, only to advise and encourage. But it was the first organization of any kind outside the corps of professional US Army surgeons to attempt a program of preventive healthcare in American military history.

The Sanitary Commission also was the first organization in America to attempt a comprehensive evaluation of army camps, soldier health, and military effectiveness by assembling a huge number of camp inspection reports from 1861 to 1864. Those reports, which commission officials called "returns," amounted to more than 1,400 documents when the program began to decline a year before the war ended. The purpose of these returns was not only to understand actual camp conditions among the hundreds of volunteer regiments but also to gauge whether volunteer officers and regimental surgeons took seriously the commission's wise sanitary principles, some of which regular officers had long tried to enforce in the small, prewar US Army. The question was could the hastily raised volunteer regiments, led by men from the same community and similar social conditions as the rank and file, meet the challenges inherent in camp life during wartime and create environments that would promote soldier health. A related question was could the civilian physicians who joined those volunteer regiments as surgeons learn how to become military healthcare providers, cooperating with regimental commanders to implement preventive healthcare measures. Civil War sanitarians in civilian society and professional army surgeons thought the answers to these questions had a direct effect on whether the young volunteers in blue would survive the war. They knew that disease of all kinds sent more soldiers to hospitals and to their graves than did combat. The volunteers themselves were hardly aware of these problems when they enrolled for army service, and thus a hefty load of education fell on the shoulders of the commission officials and inspectors as well as the professional army surgeons.

The sanitarian movement, relatively recent and limited in the United States before 1861, had a potent example in the Crimean War of 1853–56 in its efforts to improve military health during the Civil War. In that recent conflict, British and French armed forces had suffered horribly because of poor camp sanitation. The experience of the Crimean War not only spurred a major effort in both Britain and France to clean up camps and barracks but also served as a warning for what could happen to young American volunteers if some effort to avert medical disaster was not attempted.

Thus, the US Sanitary Commission was created in 1861. Among its most important goals was to employ the knowledge of its physicians as well as the Crimean example to spur the Union army to new efforts at camp sanitation. The primary method of achieving this was to institute a large and ambitious camp inspection program. Hiring inspectors (typically physicians), sending them to semipermanent army camps, and requiring them to consult with regimental commanders and unit surgeons, the program charged inspectors with completing a standard return that covered fifteen subject areas. The return thus became a snapshot of one regiment's state of camp sanitation, allowing the commission to understand how far it had gone toward the ideal level of clean and healthy soldiering. The inspection process also introduced ideas about camp sanitation to unit officers who were charged by the army with responsibility for supervising their men's health. In many cases the inspector was the first person to tell these volunteer commanders that they had to pay attention to something more than just drilling their men and ensuring they had proper weapons and ammunition. The commission operated this program with the consent of the government, but it was not given any powers to force its standards on regimental officers. Camp inspectors arrived at regimental camps as visitors and advisors, not as enforcers.

The fifteen subject areas on the standard camp inspection form constituted a list of the most important factors in preventive healthcare for soldiers.

1. Camp situation: This subject area dealt with how the semipermanent camps were situated in relation to the environment. It related to the careful selection of campsites in consideration of different types of soil, the grade of landscape, and the arrangement of tents. How much fresh air was available, the type of soil in the area, and how the camp was situated in relation to tree and brush cover were key elements in the principles of camp hygiene. The idea was to keep the camp clean, exposed to good air flow, placed away from tree cover, and planted on soil that easily drained.

2. Shelter: Inspectors evaluated the quality of living quarters, whether that was tents, huts, barracks, or civilian structures. The area around the quarters had to be dry, allow fresh air to enter and bad air to leave, and not be overcrowded. While huts, barracks, and even some quartering in civilian houses can be seen in the Civil War, most soldiers lived in tents. Sanitary principles stressed air flow inside the tent, lifting up the sides for circulation, and urged soldiers to move the tent a few feet every now and then to remain on fresh ground as often as possible. Barracks were unhealthy places for many reasons as far as sanitarians were concerned; huts were halfway between a good tent and a bad barracks in their view.

3. Clothing: Military sanitarians felt strongly about army clothing and discussed it in detail, stressing the need to avoid tight-fitting, colorful uniforms,

but they argued over exactly what type of material was best for soldier wear. Nevertheless, the camp inspection returns generally focus on whether all the clothing items a man was supposed to receive were actually given to him and the durability of the cloth, avoiding much of the arguments over color, style, and material that one can find in the sanitary literature.

4. Personal cleanliness: This subject area ranked high on the list of priorities for camp inspectors. It remained somewhat delicate because of the inherent invasion of privacy, but inspectors relied on the testimony of regimental officers and surgeons for their perspective on the topic. The emphasis was on how often to wash underwear, how often to bathe, and whether the men dusted and washed their clothes and washed their hands, faces, and necks regularly.

5. Slops: This term was used in the Civil War era to refer to the disposal of kitchen and food waste along with other trash. Slops related directly to the need for maintaining a clean camp and avoiding the intrusion of insects and other pests that would be attracted to the waste. Typically, regiments set up barrels for the men to collect the waste before dumping it outside the limits of the camp.

6. Sinks: The military culture of the Civil War era assigned the word *sinks* to the need for disposing of human waste. There was a prescribed army way to dig sinks, more commonly called "latrines" in the twentieth century. It involved creating a trench with a railing along the edge and placing some brush along the side to screen the men who used it. Most units dug sinks, but few covered the contents with a daily layer of fresh dirt or with disinfectants. A number of them had no sinks at all, forcing the men to relieve themselves wherever they wished. Even regiments with sinks had difficulty forcing the men to use them consistently.

7. Food: Inspectors focused on the quality of army rations, not just in terms of quantity and lack of spoilage but also in terms of a relatively balanced diet of meat, vegetables, and fruits. How often were different items on the ration actually issued? Army regulations stipulated that officers and surgeons were to superintend the rations and the cooking by their men, and most regiments had some oversight of those aspects. But this was inconsistent, and in some units such supervision did not exist at all.

8. Cooking: How well did the men cook their rations to achieve a healthy way of consuming their food? How was cooking organized in the army, and did the cooks maintain good care of their utensils for health purposes? Sanitarians strongly urged collective cooking by designated company cooks who prepared rations for everyone as the most efficient and best managed

system. But most Northern soldiers much preferred to cook individually or in small, self-constituted messes so they could exercise more freedom in how and when to cook. This was the worst way to prepare food in the eyes of the sanitarians, especially when soldiers failed to properly clean utensils.

9. Water: Good water was just as important as good rations, and the camp inspection returns included this need as one of its subject areas. Did water used for drinking, cooking, bathing, and laundering come from springs, streams, rivers, or municipal facilities? How clean was it, and how near were sources of contamination? A camp needed to be located near a good source of water, which by sanitary standards meant any flowing and clean source, such as a spring or a stream. The worst source was runoff water draining from the surface into a brook because it brought with it all the contaminants laying on the ground.

10. Alcohol: The inspectors were charged with gauging the extent to which liquor was a problem in a unit's semipermanent camp. Did the men have access to it, and if so did it lead to significant disciplinary issues as well as health problems? While historians have generally assumed that alcohol posed a major problem in the army, the results of the camp inspection returns give us reason to question that assumption. The picture they reveal is that uncontrollable alcoholic consumption was restricted to a handful of men in each regiment, with a considerable proportion of soldiers joining the temperance movement and the rest gravitating toward only occasional drinking.

11. Morale: Inspectors introduced what was to many regimental officers a new idea—that they should try to shape the morale, or the sense of well-being, among the rank and file. Officers could do this by creating regimental libraries, encouraging games and athletic exercises, and maintaining a regimental band. The camp inspection program focused on institutional efforts to shape soldier morale, but the returns reveal that beyond supporting a band and a library in a few regiments, very little was done to address this issue.

12. Recruit examination: The US Army required a thorough physical examination of all recruits before the Civil War, demanding the same of the volunteer regiments raised by state governments for temporary service during the conflict. But whether the volunteer regiments had undertaken that task when organized, and whether they followed up with subsequent examinations, were questions asked by the camp inspectors. Volunteer officers had a vested interest in getting as many men into the regiment as possible and usually did not allow the surgeon to properly examine each

before muster in. This caused problems when a certain percentage of all men in every regiment had to be hospitalized for health problems related to their civilian lives within weeks of entering the army. Many of them had to be discharged for disability, causing much unnecessary expense and trouble for the army healthcare system.

13. Vaccination: Camp inspectors wanted to know if a thorough system of inoculation to prevent the spread of smallpox had been undertaken at regimental organization or after the unit's creation. This also was official US Army policy before the war and was supposed to be followed by the volunteer regiments as well. But the returns show that most volunteer surgeons failed to properly vaccinate the men on enlistment. Yet they reacted vigorously at the first sign of an outbreak of smallpox within the ranks by quarantining the affected men and fully vaccinating everyone within reach. Vaccination had been so widespread in pre–Civil War America that many people thought the threat of smallpox had receded by the 1860s, which was not really the case. Many outbreaks of the disease occurred in the Union army, but all of them were contained by quick and decisive action before they got out of hand.

14. Regimental hospitals: Camp inspectors did a thorough job of evaluating the regimental hospitals they visited. It was important to find out whether the facility was under proper shelter (usually tents or civilian houses), whether it had all the medicines and medical equipment allowed by the army, and whether the regimental surgeons had it well organized. The regimental hospital was the first step in the massive hospital system created by the Union army, and camp inspectors were told to pay detailed attention to each. The problems discovered largely revolved around lack of proper equipment and shortages of the full range of medical supplies, poor housing (bad tents or inadequate civilian structures), and poor administration by inadequate medical staff.

15. Officer supervision: Last but not least, the commission wanted to know about officer supervision in general. That applied to regimental and company commanders as well as regimental surgeons. Did they all understand their duty in regard to preventive healthcare? Did they exercise due diligence in trying to fulfill that duty? This last meant, among other things, seeing that equipment and supplies were on hand, inspecting the men's rations and cooking methods, thoroughly inspecting living quarters and personal cleanliness, making sure inoculation for smallpox had been thoroughly pursued, and limiting the men's access to alcohol, among many other things on a long list of responsibilities.

These fifteen subject areas reflect the broad vision of Civil War sanitarians. They fully understood their job as being far more than just encouraging the army to clean up its campsites. Their approach to preventive healthcare was comprehensive, complicated, and demanding. But a significant divide clearly existed between the civilian sanitarians and the regular-army surgeons on issues of sanitation, even though both healthcare groups were trying to work toward a common goal. Civilian sanitarians, especially those working within the Sanitary Commission, had very high standards in all these subject areas. In contrast, the professional army surgeons paid much attention to some of them, such as camp situation, physical examination, and smallpox inoculation, but paid little if any attention to others. The surgeons also tended to be practical and realistic; they knew from experience the difficulties of making men and officers toe a strict line regarding conditions that affected soldier health, and they tended to accept something less than ideal efforts and results. The civilian sanitarians worked from a standpoint of virtually no experience in army life or in war, and thus they often did not understand the attitude of the army personnel they encountered. Both groups were similar in their composition—they were dominated by men. Although women played a significant role in the creation of the Sanitary Commission and worked for it in many endeavors, they did not participate in the camp inspection program. That was an all-male effort both by the commission and, of course, by the army.

Nevertheless, the Sanitary Commission's camp inspection program was unprecedented. The returns are filled with detailed information on the fifteen subject areas across hundreds of regiments over two years of time. Historians have long known of these returns but have not mined them for details about camp conditions. Bell Irvin Wiley in his *The Life of Billy Yank*, originally published in 1952, devoted only 4 pages (out of 361) to a brief survey of some of the subject areas described above. Rather than looking at the returns, Wiley based that discussion on a couple of documents published by the commission that summarized the findings of a small set of returns. Four years later William Quentin Maxwell expanded a bit on using the returns when he wrote *Lincoln's Fifth Wheel,* a study that mostly focused on the political history of the US Sanitary Commission. Maxwell summarized the findings of Frederick Law Olmsted, an important commission official, who looked at the returns from two hundred regiments and wrote up a report published by the organization in December 1861. Olmsted concentrated on simple statistics early in the war designed to alert policymakers to the current state of camp sanitation. For example, he stated that 80 percent of the sinks were in good shape and the rest were terrible. The limitations of the report lie in the fact that they cover only the first few months of the war, and one cannot know if the returns Olmsted used represented the different theaters of operations or were concentrated on the Virginia theater, which was most easily accessible to commission inspectors.[2]

Even though Maxwell's use of the Olmsted report was limited, and the report itself also was limited, no subsequent historian touching on these issues has utilized the contents of the camp inspection returns as far as Maxwell did. Suellen Hoy, in her study of the personal cleanliness movement in America, briefly mentioned the returns without discussing their contents. Margaret Humphreys, in her general study of soldier health in the Civil War entitled *Marrow of Tragedy,* also discussed the camp inspection program but without looking at the content of the returns. Kathryn Shively Meier examined the contents of a few early returns to bolster several of her points in *Nature's Civil War.* But she was not able to investigate a significant number of them, fully analyze the contents of those she consulted, or arrive at statistical conclusions. Yet both in her book and in one article, "Organic Armies," Meier pointed to the relationship between the environment and soldier health, especially on campaign. Judkin Browning and Timothy Silver, authors of the standard environmental history of the Civil War, also point to that important relationship by briefly discussing camp cleanliness but without delving into the contents of the returns.[3]

No historian has yet probed the camp inspection returns deeply or comprehensively for their valuable information on soldier healthcare during the Civil War. No one has attempted a statistical analysis of their content by which we can gauge how effectively the army practiced preventive healthcare for its soldiers. How these returns can inform us about the military effectiveness of the volunteer army of the Union also is a question as yet unanswered.

To fill this gap in the historiography, I undertook a careful study of the camp inspection returns preserved in the US Sanitary Commission Records in the New York Public Library. The sheer size of the Sanitary Commission's work was daunting. The commission collected 1,465 returns from dozens of inspectors beginning in the spring of 1861 and extending into the early months of 1864. It would have taken several years to fully study all the reports. Perhaps that is a reason no other historian has examined them. To make a study of these returns manageable, I selected 280 of them spread across the spectrum of time (1861–64, the span of the collection), geographic location (East, West, and Trans-Mississippi), and unit types (infantry, cavalry, artillery, engineers, and Black units in rough proportion to their size in the Union army) to make my sample as representative as possible. Another reason for spreading the returns across these various categories was to allow an examination of similarities or differences among groups over time, location, and unit types—for example, whether camp sanitation altered over time.

Statistical analyses are usually run with a 5 percent sample to draw valid conclusions, but I felt more comfortable with almost 20 percent of the whole. It took nearly two years to study and analyze these 280 returns, which had been filled out by thirty-four inspectors. But they offer a gold mine of information about camp sanitation, serving as a diagnostic tool to gauge the level of preventive healthcare in the Union army. Supplemented by information from official army documents, personal accounts by soldiers, and the writings of Civil War sanitarians both in and out of uniform, this study focuses on the concept of preventive healthcare within the military system for the largest armed force the United States had created thus far in its history. It also assesses the level of effectiveness the commission's camp inspection program achieved and sets Civil War preventive healthcare within its larger American and European context before 1861 and after 1865. Delving into the details contained in these returns allows us to craft the deepest and most comprehensive picture of camp life in the Civil War yet presented.

Just as importantly, this study addresses the level of military effectiveness to be seen in the area of officer and surgeon care for their men. Studies of military effectiveness too often focus primarily on performance on the battlefield. While that is an obviously critical component of an army's work, it is not the only topic of importance.[4] Maintaining troop strength through preventative measures to avert disease is one of many other areas of military effectiveness that historians need to explore.

The value of diving deeply into the content of the camp inspection returns is that it offers a database for hard information on the fifteen subject areas. Instead of relying on personal accounts to understand any of those topics, one can find pointed commentary by camp inspectors buttressed by statistics emerging from the 280 returns selected for study. For the first time, this volume provides solid and deep information about camp life in the Civil War that sheds new light on many aspects of soldier health.

In addition to the Sanitary Commission inspection returns, there are other useful sources of information on camp living in the Civil War. The first of these are reports by medical inspectors. By 1863, the Union army mandated the appointment of medical inspectors at the higher levels of army organization, from the division up to the field army. Many reports by Fifteenth Corps medical inspectors were donated to the US Sanitary Commission and are preserved in the commission's papers at the New York Public Library. These reports cover a much more narrow range of topics relating to camp sanitation than do the commission's own returns, but they are valuable in their own way. Another source is personal accounts by soldiers. A third source resides in *The War of the Rebellion: A Compilation of the Official Records of the Union and Confederate Armies,* which illustrates the army's effort to promote camp sanitation. A fourth source consists of books and articles by Civil War sanitarians that greatly illuminate their vision for preventive healthcare measures as applied to the army. My purpose in the following chapters is to use all types of useful sources to set the context of each subject area covered by the commission's camp inspection program. For some subject areas, there are more contextual sources available than for others, but the end result for each is a miniessay on that topic. But in every subject area, the Sanitary Commission camp inspection returns provide the heart of the discussion and represent the most unique source type undergirding that discussion.

In the following chapters, one can see that soldier life in semipermanent camps was in many ways different than what we have thought. Examining the content of the camp inspection returns complicates and broadens our understanding of the complexities of soldier health. For example, the quick take on cleanliness was that camps were dirty. The returns do not support this superficial and casual conclusion. One can find many filthy camps in those returns, it is true, but one can also find just as many camps that were models of cleanliness. Every gradation in between also becomes apparent while looking through these 280 returns. Another misconception is that the Union army was well supplied. The returns illuminate this issue too. In terms of food, the overall answer is yes, Union forces were well supplied, but even this requires a more complex response. The army ration was plentiful, but it also was unbalanced, with too much emphasis on meat, too little on fresh vegetables, and almost none in the way of fruit. In terms of medical supplies and equipment for regimental hospitals, the overall answer is a surprising no. Historians have always assumed, based on colorful stories in soldiers' personal accounts, that the Union army was awash with liquor—well, not according to the camp inspection returns. The picture regarding alcohol is that a small percentage of men were addicted to drinking, and they often crowded the regimental guardhouses, but the problem was considered manageable by regimental commanders and surgeons. In fact, the returns document just as much sobriety as inebriation, proving that the temperance movement had an important influence on the young men who joined the army. Another assumption has been that junior-level officers, such as those who commanded companies and those who led regiments, were generally competent in performing their military duties. Perhaps that was so when it came to fighting on the battlefield, but it was not the case when it came to the varied aspects of preventive healthcare in camp. Generally, they did a middling to poor job of performing those duties, even though some officers and surgeons were models of effectiveness.

While this book concentrates on the Union army, the question of sanitation in the Confederate forces naturally grows out of its findings. Neither Southern society nor the Confederate army had anything that could be considered a sanitarian movement, although some individuals in and out of the government and military wrote about how camp life could be made less dangerous to soldier well-being. I have devoted one chapter to Confederate sanitation based on the limited sources available on the subject. The picture was more grim in the Confederate army than in the Union forces, despite genuine efforts by the authorities in impose sanitary principles on Southern young men.

Simple answers to complicated questions do not work if one wants to get an accurate understanding of the topic. Healthcare actually is one of the most complicated topics imaginable when studying armies at war, with military effectiveness perhaps only slightly less complicated. I can think of no better way to approach both topics than by studying detailed reports on important issues filed by men who actually visited Union army camps with the assignment of finding out how the troops lived.

Despite the unusual amount and type of information contained in these camp inspection returns, they do have some limitations as sources of historical inquiry. The inspection program was developed to evaluate semipermanent camps, which were occupied for an extended period of time (anywhere from days to months). No Sanitary Commission inspectors accompanied the troops when they were on active campaign and bivouacked for one night before moving on the next day. In fact, campaign and battle offered a very different set of health challenges to the soldier that the returns did not address.

Another small limitation is that the camp-inspection-return form changed over time, and not necessarily for the better. Fortunately, the best form was used for most of the 280 returns examined for this study. Also, a couple of the thirty-four inspectors who filled out these returns did not do their job as conscientiously as the rest, leaving out some information. But considering the unusual amount and kind of information that does appear on the returns, these small limitations pale in comparison to the opportunity the reports offer to understand preventive healthcare in the Union army. In fact, there is no other source that is so packed with detailed information on camp sanitation as these inspection returns; they are a unique set of documents.

Preventive healthcare was based largely on evaluating and changing the environment within which soldiers lived. Sanitarians saw the relationship of men to that environment, both natural and artificial, and sought to alter that relationship for the better. The Sanitary Commission operated within a medical culture that embraced the idea that most diseases had important environmental origins, that medical personnel should strive to prevent disease, and that there was an important link between a person's emotional well-being and their physical well-being. Historian Kathryn Shively Meier has consistently pointed to the environment as a key element in soldier health.[5] My study of the Sanitary Commission's camp inspection program thus contributes to that developing aspect of Civil War history by deepening our understanding of the human-centered environment of semipermanent camps.

After the conflict, sanitarians assured Americans that their efforts had worked wonders in saving Union soldiers from unnecessary health problems. But the evidence arising from a study of the camp inspection returns does not support that glowing assessment. It reveals that camp problems were only partially resolved during the conflict. One can say that Civil War sanitarians achieved greater success than had been achieved by their counterparts in most previous wars, but in other conflicts to follow, many other armies achieved more. Nor can one argue, as Civil War sanitarians did, that their efforts taught the country how to take care of soldiers. The horrible problems associated with camp filth and the spread of typhoid fever in military camps during the Spanish-American War (1898) destroyed that self-satisfying idea forty years after Appomattox.

Despite its limited success, the Sanitary Commission's camp inspection program was a milestone in the history of American military healthcare. It represented the first effort by any group of civilians to address the problems associated with soldier health, aided the army's limited effort at preventive healthcare, and provided a rich documentation of camp life in the Civil War. Within half a century after Appomattox, the army would surge ahead, spurred on by the horrible problems of camp sanitation in the Spanish-American War, to address far more fully and effectively the many challenges to soldier health. By World War I, it had managed to bring disease-related soldier fatalities down to about the same level as combat-related deaths. It further improved that ratio during World War II. While it is wrong to credit the US Sanitary Commission for this long-range improvement in soldier healthcare, it would be equally wrong to argue that it had nothing to do with it as well. The commission was very much on the right path when tackling the problems of camp sanitation in the Civil War, achieving some degree of success in that effort. The US Army did not build on that limited success in an explicit way afterward because it had its own, much more limited program of camp sanitation that proved as inadequate in 1861 as it would in 1898. If the Federal government had given enforcement powers to commission inspectors, it is likely that much more would have been accomplished by 1865, and the enlarged success of the commission's efforts might have carried over into 1898 as well. The commission and the military worked as two separate entities with inconsistent cooperation during the Civil War, so the lessons learned by the camp inspectors were not institutionalized by the army after 1865. An opportunity was missed to avoid the suffering of the Spanish-American War camps, which were filled with similarly eager but naive volunteer officers and men as had filled the army camps of the Civil War.

In short, it would be as wrong to argue that the Sanitary Commission camp inspection program was fully successful as it would be to argue that it was a dismal failure. Its limitations were mostly institutional in nature. The commission had no power within the army structure, which itself was overwhelmed by a multitude of responsibilities to the point that it could pay only limited attention to preventive healthcare. The army would have had a better chance of doing so if the volunteers had been funneled directly into regular units, as was to happen in twentieth-century wars. The chief institutional problem lay in the fact that the volunteers served in their own regiments, raised by the state governments in a perfunctory and hasty manner, before they entered Federal service. Those volunteer regiments thus maintained an existence apart from the regular army while serving the central government, and their internal administration was never fully controlled by the professionals. All depended on whether the volunteer officers and volunteer surgeons were willing to take regular-army regulations seriously enough to implement them in a conscientious manner. Some of them did so in spectacular fashion, while others callously neglected those wise instructions. The rest paid only middling respect to those rules. Much the same took place in the Spanish-American War.

Camp living in the Civil War was, therefore, a mixed bag containing a complicated set of circumstances that threatened soldier health. Sanitarians deserved a great deal of credit for trying to meet those challenges, and whatever degree of success they achieved was better than not trying at all. In many ways their efforts worked against the current of American culture. It represented a higher level of influence in shaping the living environment and thus the lives of nearly 3 million young men, most of whom gave little thought to the fifteen subject areas that were so important to the Sanitary Commission. Half a century after Appomattox, the developing corporate culture of the United States was much more conducive to the environmental engineering attempted by sanitary physicians of the Civil War era.

I wish to thank several people. My sincere gratitude goes to Angela Zombek for her appreciation of and support for this book project. I also wish to thank Kathryn Shively Meier for reading an earlier draft of the manuscript and offering good suggestions for improvement. Finally, I thank my wife Pratibha for her meticulous reading of the manuscript and her insights about making it better.

I

War and Soldier Health

As the North began to prepare for war following the fall of Fort Sumter in April 1861, a number of thoughtful people drew on an international heritage of soldier health in Western military history. They knew an important fact: the greatest threat to a fighting man's health was not bullet and shell but camp life itself. Simply living in the army exposed a recruit to a wide range of health threats, and sending him out on a field campaign exposed him to yet another set of threats to his well-being that had little to do with combat. Awareness of those facts was restricted to a relatively small group of people, many of whom were quite vocal in their advocacy of preventive healthcare in the army. Unfortunately, the overwhelming majority of volunteers who flocked to the colors were utterly unaware of those health threats, and most of them were not receptive to the news that they had a bigger chance of dying from disease than from bullets. Healthcare advocates had a big job ahead of them as the enthusiasm to save the Union swept the Northern population in those early months of the conflict.

For those who wanted to read it, there existed a considerable body of published work on the subject of army health, and for the historian, this has been significantly supplemented by recent scholarly studies. Reliable statistics for soldier deaths due to disease arising from living conditions date back to at least the late seventeenth century. Finnish garrisons in the Baltic region lost more than 37 men per 1,000 from 1662 to 1674, which scholars estimate was a ratio about twice as high as the mortality rate of civilians in that area. Similar disparity between the death rate in French regiments and the civilian population in the 1780s is documented.[1]

The Napoleonic Wars (1803–15) increased awareness of this persistent problem, not only for units in garrison but also for those campaigning in the field. British regiments on home station during 1801–5 suffered a death ratio estimated at between 50 and 100 percent above civilian rates. On average, British forces serving in the Peninsular War (1807–14) had 209 men sick in hospitals per 1,000, while their French opponents averaged 130 per 1,000. During a three-year period, more than 22 percent of all British forces in Iberia were "constantly sick." Hospital care during the Napoleonic Wars diverged into two systems: one based on regimental hospitals followed by the British, and the other based on general hospitals followed by the French and most Continental armies. Both systems had advantages and disadvantages. The general-hospital system required fewer medical staff by concentrating patients into larger groupings, which provided more uniform treatment and lowered administrative costs. But the regimental system provided closer attention to the individual, allowed more emotional support because the patient was among comrades, and produced less hospital gangrene because of the smaller groups of patients.[2] The Union and Confederate armies would maintain both systems of soldier healthcare during the Civil War.

The illnesses that brought so many soldiers to both hospital systems during the Napoleonic era ranged widely across the spectrum. Insect-borne diseases included yellow fever in Haiti, which killed one-third of a force of 20,000 men in 1802. Typhus and other diseases during the Russian campaign of 1812 killed 220,000 men on both sides. Bubonic plaque killed 92 percent of the soldiers who contracted it during the Middle East campaign of 1799, taking out of action at least 2,000 men of a force of 13,000 French troops.[3]

EUROPEAN SANITARY LITERATURE

The Napoleonic era also produced an increased desire to study the limitations of military medicine from the standpoint of preventive care. One of the earliest books on the subject came from Dr. Robert Jackson, a Scots-born physician who had served in the British forces during the southern campaigns of the American Revolutionary War (1775–83). After that conflict, he traveled extensively in Europe and became inspector general of army hospitals in the British Army during the Napoleonic Wars. Jackson was well placed to write a treatise on disease, preventive healthcare, and the military system, which was originally published in 1804 and reached its third edition by 1845, eighteen years after his death. Jackson's *A View of the Formation, Discipline, and Economy of Armies* influenced the Civil War generation's awareness of preventive healthcare issues in military life.[4]

Jackson began his treatise with a thorough discussion of martial races, having acquired, he thought, information on various nationalities and their aptitude for army service. Some of these ideas seeped into the American consciousness. Based on his personal experience, Jackson argued that the United States had won its independence more from British mismanagement than from American prowess. "They are not in general bold and resolute," he wrote of the colonists, although he thought they liked to boast of being so. Jackson believed in the concept of national character and thought that prewar occupations and the anatomy of the individual played large roles in a peoples' ability to become good soldiers. He believed that purer races produced men of greater endurance who were less susceptible to disease. Warmer climates produced men who grew to maturity faster, while in very cold climates men did not even reach their fullest physical development. Jackson therefore asserted that middling climates produced "physical and moral powers" because of the influence of both cold and hot climes. "The inhabitant of the temperate region has the best chance of attaining eminence in war." Jackson also argued that other environmental aspects influenced human ability and development, with damp or heavy air, flat or hilly terrain, and soil type all having their effect. A combination of rich soil and moist air was conducive to big physical development, while hilly and arid regions produced smaller and less powerful men.[5]

This heavy investment of race and environment in producing war-worthy specimens of humanity contradicted the other major theme of Jackson's book, a detailed discussion of how one could minimize the health threats to soldiers. The doctor did not seem aware of this basic contradiction as he pioneered in the discussion of preventive healthcare for armies. If it was true, as Jackson firmly knew, that the army environment was unhealthy and that one could change it to improve well-being, then one need not worry about the tortured logic and racist-tinged discussion of what kind of man made a healthy soldier. That is why this second emphasis of his book, preventive healthcare, was more influential to the Americans of the Civil War era than his discussion of race. Although William A. Hammond, the surgeon general of the US Army, included a similar discussion of racial types and martial aptitude in his *Treatise on Hygiene with Special Reference to the Military Service*, published in 1863, he was the only Civil War–era sanitarian to advocate this connection.

Jackson suggested a drastic alteration in the training regimen of British troops. He thought the recruit should first be instructed in how to take care of himself for six months, which included lessons in how to cook his food, how to wash and mend his clothes, and generally how to protect his health. He found that throughout Europe, military training neglected physical exercise as a way to toughen the recruit against disease and the stress of field campaigning. After this initial six-month period, Jackson advocated another six months of training in weapons use before the new soldier was sent to his regiment for duty. Even then he should be given a third six-month period to learn how to cooperate with his officers and comrades.[6] Jackson's suggestion for such an extended training period in preventive healthcare was farsighted, but it fell on deaf ears.

Living conditions while in the army drew intense scrutiny from Jackson. These fell into two categories—barracks while on permanent station and tents or huts "for moving armies." Jackson identified special health concerns in each grouping. "Where many men are collected together and confined within narrow limits, the atmosphere of the confined circle is liable to be corrupted." The key here was good ventilation for free circulation of fresh air. Barrack windows should extend all the way to the floor, and the lower part should swing open like a door. The ideal occupancy of a barrack room was twelve to fourteen men, with a partition for the sergeant's sleeping quarters. Jackson did not like tents because the moisture arising from the earth, coupled with the "poisoned emanations" from the men's breath, produced health risks. Still, this could be lessened by a wooden floor and good ventilation.[7] His discussion of these issues foreshadowed that of Civil War sanitarians.

Jackson correctly identified several major purposes for the soldier's uniform, which included offering a striking appearance to attract attention and encourage recruitment, conditioning the soldier to think of himself as part of a larger organization, and the utilitarian purpose of protecting health. This third purpose was the most important, in his view, and the least well served by British Army clothing, necessitating a gradual shift from woolen to flannel uniforms. Jackson felt that the feet were among the most important parts of a soldier's anatomy and needed special care. He advocated the issue of a flannel sock because "flannel preserves more equal temperature of heat than linen or cotton" and better protected against blistering. Army shoes needed to have "thick and firm outer soles," with "an inner sole which has an obscure sliding motion—the quarter short and high, so that mud or sand do not easily enter." The leather should be "well tanned" and coated with oil, wax, or tallow for water resistance. Hats should have big brims and deep crowns, and the soldier should be encouraged to change clothing for sleeping. It was good, he thought, to expose the body to air while undressing, and using a night shirt for sleeping reduced wear and soiling of the daytime clothes. Jackson listed what he considered to be the ideal issue of clothing to a soldier, comprising two linen, cotton, or flannel shirts; two pairs of socks; two pairs of underwear made of linen or flannel; two pairs of shoes; a foraging cap; shoe brushes and blacking; razor and strap; hair brush; soap and sponge to wash his body; towel; handkerchief; night shirt; and knife, fork, and canteen.[8]

Good clothing had a direct connection with a clean body, and in Jackson's view, "nothing contributes more to preserve health than personal cleanliness." It provided "an accession of physical force and vigour" in addition to making the man feel good about himself. The soldier should be taught to wash himself fully every day and wash his hair frequently. He needed to remove dirt from his body and clothing and avoid the temptation to just cover it up with colorful clothing on his body and grease on his hair. "Where a man is perfectly clean in person as freed from all exterior impurity, he might be said to live at every pore, and to be animated in every fibre."[9]

Jackson's views on diet ran counter to the prevailing ideas of British society. He recognized that the English ate more animal food than any other nation (except the United States) yet did not believe that this contributed to their military prowess. Jackson knew that many nations of military greatness ate far less meat, and he understood that vegetable diets gave the human body strength more than any other diet. "The quantity of physical force best adapted to the purposes of war may be derived from a plain and homely diet, of comparatively small measure." Vegetable food might offer less brute strength, but it afforded "more endurance of toil" than meat-based fare. Jackson found that tea and bread was healthier than eating beef for breakfast. He also advocated individual cooking, but if group cooking in a mess had to be conducted, then it was best to alternate men for kitchen duties rather than making one man a perpetual cook. When it came to water, Jackson urged that soldiers be taught to take it from running streams whenever possible. They should have a small supply of alum to settle muddy matter before using it; vinegar, which the Romans used to improve the taste, also could be used. In the British Army, far too much rum was available. In fact, the doctor thought its use was out of control.[10]

Although Jackson's book received limited attention by Civil War–era sanitarians, the ideas he outlined were repeated by them in their own writings. In part, this was because no one had a monopoly on insights as to how to make life healthier for soldiers. Most of those ideas were common among knowledgeable people who studied the problem. They may have differed in solutions—for example, Civil War sanitarians generally thought tents were healthier than living in barracks, in contrast to Jackson—but everyone was on the same page when it came to identifying all the important factors that affected soldier health.

In addition to Jackson's treatise, Civil War sanitarians had ample evidence from the American past in how military service affected the health of soldiers. Unfortunately, they were not well tuned in to their lessons. The American Revolutionary War, the War of 1812 (1812–14), the Second Seminole War (1835–42), and the Mexican War (1846–48) all had witnessed severe military health issues, but none of those conflicts produced a significant awareness of how to deal with such problems. To take the most recent American conflict prior to the Civil War, more than 100,000 troops served in the Mexican War. More than 1,500 of them were killed on the battlefield, while over 10,000 died of illness. Moreover, death by disease was more than ten times greater in the US Army than among civilians on the home front during the conflict.[11] Yet no special protest was raised in the wake of the Mexican War, with no effort made to improve conditions.[12]

To a degree, Civil War sanitarians could draw on a limited corpus of published works by those who paid attention to civilian problems of healthcare in the years before the firing on Fort Sumter. For example, Lemuel Shattuck's *Report of a General Plan for the Promotion of Public and Personal Health,* focused on Massachusetts, was published in 1850. It presented a plan for a major sanitary survey of the state, citing the advanced policies for public sanitation to be seen in Prussia and many German states, with Britain's public-health policies following behind those Continental nations. Shattuck characterized the health status of Massachusetts as far worse than most of its citizens believed.[13]

But by far the biggest influence on Civil War sanitarians regarding preventive healthcare in the army was the Crimean War. "That experience was a complete chapter by itself on sanitary science," wrote Charles J. Stillé in his 1866 *History of the United States Sanitary Commission.* The problems were legion, ranging from a lack of fresh bread and vegetables, which eventually produced scurvy, to poor camp sanitation, which led to rampant cholera at the siege of Sebastopol. The British and French armies, in addition to the civilian populace of both nations, were highly aware of those unusually severe problems. That awareness produced both shock and a movement to ameliorate the issues in the short run. In the long run the Crimean experience led to significant reform of the British military health regimen that bore fruit by the 1860s. Among the 90,000 troops on home station in 1859, the death rate had dropped from 17 per 1,000 to only 8 per 1,000, although the troops stationed overseas had not yet experienced such a dramatic improvement.[14]

France's army suffered on the same level as its British allies at Sebastopol, which sparked a similar reaction from that nation's military health establishment. Jean-Baptiste Louis Baudens, a French military physician sent to inspect hospitals in the Crimea, noted in his *On Military and Camp Hospitals,* published in an English edition in 1862, that those French regiments that suffered the least were commanded by officers who were "careful of their men." Baudens cited as a model the camp of the Eighty-First Regiment of Infantry, with its wide and clean streets lined by fir trees planted by regimental members. For shelter, he supported the conical tent with walls that could be raised two feet to provide ventilation in good weather. It was made of cloth woven in open texture that allowed the fabric to breathe, although this also let rain sift through. Tents with vertical walls did not resist the wind as well as conical shapes, although they were roomier and more comfortable. It was typical of French soldiers to dig an excavation a foot deep and place their tents over it, a practice that all Civil War sanitarians condemned heartily as promoting disease because rainwater would collect in the hole. Baudens admitted that French soldiers at Sebastopol were not as clean as English troops, who washed their underclothing in warm water and changed it twice a week. "Our soldiers were not so careful," he wrote. "Filthiness checks the functions of the skin, and engenders vermin."[15]

Fresh meat remained a significant part of the French military diet in the Crimea, but preserved meat became an additional part of the army ration. It was packed in hermetically sealed tin cans and was "of excellent quality," according to Baudens. But the men did not like it because it was of a smaller quantity due to having no bones. Powdered meat was issued on occasion but never won favor among the troops. This product "had a suspicious odor, and the men were always in doubt whether animals of all kinds were not used in its manufacture." They "manifested a great repugnance and disgust toward it." Baudens advocated the issue of horse meat on a regular basis, but few others agreed with him. On the other hand, he argued that French troops received too few fresh vegetables at Sebastopol, a point most sanitarians could support. Preserved vegetables were issued but, toward the end of the war, were increasingly of poor quality as fermentation set in; the men often threw them away. "Man has need of vegetables as much as of meat," Baudens correctly asserted. "The necessity of a varied nourishment has been established as a practical fact."[16]

In addition to the details of how to keep troops healthy in the field and in barracks, the Crimean experience offered British and French observers a more fundamental lesson. It was imperative to teach soldiers that it was vital for them to learn how to take care of themselves. Even more important was to teach their officers how to care for the troops placed in their charge. Surgeons and sanitarians were the teachers, soldiers and officers the students, in a life-or-death scenario every time a major war broke out. Edward Barrington de Fonblanque, the assistant commissary general of the British Army, argued that preventive healthcare should be commonly understood by everyone rather than remain the preserve of a specialized coterie of experts. "Our daily experience and observations suffices to teach us its broad principles," he wrote in a general study of the British military system published in 1858. The army had an arduous task in this regard because it tended to draw recruits from class levels in which people lived in tightly confined spaces, urban or rural. They had little education and hardly any awareness of how important it was to have fresh air flowing through their living quarters, to eat a balanced diet, and to keep their bodies clean on a regular basis.[17]

Americans interested in preventive healthcare for the army were keenly aware of the Crimean War and its problems. They also were highly aware that this conflict had jumpstarted successful efforts in Britain and France to ameliorate the age-old military threats to soldier health and life. The British government had created a sanitary commission and sent it to the Crimea in April 1855 with "plenary powers to do anything," as Charles Stillé put it. This remained a powerful incentive for American sanitarians to create a sanitary commission of their own as soon as the Civil War broke out. Stillé praised the British commission as achieving "the grandest contribution ever made by science to the practical art of preserving health among men required to live together in large masses."[18]

Moreover, the Delafield Commission, consisting of three US Army officers dispatched to observe the Crimean War, produced detailed information relevant to preventive healthcare among the allied forces. Cavalry Capt. George B. McClellan praised French infantry officers for bestowing "the utmost care upon the comfort and well-being of the men, rightly regarding that as probably the most essential element to insure efficiency, contentment, and willing obedience. This example cannot be too strongly urged for imitation." Ordnance officer Maj. Alfred Mordecai provided a long excerpt from the report of the French minister of war to Napoleon III describing the logistical system that kept French troops fed with a variety of rations, including processed foods. Engineer Maj. Richard Delafield, the head of the commission, also provided details about processed foods and endorsed its potential for American military use. All three commission members were alert to the many health-related problems of campaigning and eager to see how the allies dealt with them, in addition to covering a wide variety of other topics relating to current and future military hardware, tactics, and operations.[19]

In many ways, due to the horrible suffering at Sebastopol, the Europeans were well ahead of the Americans in military preventive healthcare by the time the Civil War broke out. English nurse Florence Nightingale popularized the concept of a pavilion arrangement for large military hospitals, something the French had initially developed for civilian hospitals near the end of the previous century and the British had taken up early in the nineteenth century. This idea arranged the buildings of a general hospital in patterns to spread them out within short distances of each other, all of which was designed to limit the number of patients in any individual building and create a flow of fresh air not only through each one but between the buildings as well. The most commonly noted layout was that of a wheel, with individual buildings serving as spokes, but there were other patterns too. Nightingale's *Notes on Hospitals,* published in 1858, helped bring the concept to the United States in time for implementation during the Civil War. For her, the most important advantage of a pavilion scheme was that each ward would essentially have a separate ventilation system, diffusing its polluted air into the atmosphere instead of into another ward.[20]

By 1861, not only in military medicine but even in the public-health movement, the United States was behind more advanced European nations, such as Britain, France, and many German states. Despite well-publicized health problems in major cities, such as New York and Boston, and the unusual proposal for a sanitary survey of a state (Massachusetts), most Americans were lagging well behind the forward curve in ideas and actions concerning ways to prevent disease. In many ways the outbreak of the Civil War spurred greater awareness of this issue.[21]

AMERICAN SANITARY LITERATURE

There quickly developed a relatively small but very vocal coterie of military sanitarians after the firing on Fort Sumter. They included civilians in varied walks of life, largely medical and legal, as well as a number of military surgeons. They were not shy about publishing their views in strident tones. While some worked through the newly created US Sanitary Commission, many of them had little if any connection with that nongovernmental agency. They sometimes disagreed on details but largely united on most of their recommendations for improved healthcare of soldiers to prevent disease from exacting the kind of death toll that had tragically occurred at Sebastopol only six years earlier.

John Ordronaux contributed a major voice to this educational effort. Born in New York City and a graduate of Dartmouth College, he earned a degree from Harvard Law School and a medical degree from the National Medical School. Ordronaux became a professor of medical jurisprudence at Columbia Law School in New York City in 1860, the year after publication of the first of his fifteen books on a variety of topics. The first edition of his second book, *Hints on Health in Armies, for the Use of Volunteer Officers,* was published soon after he penned the preface on May 23, 1861. A second edition came out in July 1863. "All that can be done, should be done to protect troops against preventable disease," he wrote. "Officers and men need an insight into the general principles of hygiene, in order to be able to assist, themselves, in furthering prophylactic measures." He considered his book "a popular synopsis of the leading principles of Military Hygiene, as designed for laymen rather than surgeons."[22]

Ordronaux relied on published statistics arising from the Crimean War to assert that disease was "nearly *four times* more formidable to armies than bullets." He drew on another set of published statistics to show that even in barracks armies suffered mortality rates twice as high as civilians. "The general negligence of preventive measures which prevails in most armies" was the cause. Ordronaux partly blamed an attitude that bad health was a natural condition of life for this neglect. He argued that sanitarians needed to enlighten everyone, both in and out of the army, that good health was "our natural state" and that it could be encouraged by the proper measures. As indicated by the title of his book, Ordronaux focused on officers of the volunteer army as the key to health improvement. "It is upon officers, therefore, of every grade, that rests the responsibility of preserving the health of their men." He argued that good health was an important weapon in winning the war, and officers should be punished for neglecting their duty to foster it.[23]

Published statistics relating to the peacetime French army indicated that the first year of a man's service tended to be the most dangerous. The mortality ratio was 6.5 per 1,000 men for the first year but steadily dropped to 2.0 for the seventh year of service. Part of this problem stemmed from the need to get as many recruits as possible, which led to enlisting boys in their teens. Ordronaux thought that anyone under twenty years of age should be rejected. Napoleon himself would have agreed, having been quoted as saying, "I must have grown men; boys serve only to encumber the hospitals and roadsides." Ordronaux went much further and advocated a comprehensive system of selective service in which recruitment officials thoroughly gathered information about the personal history of each man, held them to high health standards, and then assigned them to positions in the army suited to their skills and physical development. The French had developed something like this system; at least they carefully measured and classified a recruit's manual strength to determine whether to assign him to particularly strenuous army positions, such as those in the artillery and engineer services.[24]

After matching the recruit and his abilities with the demands of army life, Ordronaux warned that the man had to gradually acclimate to the new military environment over time. The suddenness of that transition produced the kind of disturbance to his health that contributed to the elevated death rate noted in the French statistics for the first year of service. He was plucked from "the comforts of home, and the moderate, generally self-imposed and self-regulated duties of civil life, to the extremes of diet, (quantity and quality,) fatigue and exposure, incidental to active operations in the field." Ordronaux advocated a kind of modern basic training, unheard of in the US Army of that time, in which medical officers had a role. It would include plenty of physical exercise in addition to moderate sessions of drilling. A month seemed long enough for some recruits, but Ordronaux was sure it was too short for others. He envisioned that the men would be taught habits of personal cleanliness in addition to practicing long marches, creating entrenchments, and participating in sham battles, all of which was not only to teach him his military craft but to physically and mentally condition him as well.[25]

It is ironic that even as Ordronaux penned the preface of his first edition, the Union military system was gorging itself with thousands of completely raw volunteers in a tremendous burst of patriotic enthusiasm. This would be repeated numerous times over the next couple of years as the

Federal government issued call upon call to the states for more troops. As it did so, the Union army adopted none of these wise suggestions. In fact, few of them were even possible to follow given the emergency facing the country, for which a large army was needed immediately. The existing military system was hardly able to clothe, feed, and arm these raw recruits, much less carefully select them, slowly acclimate them to army life, and teach them military hygiene.

Ordronaux was not naive about any of this. "Overcrowded, ill-ventilated barracks, small, foul tents, indifferent provisions, [and] badly organized hospitals, will continue to do their work of silent destruction, until medical men are allowed some power and discretion in the housing, feeding, and superintendence of troops," he admitted. Until medical officers had an opportunity to exert some influence, "we must expect to see the flower of every army cut off, and the state shorn of its most useful members in times of direst necessity." His final plea was to the enlisted soldier himself, who, the professor asserted, had a patriotic duty to his country and to himself to take care of his health even if his officers and the army failed to do everything they could to help him.[26]

An important aspect of this problem lay in the fact that the military policy of the United States relied on a tiny professional army, with its small corps of professional military surgeons, and the massing of volunteers directly from civilian life to meet national emergencies. This essentially negated any chance that the bulk of the wartime army could be trained or acclimated in any sensible way other than the fastest, most crude, and incomplete fashion. That was why Ordronaux specifically identified volunteer officers as his main audience. They typically had no more military experience than the enlisted men of their regiments and were just as ignorant of health concerns in the army as their charges. Teaching both officers and enlisted men the importance of camp sanitation, good food, and plenty of rest when they were far more interested in the most advanced small arms available, learning how to drill, and hoping for a chance to see the war was extremely difficult to do.

Fortunately, the professional medical men of the regular army generally were aware of the need for preventive healthcare and supported efforts to instill these principles in the volunteers. Surgeon General Hammond, for example, authored a book on the topic, which was published soon after he penned the preface on June 25, 1863. At that point, halfway through the war, Hammond felt certain that great progress had already been made in teaching the volunteers the importance of preventive healthcare. But he was unable to cite any statistics to support his optimism. In the preface of *A Treatise on Hygiene with Special Reference to the Military Service,* he noted "that the curative influences of hygienic measures have been too much neglected," but he was sure that "a growing attention to the subject of sanitary science" would help alleviate the problem. In part, he was led to this belief by the improvements in British soldier health since the traumatic experience of the Crimean War. Hammond cited published statistics indicating that mortality in the British Army dropped from 14 per 1,000 men in the 1830s to 5 per 1,000 by 1860. The improvement in some especially dangerous colonial postings was even more impressive. For example, in Jamaica the death rate dropped from 128 per 1,000 during 1837–56 to only 17 per 1,000 by 1861.[27]

Hammond added another perspective to the problem of army hygiene not noted by Ordronaux. He was not surprised that soldiers were sicker than civilians because army life concentrated men into smaller, more densely packed accumulations than was typical even of large urban areas. Hammond studied the arrangement of an army camp as laid down in the regulations and calculated it to be large enough to hold the population of a big city. If enlarged to the size of a city, the camp would accommodate 86,448 men per square mile—in contrast, London held 50,000 people per square mile. In fact, using the same method, Hammond estimated that British camp density at Sebastopol amounted to 347,000 men per square mile when computing the entire ground of the camp. When looking only at the area covered by tents and huts, it rose to 1,044,820 men per square mile.[28] How accurately he came to these figures is an open question, but there can be little doubt that public sanitation was even more important in the army than in civilian life because of the heavy concentration of men in small areas.

Like Jackson, Hammond believed in a race-centered view of mankind, but he was far less dogmatic in his conclusions. He considered only Europeans, Americans, and Africans in his discussion, noting that Europeans were better developed physically and in the capacity of the cranium than Africans, African Americans, or Native Americans. Race mixing produced physical degeneration in Hammond's view. He thought Europeans and North Americans who were descended from Europeans made the best soldiers in all ways, physical, emotional, and intellectual. But Hammond felt that this was due more to environment than biology. He rejected the notion that a Black man made a poorer soldier because of his race or the development of his cranium and admitted in his book that African American recruits had proven their ability to adjust to army life thus far in the conflict.[29]

While Ordronaux and Hammond authored some of the salient sanitary publications of the Civil War, other authors weighed in as well. Jean Roemer, a former cavalry officer of the Netherlands who wound up in the United States at the time of the war, wrote a treatise on cavalry that was published in 1863. "Men congregated in masses, and in small areas, overtasked, uncleanly, and improperly fed, whether they be soldiers or artisans, are subjected to precisely the same laws of health and disease, and the violation of those laws always entails the same fearful penalty upon all." Like Ordronaux and Hammond, Roemer found the remedy in granting medical personnel more power to act in correcting sanitary abuses and in making officers aware of these problems and how to deal with them. Another officer named James A. Congdon, a major in the Twelfth Pennsylvania Cavalry, authored a book published in 1864 addressed to his fellows in the mounted arm. Part of his message was to raise their awareness about health issues centered on "cleanliness, clothing, and diet."[30]

THE UNITED STATES SANITARY COMMISSION

In short, there was an ample supply of advice about soldier health available to Civil War participants, a combination of European historical example mingled with civilian experience at public-health concerns and topped off by a small but knowledgeable group of American sanitarians who largely worked though the US Sanitary Commission. This organization began in a meeting called by Elizabeth Blackwell, the first American woman to earn a medical degree, to mobilize women in support of the Union war effort through an organization she called the Women's Central Association of Relief. Blackwell was aided by Henry W. Bellows and other men who, after the meeting took place on April 29, 1861, in New York City's Cooper Union Hall, became convinced that a larger organization was needed. The men, who were prominent in the health professions of major Northeastern cities, created the US Sanitary Commission to serve as an interface between the government and grassroots efforts to care for soldiers. Blackwell's relief organization, which had given birth to the Sanitary Commission, was later absorbed by it as a branch group. Bellows's commission soon grew to address a wide range of efforts that included providing food and medical stores to supplement army supplies in military hospitals, donating antiscorbutic foods to units suffering from scurvy, and offering advice to government and army officials about needed reforms in the area of preventive healthcare. For our purposes, the most important effort of the commission was a major program of evaluating the health conditions of army camps and trying to persuade volunteer officers to improve them.[31]

The US Sanitary Commission, heavily inspired by the British Sanitary Commission of the Crimean War, differed markedly from its predecessor. The British organization had been created by the government with extraordinary emergency powers not only to investigate but also to correct sanitary abuses in the field. The American version was a grassroots, nongovernmental organization with no such powers. Its leaders had to convince the government to at least sanction its legitimacy, which was easily done, but the government could not give it any teeth—to do so would have entailed imposing a group of civilian experts on the judgment of military experts in the army medical system. This was not just a turf battle, but a real concern; such a situation would have been fraught with tension, infighting, and probable lack of success in bettering sanitary conditions. All the sanitarians could do was to advise and try to have an influence. They would have far less trouble in this goal with medical personnel in the regular army, most of whom were already aware of sanitary science. The commission's main target, however, was the huge number of regimental commanders and surgeons of the volunteer regiments, very few of whom had any exposure to army ills or sanitary principles. The commission received no government funds, relying entirely on private contributions, but it achieved a national presence that was impressive considering all the roadblocks to its success. Its accomplishments were many, but its limitations and failures also were a fact of its well-meaning existence.[32]

Charles J. Stillé, who authored the official history of the commission right after war's end, stated that its main purpose was "to popularize the general elementary truths of sanitary science, and to enforce their application by a picture of the terrible results which had followed the violation of sanitary laws in the British Army during the Crimean and Indian campaigns." He thought, along with his fellows in the commission, that these sanitary principles were "so obvious and simple" that they had been known for at least a hundred years. Stillé recognized that his compatriots had an uphill struggle.[33]

In June 1861, soon after the Sanitary Commission was organized, its executives felt that their first job should be to obtain information on the condition of the new troops being raised, not only for the initial call for three-month volunteers but also for subsequent calls for three-year men. They wanted to determine "what sanitary measures were most essential" to protect soldier health. The president, Dr. Henry W. Bellows, and Dr. John S. Newberry went to inspect the western troops while others were dispatched to Washington, DC, and to Fortress Monroe on the Virginia coast. This initial effort was also spurred by the knowledge that the US Army had no real system of inspecting camps and hospitals before the outbreak of the war.[34]

The results of these initial inspections staggered the commission leaders. Bellows took a mature view of the situation when he admitted that the soldiers were "officered in the semipolitical and semi-accidental fashion of most volunteer regiments," implying that one could not expect much from a mobilization system that relied so heavily on rank amateurs leading green recruits. The frenzied nature of the mobilization caused enormous sanitary problems. As Bellows and Newberry toured the West, Dr. Robert Tomes and Mr. Elijah J. Dunning looked at camps around Fortress Monroe. Landscape architect Frederick Law Olmsted, with the help of Dr. Elisha Harris, inspected twenty camps of volunteer regiments at Washington in early July. As all of these reports filtered in, the commission leadership came to the conclusion that one of their greatest challenges was to alert the government to camp sanitation problems and push to have the issues corrected.[35]

Thus was born one of the most salient efforts of the US Sanitary Commission: the creation of a corps of camp inspectors who filed more than 1,400 reports of conditions in army camps. As Dr. Alex McDonald explained, this corps consisted of "regimental visitors or inspectors" recruited mostly from among Northern physicians and surgeons. The commission started with only six inspectors, hired soon after the First Battle of Bull Run in late July 1861, and sent them to various parts of the theater of war. It then supplemented the inspection program with a blizzard of publications to educate volunteer officers and surgeons. For example, Dr. William H. Van Buren authored a short pamphlet titled *Rules for Preserving the Health of the Soldier.* Its preface was signed on July 12, 1861, and the work went through at least five editions during the war. Van Buren laid out in simple terms a number of important points: men not physically capable of enduring military life should be discharged as soon as possible; all recruits should be vaccinated against smallpox; all medical officers should become closely familiar with army regulations; the army ration was generous in quantity, and a good commissary could save up to 30 percent as a way to create a company fund for purchasing fresh vegetables, milk, butter, and other delicacies for sick soldiers; the best way to cook rations was by dedicated cooks and by messes rather than individually; officers should follow regulations to superintend their men's cooking, taste their food, and ensure they cleaned utensils properly; and the soldier should drink water in moderation, especially when overheated. "It is, then, one of the highest duties of an army surgeon to make himself well acquainted with the correct principles of military hygiene," concluded Van Buren and Dr. Alfred C. Post in another publication, *Report on Military Hygiene and Therapeutics,* which appeared in its fourth edition by the end of the war.[36]

The combination of camp inspections coupled with vigorous efforts to educate the volunteers through publications became, in some ways, the main focus of the Sanitary Commission. The inspections certainly were "a distinguishing feature" of the organization's work, as Stillé put it. In fact, one could go further and characterize the camp inspection returns, as they were called, a wholly unique feature of Civil War medical history. In no other conflict in America had anything like it been attempted by an organization outside the confines of the army medical system. The commission leaders judged, after only six months of inspections, that the returns were "of inestimable value," and they pursued the program until early 1864. Army camps became the focus of sanitary reform in the Civil War.[37]

The Sanitary Commission gave detailed instructions to its camp inspectors. They were to personally observe conditions, interview regimental commanders and medical personnel, offer pertinent advice, and try to support any influence regimental surgeons had in regulating the health conditions of the camp. Above all, the inspectors needed to be mindful of army protocol and etiquette; as civilian advisors they only had the opportunity to persuade, and that task could not be accomplished if they offended officers. In fact, the instructions, which were signed by Olmsted, placed great emphasis on establishing fruitful relations with regimental officers and surgeons. Olmsted encouraged inspectors to meet and discuss not only with the colonel but also with company commanders and the regimental quartermaster and commissary about all issues relating to preventive care. And they should contact the commission if they felt something special could be done to help a regiment, such as supplying it with unusual equipment or with extra food not provided by the army supply system.[38]

If an inspector followed these instructions faithfully, he had to invest a good deal of time and energy into each visit to a regimental camp. Some did so and with encouraging results. Dr. Newberry, for example, reported a visit by Dr. A. N. Read to Camp Nevin in Kentucky, where regiments assigned to the Department of the Ohio were wintering during 1861–62. Read first introduced himself to the regimental commander and the two surgeons, then asked their permission to visit each company captain and to minutely inspect the men's lodging. Accompanied by the captains, Read went through the tent areas. He found the officers took his visit seriously. "They were always courteous, and usually showed a commendable desire to learn their duties more perfectly. They often asked me for a copy of the inspection returns" to learn from them. Read also inspected the latrines, hospitals, and commissaries with the regimental surgeon.[39]

Read's experience was entirely positive, but it landed on the upper end of a spectrum. Some officers and surgeons, like those at Camp Nevin, eagerly cooperated with and respected the advice of the visitor while others looked on him as a nuisance. As will be developed throughout this book, inspectors found a wide variety of responses to their efforts, and by no means were all of them positive.

Regardless of the reception, the camp inspector was hired to inspect, and he was required to fill out a standard form issued by the commission. This standard form was the only opportunity to impose some sort of uniformity on the process of inspection, and commission executives spent a good deal of time and energy in making it comprehensive. In fact, they threw everything they could think of into it, coming up with 179 questions on the first of five versions of the printed standard form used during the war. Many of those questions were merely different aspects of a major topic. This first form, identified as No. 19 to indicate how many publications the commission had thus far issued, came out soon after the inspection program began in the late summer of 1861. In fact, a handful of the earliest reports were handwritten by the inspector because the form had not yet been published. But not long after Form No. 19 was issued, it was revised and reissued as Form No. 19a about March 1862. On this second edition the questions were more conveniently grouped into twenty-one "subject areas" for easier comprehension and the total number of questions slightly increased to 180. "Inspectors will be careful to remember that the answers of the Return are expected to present evidence of INVESTIGATION. Except in a few necessary cases, the answers are not intended to be those of the persons whom the inspector examines, but to express his own conviction after due inquiry and reflection."[40]

Most of the camp inspection returns wound up being filled out on either Form No. 19 or Form No. 19a, especially the latter, which was longer than any of the others. In fact, 19a was by far the best of the five versions ultimately used by the Sanitary Commission. For unexplained reasons, commission executives tinkered with it, producing a version simply known as Form A. It had more questions, totaling 191, and included two new subject

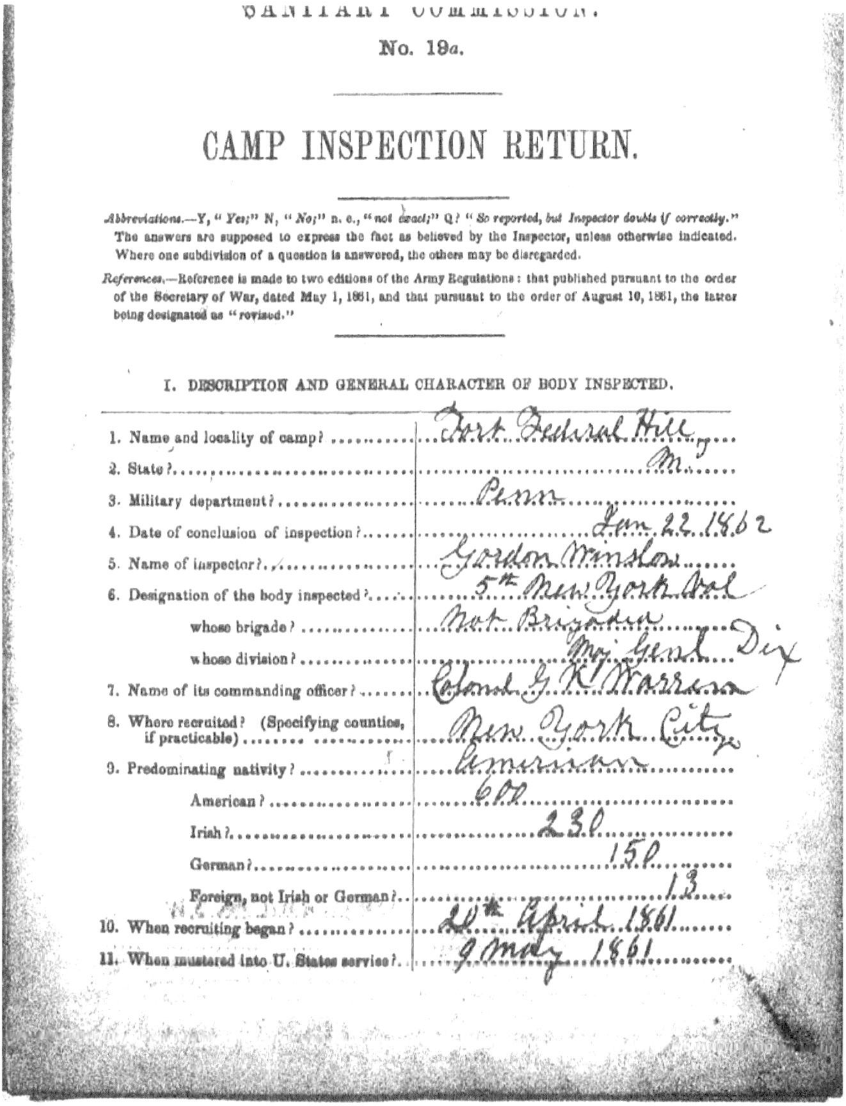

SANITARY COMMISSION.

No. 19*a*.

CAMP INSPECTION RETURN.

Abbreviations.—Y, "*Yes;*" N, "*No;*" n. e., "*not exact;*" Q? "*So reported, but Inspector doubts if correctly.*" The answers are supposed to express the fact as believed by the Inspector, unless otherwise indicated. Where one subdivision of a question is answered, the others may be disregarded.

References.—Reference is made to two editions of the Army Regulations: that published pursuant to the order of the Secretary of War, dated May 1, 1861, and that pursuant to the order of August 10, 1861, the latter being designated as "revised."

I. DESCRIPTION AND GENERAL CHARACTER OF BODY INSPECTED.

1. Name and locality of camp?	Fort Federal Hill
2. State?	Md
3. Military department?	Penn
4. Date of conclusion of inspection?	Jan 22. 1862
5. Name of inspector?	Gordon Winslow
6. Designation of the body inspected?	5th New York Vol
whose brigade?	Not Brigaded
whose division?	Maj Genl Dix
7. Name of its commanding officer?	Colonel G. K. Warren
8. Where recruited? (Specifying counties, if practicable)	New York City
9. Predominating nativity?	American
American?	600
Irish?	230
German?	150
Foreign, not Irish or German?	13
10. When recruiting began?	20th April 1861
11. When mustered into U. States service?	9 May 1861

Camp Inspection Return for the Fifth New York, Page 1. Gordon Hubbard Winslow not only served as chaplain of the Fifth New York but also acted as a US Sanitary Commission camp inspector, based on his prior occupation as a physician. On January 22, 1862, he inspected his own regiment's camp and filed this report to the commission on the standard Form No. 19a. The regiment at that time was commanded by Col. Gouverneur K. Warren, a graduate of West Point who later gained fame for his actions at Gettysburg, which catapulted him to command of the Second Corps and later the Fifth Corps, Army of the Potomac. This is the cover page of a typical camp inspection return filled out in legible handwriting. (Gordon H. Winslow return, Fifth New York, January 22, 1862, Series 7, US Sanitary Commission Records, NYPL)

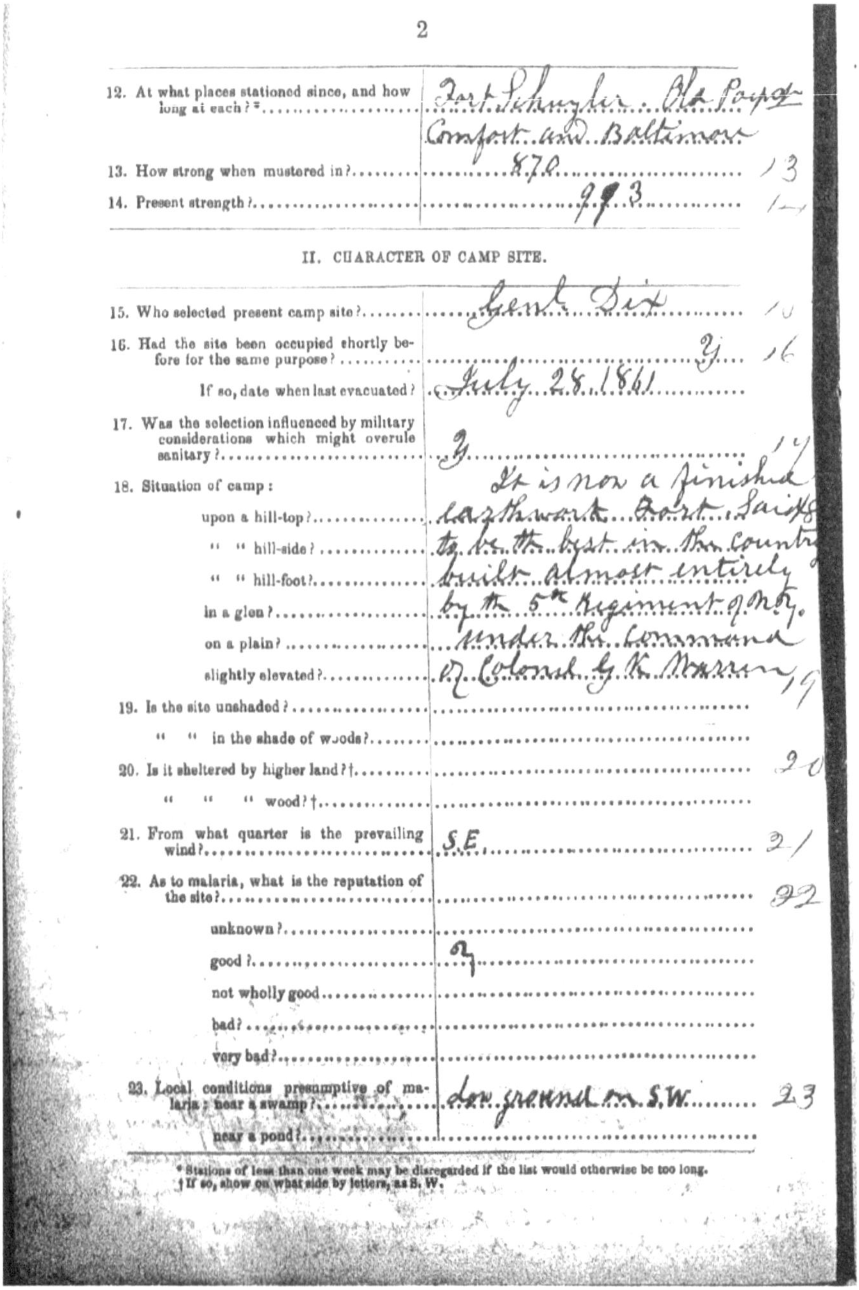
2

12. At what places stationed since, and how long at each?* — Fort Schuyler .. Old Point Comfort and Baltimore

13. How strong when mustered in? — 870 — 13

14. Present strength? — 993 — 14

II. CHARACTER OF CAMP SITE.

15. Who selected present camp site? — Genl. Dix — 15

16. Had the site been occupied shortly before for the same purpose? — y — 16

If so, date when last evacuated? — July 28. 1861

17. Was the selection influenced by military considerations which might overrule sanitary? — y — 17

18. Situation of camp: — It is now a finished

upon a hill-top? — earthwork Fort said

" " hill-side? — to be the best in the country

" " hill-foot? — built almost entirely

in a glen? — by the 5th Regiment of N.Y.

on a plain? — under the command

slightly elevated? — of Colonel G. K. Warren — 18

19. Is the site unshaded?

" " in the shade of woods?

20. Is it sheltered by higher land?†— 20

" " " wood?†

21. From what quarter is the prevailing wind? — S.E. — 21

22. As to malaria, what is the reputation of the site? — 22

unknown?

good? — y

not wholly good

bad?

very bad?

23. Local conditions presumptive of malaria: near a swamp? — low ground on S.W. — 23

near a pond?

* Stations of less than one week may be disregarded if the list would otherwise be too long.
† If so, show on what side by letters, as S. W.

Camp Inspection Return for the Fifth New York, Pages 2–3. Winslow conscientiously provided all the information he could, adding extended comments where he felt it would help the commission in its assessment of camp conditions in his regiment. (Gordon H. Winslow return, Fifth New York, January 22, 1862, Series 7, US Sanitary Commission Records, NYPL)

23. Local conditions presumptive of malaria:		
near a river?	Y	23
near a river delta?	Y	
24. Soil of camp site:		
sandy?	Y +	24
loose gravel?		
loose loam?		
firm loam?	Y +	
agglomerated pebbles, gravel, or sand, (hardpan)		
impervious clay?	Y	
25. Sub-soil:		
sandy?	deep white Sand	25
loose gravel?	+ ferruginous Strata	
loose loam?	Sand + rock +	
firm loam?		
agglomerated pebbles, gravel, or sand, (hardpan)		
impervious clay?	Y	
26. Is the site favorable for surface drainage? (as to inclination)		26

III. ARRANGEMENT AND CONDITION OF CAMP.

27. Is the camp arranged mainly in accordance with the "army regulations?"	The Regt. is now in Barracks
more crowded?	which form three sides of
more open?	a hollow Square. One Mens qu-
28. How far apart are the tents in the rows?	ters on the left of Sally Port 195 ft
29. How is the artificial drainage?	long 24 ft wide 27 ft high to
systematic and complete?	ridge. Two Stories 10 ft each
partial, and with no general system?	giving to each company 65+24 10 ft – Piazza extends the whole
entirely neglected?	front with Stairs on the end
30. Are the drains mainly straight?	out side to the upper Piazza
Are the drains very sinuous?	On the end at right angles is
31. About how deep are the drains generally?	the same style of building 185 ft

long Piazza accommodating four companies. The Kitchens on each end 25 ft + 24 the musicians rooms over the kitchen drummers at one end, Band at the other 25+24 ft – The areas that dealt with courts-martial and inspections conducted by army personnel. This was further altered with the issuance of Form C late in 1863, which reverted to 180 questions and a "more streamlined appearance . . . by consolidating information about camp locations." As if that were not enough, executives issued their fifth and final edition of the form, K, sometime early in 1864. Form K was by far the most different of the five versions with only eighteen questions, eliminating all subject areas. Fortunately, only the last half-dozen returns on file in the commission archives were made using Form K.[41] It was almost useless as a gauge for the wide range of sanitation issues included in previous versions.

The changes in the camp-inspection-return form pose something of a limitation on the historian, and one cannot help but conclude that they imposed limitations on the work of the commission as well. Form No. 19a was by far the best, and fortunately it represents the majority of returns on file. But the quality of information on versions A, C, and K declines significantly, offering less information on late-war camp conditions than are available for early and mid-war periods. Form A deleted important subject areas, including the physical examination of recruits and smallpox vaccinations, and severely reduced the number of questions concerning the disposal of camp garbage and the conditions of latrines. In these last two subject areas, inspectors went from several questions regarding each subject area on Form No. 19a to just one yes-or-no option on Form A. Form C did not add anything material, and Form K was of practically no value in gauging those two subject areas. There appears to be no explanation for these disruptive changes in what had been a very good standard form. The only insight may come from an assertion by Dr. McDonald, written soon after the conflict, that by 1864 and 1865, commission executives considered the camp inspection program less necessary.[42] Judging by the returns, however, it is difficult to understand why they thought so, for there is no clear evidence that camp conditions had significantly improved. Moreover, even if inspections were less important by the last year of the war, there was no logical reason to change the standard form so drastically.

Despite these concerns about the standard inspection form, the results of the camp inspection program were impressive. A total of 1,465 returns were filed between August 20, 1861, and February 10, 1864. Of that number, more than 1,400 wound up in the US Sanitary Commission Records in the New York Public Library.[43] The camp inspectors did not assign numerical evaluations; they simply wrote "yes" or "no" on many questions and often made explanatory notes for others. Some method of assigning numerical evaluation was necessary to create an objective measure of success or failure in camp sanitation, and this came from another, similar source. The army began to methodically inspect camps by early 1863, when it issued general orders requiring commanders in the field to appoint medical inspectors on the corps level. Fortunately, Surg. John M. Woodworth of the First Illinois Light Artillery sent copies of the Fifteenth Corps camp inspection reports (and other medical documents) to the Sanitary Commission right after the war. They provide a wonderful source of detailed information on health conditions in the corps. These army reports share many similarities with the commission camp inspection returns, although they address far fewer subject areas. They also are far more streamlined than the commission forms because the corps medical officer was required to inspect camps every week. They assigned a rating system consisting of "Good," "Fair," and "Bad" to each category for each report.[44]

This was a sound system, and I adopted it for my evaluation of the camp inspection returns of the Sanitary Commission, judging whether the inspector's yes or no and qualitative comments should be listed as good, fair, or bad. This allowed me to express the percentage of good, fair, and bad results for every subject area covered by the return. I was guided in my evaluation by a careful reading of the literature produced by Civil War sanitarians and what they saw as sanitary principles. After completing my comprehensive evaluation of all the subject areas on all 280 returns, I went back to the first 4 returns and reevaluated them to doublecheck if my judgment had altered following the monthslong processing of the 280 forms. The second evaluation of these first four forms was so close to my original evaluation as to lend confidence in the consistency of transferring qualitative answers into specific groups (good, fair, and bad) that could then be quantified.

14

160. If so, has it been impracticable to remove them to the general hospital?	not necessary	160
161. Are there any contagious or infectious cases?	no	161
162. Are they kept in a separate tent or house from the others?		162
163. Are the discharges from the latter placed in the privy used by others?		163
164. What has been the daily average number on the sick list during the last two weeks, as by morning reports?	125	164
in general hospital?	8	
in regimental hospital?	25	
sick in quarters?	92	
165. Have there been any deaths in that time?		165
how many?		
from what causes?		
166. Are the dead buried near the camp, and at what depth?		166
167. Is the general health of the regiment improving or deteriorating?	Improving	167

XXI. PREVENTIVE DUTY OF SURGEON.

168. Does the surgeon understand that he is responsible for all conditions of the camp or regiment unfavorable to health, unless he has warned the commanding officer of them?	y	168
169. Does the surgeon make a daily inspection of the camp, with reference to its cleanliness?	y	169
170. Does he inspect the food, and see how the cooking is done?	y	170
171. Does he report on these matters, and urge remedies upon the company officers, and, when necessary, upon the commanding officer?	y	171
172. Is anything administered to the well men to guard against the effects of malaria? (Prophylactics)	In some instances	172
173. Is there a drill before breakfast?	no	173
174. If so, does the surgeon approve of it?		174
175. If not, has he remonstrated against it with the commanding officer?		175
176. What is the length of time the men are on drill daily?	5 hours	176

Camp Inspection Return for the Fifth New York, Pages 14–15. The last page of Form No. 19a allowed the visitor to make any comments on any topic, and Winslow took the opportunity to write glowingly of Warren's care for the regiment. (Gordon H. Winslow return, Fifth New York, January 22, 1862, Series 7, US Sanitary Commission Records, NYPL)

XXII. ARMS AND ACCOUTREMENTS.

177. What is their arm?	Sharps Rifle 2 Companies, rest
177¹. Have the men confidence in it?	[illegible] rifles Ry
178. Is there any limit placed upon the weight of the knapsack for heavy marching order?	n
179. If so, what?	
180. Is the cartridge-box sustained only by a belt?	belt only
or, has it the additional support of a shoulder strap?	
if, by belt alone, what effect has the surgeon observed, if any?*	

* It is alleged to induce hernia.

There is a school of instruction for officers every evening, in all the arts of war. The Colonel who was formerly tactitian at West Point is indefatiable in his efforts to raise the Regi ~~to the hig~~ highest state of perfection attained in the regular army, and has succeeded to the admiration of all. I doubt if the army presents a better specimen of well drilled, well disciplined and effective officers & men

The bayonet exercise is receiving special attention. There are drills also in both heavy and light Artillery. Should the Govt. desire to transfer a Regiment fully prepared for any Service, into the regular army, they could not do a better act or to a more deserving body than to the select 5th N.Y. vol

THE INSPECTORS

A total of thirty-four inspectors filled out the 280 camp inspection returns used in this book. They represented differing occupations and professions because, as the Sanitary Commission expanded its corps of inspectors, it also expanded the list of acceptable backgrounds and training of those men. Although many of the thirty-four inspectors remain obscure due to a lack of biographical information, the rest enjoy some degree of presence in the literature (and on the internet) so that we can get a good flavor of their lives and activities before, during, and beyond their service to the commission.

As seen from the table, sixteen of the thirty-four inspectors were physicians or surgeons. Four of the thirty-four were ministers, but three of these were physicians as well. There were three teachers, but two of them were also physicians. One of the thirty-four was a landscape engineer. For the fifteen remaining inspectors, their occupation is unknown.

Godfrey Aigner was the house physician of the New-York Dispensary, a charitable hospital operating since 1790 in the heart of Manhattan that treated more than 44,000 people in 1859. Aigner, who completed nine of the camp inspection returns, often had his name misspelled. After examining Flag Officer Andrew Hull Foote's wounded left foot three weeks after the Battle of Fort Donelson (February 13–15, 1862), he was referred to in official reports as "Geofrey Aiguer." The commission, however, spelled his name "Godfrey Aigner" and relied on his thorough, professional inspection of troops at Cairo, Illinois, in 1861 and early 1862. "If an ounce of prevention is worth a pound of cure in private practice, it is surely a great deal more in military life," Aigner concluded in a report of his work.[45]

Bernard Jean Bettelheim had the most unusual life story of all the thirty-four inspectors. Born of a Jewish family in Hungary, he earned his medical degree in Padua, Italy, by 1836. Bettelheim practiced in Italy and Egypt but converted to a Protestant sect after 1840 while living in Smyrna, Ottoman Empire. For many years, missionary zeal infected his attitude, and he obtained permission to spread his version of religion to Okinawa by 1846. Bettelheim took his family with him as he carved out a dubious record as the first Protestant missionary on that island. He was rude and condescending, and he deliberately desecrated native sacred places, earning a well-deserved hatred among the very people he hoped to convert. Local authorities were able to get him transferred out of their country by 1854. When the family stopped in the United States, they made it their home. Bettelheim engaged to conduct numerous camp inspections for the Sanitary Commission by 1863,

Name	Birthplace and Date	Occupation	Place and Date of Death	Number of Reports Filled
Godfrey Aigner (also spelled Geofrey Aiguer)	Unknown	House Physician, New York Dispensary	Unknown	9
George L. Andrews	Unknown	Physician	Unknown	30
Bernard Jean Bettelheim	Hungary (modern Slovakia), 1811	Physician, Protestant missionary, surgeon of 106th Illinois	Missouri, 1870	8
George A. Blake	About 1828	Physician	About 1892	19
C. W. Brink	Unknown	Unknown	Unknown	3
M. P. Buel	Unknown	Unknown	Unknown	3
Alfred Lewis Castleman	Kentucky, 1808	Physician, President of Wisconsin Medical Society, surgeon of 5th Wisconsin, author	Oakland, California, 1877	10
William M. Chamberlain	Unknown	Unknown	Unknown	21
Robert Collyer	Keighty, Yorkshire, England, 1823	Methodist and later Unitarian minister, author	New York City, 1912	4
Edward A. Crane	1832	Physician	1906	28
John H. Douglas	Waterford, New York, 1824	Physician, throat specialist	New York City, 1892	17
E. J. Dunning	Unknown	Unknown	Unknown	2
George Granville Edgerly	Unknown, but lived in Concord, New Hampshire	Unknown	New Orleans, July 15, 1864 (while still in service to the USSC)	12
William W. Estabrook	Unknown, but lived in Clinton, Iowa	Physician, Episcopalian minister, chaplain of 15th Iowa, surgeon of 45th Iowa	Unknown	1
James Gall, Jr.	Scotland, September 1836	Landscape engineer	Paterson, New Jersey, February 17, 1910	3
Franklin B. Hough	Martinsburg, New York, July 20, 1822	Physician with an interest in botany, geology, mineralogy, history, and forestry, surgeon of 97th New York, author and translator	Lowville, New York, June 11, 1885	13
W. S. Hough	Unknown	Unknown	Unknown	1
F. U. Johnston	Unknown	Unknown	Unknown	5
Robert Jones	Unknown	Unknown	Unknown	5

Name	Birthplace and Date	Occupation	Place and Date of Death	Number of Reports Filled
Marvin M. Marsh	Pompey, New York, 1812	Teacher and Physician	New York City, 1868	5
Alex McDonald	Unknown	Physician	Unknown	2
Edward Mead	Unknown	Unknown	Unknown	7
Julius Nichols	Unknown	Unknown	Unknown	2
Henry Oliver	Unknown	Unknown	Unknown	10
Jesse William Page	Unknown	Unknown	Unknown	1
Henry Park	Unknown	Unknown	Unknown	1
W. M. Prentice	Unknown	Unknown	Unknown	16
A. N. Read	Unknown	Physician	Unknown	12
T. B. Smith	Unknown	Unknown	Unknown	3
Lewis H. Steiner	Frederick City, Maryland, May 4, 1827	Teacher and Physician	Baltimore, Maryland, February 18, 1892	4
William F. Swalm	Brooklyn, New York, 1837	Asst. Surgeon of 84th New York and 15th New York Engineers	New York City, August 27, 1909	2
Robert Ware	Boston, Massachusetts, September 2, 1833	Physician and surgeon of 44th Massachusetts	Washington, North Carolina, April 10, 1863	15
Henry W. Warriner	Hawley, Massachusetts, 1824	Teacher and Editor	Deerfield, Massachusetts, November 23, 1871	3
Gordon Hubbard Winslow	Vermont, 1805	Physician, Episcopalian minister, Chaplain of 5th New York	Potomac River, Virginia, June 7, 1864	3

filling out his returns with attention to detail and a readiness to pen qualitative evaluations of what he saw. For example, Bettelheim recorded that on inspecting the camp of the Fifty-Seventh Indiana near Murfreesboro, Tennessee, on March 17, 1863, he thoroughly advised Asst. Surg. Hosea Tillson to conduct more regular inspections of the men's clothing and washing and to get them better tents. Close attention to personal cleanliness as specified in Army Regulations No. 100 was lacking, and Bettelheim suggested ways the soldiers could remove vermin. He also pushed for more soft bread in the ration and urged Tillson to contact the US Christian Commission for help in creating a regimental library. Despite his hateful attitude toward non-Christian groups, Bettelheim was one of the better inspectors of the commission, filling out 8 of the 280 returns used here. He enlisted as surgeon of the 106th Illinois on August 10, 1863, noting his place of residence as Cayuga, Illinois, but resigned his commission the following December.[46]

Alfred Lewis Castleman has a relatively high profile among historians of medicine in the Civil War era because of his outspokenness. He received training at the Louisville Medical School before moving to Milwaukee in 1835 to practice. As president of the state medical society by 1853, he attacked quackery and advocated for the creation of a medical school at the University of Wisconsin and the establishment of a state mental asylum. On the outbreak of war, Castleman became surgeon of the Fifth Wisconsin. His experience with the Army of the Potomac during the first year of the conflict exposed him to what he considered to be many faults in the medical system. Most of them stemmed from a perceived lack of respect for the professionalism of army surgeons. Castleman vented his frustrations in *The Army of the Potomac Behind the Scenes: A Diary of Unwritten History,* published in 1863. Even before its appearance, he had resigned his commission in December 1862. Thereafter he became an avid supporter of the Sanitary Commission, filling out ten of the returns used here. He concentrated on inspecting camps in the Army of the Cumberland during 1863, producing some of the more useful information to be included in this study. After visiting the Seventy-Ninth Pennsylvania near Murfreesboro, Castleman admitted its camp was better than most. Yet he still "found many opportunities of making suggestions in small matters." His chief advice was to improve the latrines and garbage-collection regimen.[47]

Robert Collyer was among the least likely candidates for a camp inspector. Born in England, he initially worked as a blacksmith like his father but eventually moved to the United States, where he became a Methodist minister. Collyer later switched to Unitarianism and founded the Unity Church in Chicago in January 1860. Henry Bellows, minister of All Souls Church in New York City, invited Collyer to join him in camp inspection work, and the Englishman agreed despite having no medical training. Collyer toured many camps near Washington, DC, soon after the First Battle of Bull Run and then went to Missouri in October 1861. He looked back over his burst of field activity in a letter to a friend on October 29. "I came into contact with about 50,000 all told and found camp like homes, a few nearly perfect, a good many that needed to be amended, and the rest dirty, disorderly and disorganized." That was an honest assessment that could be applied to the results of virtually all camp inspectors across the country. Four of the returns used here were written by Collyer.[48]

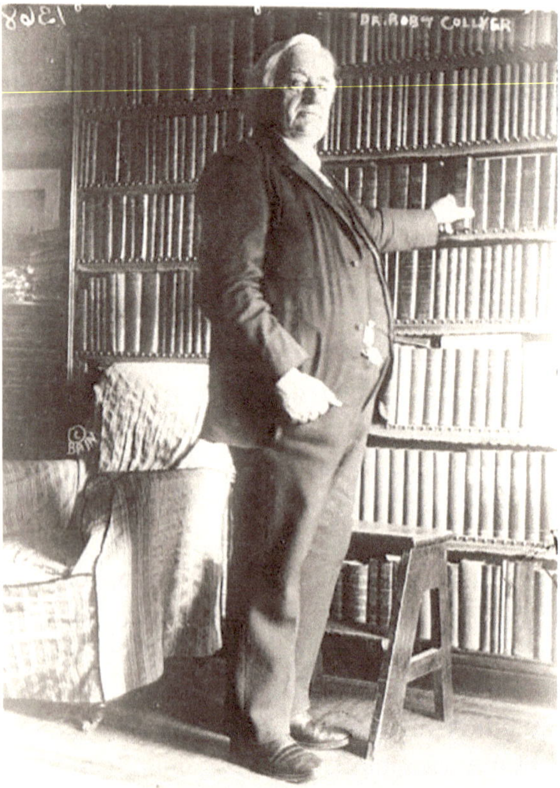

Robert Collyer. The English-born Collyer immigrated to the United States and eventually became a Unitarian minister in Chicago. He was thirty-eight years old when the Civil War began. Although having no medical training, his friendship with Henry Bellows led to his work as a Sanitary Commission camp inspector. This photograph was taken long after the war ended and before Collyer passed away in 1912. (Library of Congress, Prints & Photographs Division, LCDIG-ggbain-07414)

John Hancock Douglas achieved notice for his work beyond the Sanitary Commission. He earned a bachelor's degree from Williams College in 1843 and a medical degree from the Medical School at the University of Pennsylvania in 1847. Douglas traveled three times to Europe before settling in Manhattan as a throat specialist. He became a camp inspector in July 1861 and worked as a commission administrator in September of that year. Douglas filled out 17 of the 280 returns used here. He resigned from commission work in July 1864 and edited several medical journals in the Civil War era, resuming his practice in New York City. In fact, Douglas was called in to consult with Ulysses S. Grant when the former president developed throat cancer. He could do little more than to help relieve Grant's pain as the former general struggled to write his memoirs. After Grant's death in 1885, Douglas himself suffered a serious decline in health, probably due to a stroke, and endured financial difficulties until he died in 1892.[49]

William W. Estabrook, on the other hand, had a varied and visible career. Trained as a physician but then switching to the Episcopalian ministry, he was living in Clinton, Iowa, when the war broke out. Estabrook enlisted as chaplain of the Fifteenth Iowa in December 1861. He applied both of his professions at the Battle of Shiloh (April 6–7, 1862), where he not only acted as chaplain but also performed surgery on wounded men. Detailed to serve as chaplain of Seminary Hospital at Corinth, Mississippi, in September 1862, Estabrook resigned his commission in April 1863. He filled out one of the selected returns. Estabrook also served as surgeon of the Forty-Fifth Iowa, a hundred-day regiment, from May to September 1864.[50]

James Gall Jr., who filled out three returns, was born in Scotland. He became a landscape engineer in the United States and worked with Olmsted in creating Central Park in New York City. Undoubtedly, Gall came into Sanitary Commission work only because of his association with Olmsted. Gall also worked on Prospect Park in Brooklyn and after the war helped plan national cemeteries at Vicksburg, Gettysburg, and Chattanooga. Another of his major projects was to help lay out the Vanderbilt estate, Biltmore, in western North Carolina.[51]

Franklin Benjamin Hough, who filled out thirteen of the returns, was the renaissance man of the thirty-four inspectors. He graduated from Union College in 1843 with an interest in botany, geology, and mineralogy. Hough then took a course of study at the Cleveland Medical College before opening a practice in Somerville, New York, from 1848 to 1852. He added local history to his list of interests, writing several county histories, and also recorded meteorological observations. Hough moved to Albany to superintend the 1855 New York census, moving again by 1860 to Lowville, New York. With the outbreak of war, he became involved in sanitary efforts. Most of his camp inspections were conducted late in 1861 and early in 1862. In addition to the official form, Hough kept a diary of his experiences as a camp inspector to be read by his children, illustrating it with hand-drawn pictures. He also translated into English the French-language edition of Baudens's book on sanitary conditions of the French and British armies during the Crimean War, providing annotations to compare the conditions of that conflict with those in the early months of the Civil War. His translation was published with a dedication to the administrative and medical officers of the US Army in 1862. Hough became surgeon of the Ninety-Seventh New York from July 3, 1862, until he resigned on March 10, 1863, and agreed to write a history of the regiment's brigade, which was published in 1864. Hough achieved his greatest influence, however, right after the war. While working on the 1865 New York state census, he noticed an alarming decrease in the production of lumber in some areas of the state and its increase in others. This sparked

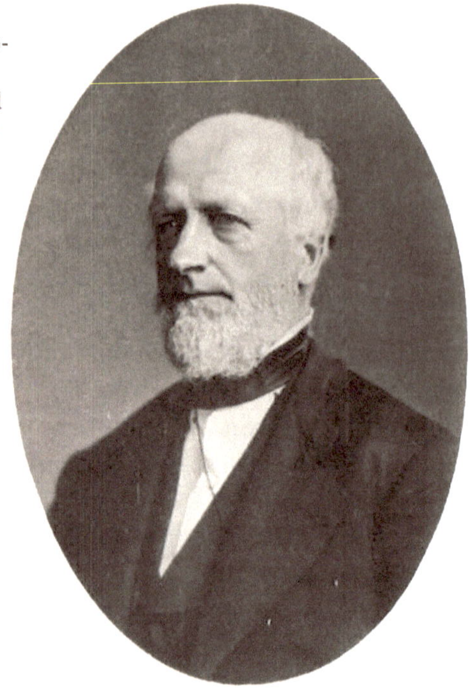

Franklin B. Hough. A polymath proficient as a botanist, geologist, mineralogist, physician, historian, and census taker, Hough was thirty-nine years old when the Civil War began. During the war, he was a Sanitary Commission camp inspector and surgeon of the Ninety-Seventh New York for a time. After the war he gained national fame as a pioneer forester. This photographic portrait was taken between 1880 and 1885. (Library of Congress, Prints & Photographs Division, LC-USZ62-11107)

his curiosity and concern, leading to a concentrated effort to study the science of forestry for the rest of his life. Hough became a prominent leader in the development of governmental efforts to study and correct problems of deforestation. He was appointed a special agent of the US Department of Agriculture for this task and later became the first chief of the department's newly created Division of Forestry in 1881. In short, camp sanitation was only one small part of Hough's busy life as an environmentalist, historian, and healthcare provider.[52]

Marvin Manville Marsh became a schoolteacher before attending Albany Medical School, from which he graduated in 1841. Marsh practiced in Onondaga County until 1857, when he once again became a teacher. The Civil War brought him out for camp inspections, and he completed five of the returns used here, all of them along the coast of South Carolina during the middle phase of the war. Marsh also collected weather observations for the Smithsonian Institution while living in the Beaufort area with his wife. Near the end of the conflict, he became superintendent of the Discharged Soldier's Home in New York City until its closure in 1866.[53]

Lewis Henry Steiner, who filled out four of the returns, was a graduate of Marshall College in Pennsylvania. He went on to earn a master's degree in 1849, the same year he finished his training in the medical school of the University of Pennsylvania. Steiner practiced in Frederick, Maryland, for a while before moving in 1852 to Baltimore, where he taught chemistry for a short time before moving first to Columbian College in Washington, DC, and then to several other colleges in the years before the Civil War. Steiner published a booklet about the Confederate occupation of Frederick during the Maryland Campaign of 1862, which he personally witnessed.[54]

William F. Swalm became a surgeon's mate in the Fourteenth Regiment New York State Militia, which entered US service as the Eighty-Fourth New York. By the time he resigned in November 1862, Swalm was listed as an assistant surgeon. He filled out two of the returns used here. In January 1865 he became assistant surgeon of the Fifteenth New York Engineers. After the war Swalm was employed as a medical officer in the Brooklyn Fire Department.[55]

Robert Ware was an unusual inspector. The son of Harvard medical professor John Ware, Robert graduated from Harvard in 1852 and studied medicine in Boston and Europe before receiving his medical degree from Harvard in 1856. He largely cared for the poor and indigent before becoming involved with the Sanitary Commission in the first year of the war at

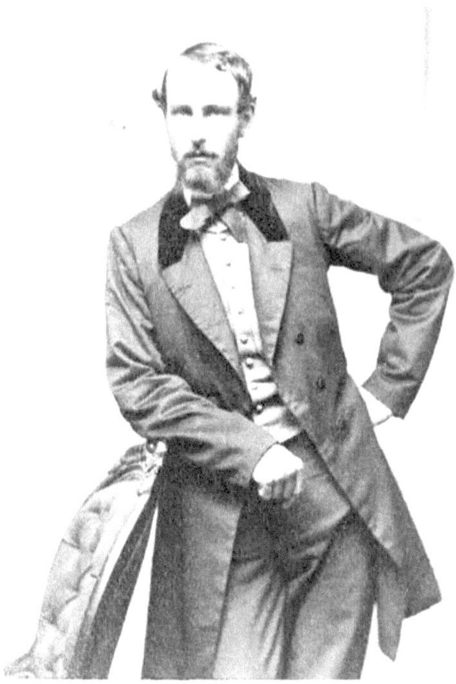

Robert Ware. This young, promising physician, the son of a Harvard professor, was one of the most conscientious camp inspectors. He also wrote letters describing his inspection experience that highly enlighten us on the job of a commission worker. Through consistently hard work along sanitary lines, Ware eventually won respect among the members of the Forty-Fourth Massachusetts, which he served as surgeon. He tragically lost his life to disease before the nine-month enlistment period of his unit ended. Ware is depicted in this carte de visite, taken by John Payson Soule, in civilian clothes before entering the army. (Wolcott Family Civil War Carte de Visite Album, vol. 1, p. 2, no. 70.23, Collection of the Massachusetts Historical Society)

age twenty-eight. Ware filled out fifteen of the selected returns. Working out of Newport News, Virginia, in December 1861, he visited two regiments each day by riding on horseback to their camps. On moving to Rockville, Maryland, Ware carried his sanitary returns in a rubber bag to keep them dry on rainy days. Then moving to Fortress Monroe in January 1862, he began to feel the strain of constant visiting. "I am so much in the daily habit of talking about dirt and bad air to all whom I meet, that when it comes to sitting down and talking to a person who isn't dirty and doesn't breathe bad air, I hardly know what to say." Ware felt that he was "nothing if not Sanitary at all times and places."[56]

The commission assigned Ware to hospital-transport service during the Peninsula Campaign, when he helped outfit government steamers for carrying sick and wounded soldiers from southeastern Virginia to hospitals in the North. He accepted a commission as surgeon of the Forty-Fourth Massachusetts, a nine-month regiment, in the fall of 1862. Ware earned the nickname "Old Sanitary" because of his assiduous efforts to weed out food delicacies from home, such as "cake, pickles, preserves, [and] canned goods," that he thought were injurious to soldier health. "With a frame compact, sinewy and nervous, Dr. Ware [was] the apparent embodiment of physical health," recalled Zenas T. Haines of the Forty-Fourth. Another regimental member described the surgeon as "pure-souled, refined, and high-minded" because he insisted on "the strictest observance of sanitary regulations." At first many men in the regiment resented his attention to their health. Haines complained that Ware's experiences as a Sanitary Commission worker during the Peninsula Campaign had led him to strip down the recruits of the Forty-Fourth Massachusetts to the bare necessities, "and we are reduced to a very bad condition indeed. We shall probably see the wisdom of this severity more clearly by and by. At present a majority of the boys don't see it at all." When a transport arrived with sutlers and their wares in late January 1863, Robert had his hands full. "Now the barracks will be filled with all sorts of mouldy trash in the shape of pies and decayed puddings, semi-putrescent sausages, and unwholesome litter general[ly]; and on Sunday inspection I shall rouse the wrath of the men by having a considerable amount of it emptied into the swill barrels."[57]

Ware died, tragically, before the regiment went home. His apparently strong constitution hid what likely was a "cardiac debility not favorable to a long life," a sign of it appearing briefly during a visit to Washington, North Carolina, in November 1862. It is possible that the heart condition made him vulnerable to a severe attack of double pneumonia, with typhoid symptoms, on April 5, 1863, during the siege of Washington by Confederate forces. For several days his mind wandered with the high fever. On April 10 a particularly heavy Confederate artillery bombardment "excited him to wildness," but later that day he died peacefully just four days before the lifting of the siege. By this time most of the regiment had accepted him despite his strict measures and felt great sadness over his death. Ware was buried on the afternoon of April 11 but disinterred on April 26 for transport to Boston. "He was a good man," concluded John J. Wyeth of the Forty-Fourth Massachusetts, a sentiment echoed by the many Black men and women who he treated and gave medicine to during his short term in the army.[58]

Henry W. Warriner, who filled in three of the returns, became a professor at Antioch College. He also edited a Republican newspaper in Louisville, Kentucky, early in the war. Warriner later became a Sanitary Commission worker and was involved in compiling material for its history after the conflict. He lived in Deerfield, Massachusetts, served in the state legislature, and taught at Plymouth until his death.[59]

Gordon Hubbard Winslow was responsible for three of the returns in this book. He graduated from Yale College and became a physician but later switched to the Episcopalian ministry on Staten Island. That is how

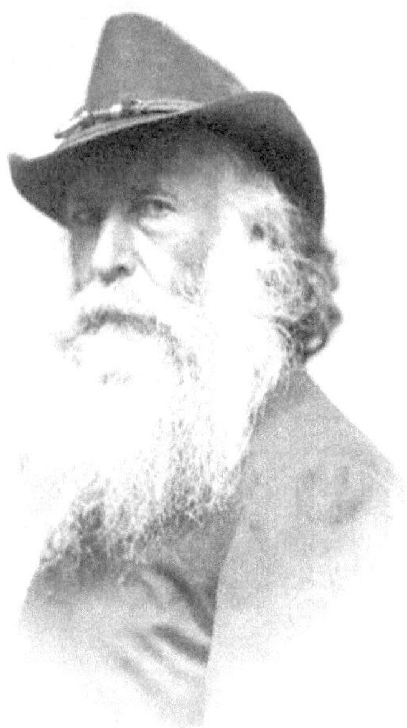

Gordon Hubbard Winslow. A physician and chaplain, Winslow was fifty-six when the Civil War broke out. While serving as chaplain of the Fifth New York, he also inspected camps for the Sanitary Commission. (Library of Congress, Prints & Photographs Division, LCDIG-ppmsca-71474)

he became chaplain of the Fifth New York early in the war and mustered out with the regiment in May 1863. While serving with the Fifth, Winslow also inspected camps for the Sanitary Commission and was assigned to the Army of the Potomac for that purpose. He drowned in the Potomac River on June 7, 1864.[60]

The camp inspectors were an eclectic lot. While the profession of medicine was the most common occupation among them, many others were represented as well. Few of these men had experience as regimental surgeons, some had no experience in medicine at all, and the background of nearly half is unknown. The quality of the returns they filled out also varied. While most of these inspectors were thorough and thoughtful, answering every question and often writing extra information, a couple never wrote anything extra and did not even provide a checkmark to indicate yes or no for all the questions. On the whole, however, the returns are a unique and reliable resource for the study of preventive healthcare in the Union army.

As Henry Bellows and the rest of the executive committee informed President Abraham Lincoln in August 1862, the US Sanitary Commission was "pledged to act with energy wherever it can, in all that concerns the health of the volunteer Army."[61] They tended to view the camp inspection program as the foundation of that worthy effort. Preventive healthcare through rational observation and smart correctives was the goal, as the commission drew on a wealth of experience in the Crimean War, the authority of published statistics concerning public-health concerns in the United States, and a strident desire to help the Northern cause by conserving its precious manpower as much as possible in the camp environment. The following chapters delve into the camp returns to see what the commission inspectors found.

2

Camp Situation

The first subject area on the US Sanitary Commission form for camp inspectors related to the camp's environment. Camp situation, as it was labeled, connected the soldier's military home with the natural environment as a unique place separate from the rural or urban environments in which most Americans lived. It concentrated hundreds of men in a small space, greatly increasing the pollution of their living area and setting up close contact for the transmission of diseases. All sanitarians wrote about this subject area as one that held obvious and fundamental influences on soldier health. The US Army also highlighted the importance of properly selecting a campsite, arranging the living quarters in an orderly way, and policing the grounds regularly to avert catastrophic diseases from spreading.

In many ways, the most fundamental topic of preventive healthcare in the army was the relation of the camp to its environment. This involved looking at the type of soil the camp was located on; examining the topography of the area, its tree cover, the presence of standing water on the surface, and the water level underneath the surface; and determining how much and from which direction wind sailed through the site. The tight connection between man and nature was obvious.

ARMY CAMPS

But first we must define what the army meant by a camp. Volunteers tended to use the term loosely, but there were various gradations of camping arrangements. George B. McClellan noted this in writing of his Delafield

Commission experience in Europe. The term *camp* could refer to "all the arrangements of the troops when halted, whether in tents, huts, bivouac, or villages, provided they are not in cantonments or winter quarters." The last two site types implied a lengthy stay in one spot, while the previous four involved temporary stays.[1]

English cavalry officer Louis E. Nolan identified two types of camps, "Marching" and "Fighting," depending on the proximity of the enemy. He noted that European armies seldom used tents except in their camps of instruction. In the field they considered them a nuisance that retarded movement and preferred to utilize the many villages that dotted the European landscape to shelter their troops. To bivouac in the open was at times necessary but dangerous in Nolan's view. Sleeping even temporarily in the open, with only a blanket as cover, exposed the soldier to cold and damp night air. The experience "destroys the health for the men," he concluded. In selecting temporary camps Nolan advised avoiding wet and low ground, choosing instead slopes so that rainwater could run away from instead of toward the camping area. Planting oneself near sources of good water and wood was smart, and preventing the men from bathing upstream in the source of water was essential.[2]

The US Army was up to date in terms of establishing standards for camps. It began in the middle of the Revolutionary War when Frederick W. A. Von Steuben created the first standard camp regulations for the Continental Army at Valley Forge. Published in 1779, it was the beginning of a long tradition of detailed information about camp selection and arrangement in American forces. The general idea was to establish the camp based on the regimental front as defined by the unit in a two-rank line of battle. Each company laid out a street perpendicular to that basic line with tents pitched so as to face each other across each street. The tents were to be put two paces from each other, with the same distance between the rear of tents on adjacent streets. Sinks were to be dug 150 paces away from camp for the men and 100 paces away for the officers.[3]

Facing page: Camp Layout. The army prescribed the way a semipermanent camp should be laid out, beginning with the color line and proceeding with the company streets placed at a right angle to that line. Two rows of tents or huts on either side of the street were separated from the company kitchens. Officers' quarters were separate from the enlisted men's quarters. Sinks for the men and officers also were separated as far as they could be—in this layout, on opposite sides of the regimental camp. (Revised Regulations, 77)

Camp of a Regiment of Infantry.

Cl.—Colonel.
Lt. Cl.—Lieut. Colonel.
M.—Major.
Surg.—Surgeon.
Ast. Surg.—Asst. Surgeon.
Adjt.—Adjutant.
Q. M.—Quarter Master.
n-c-s.—Non.-Com.-Staff.

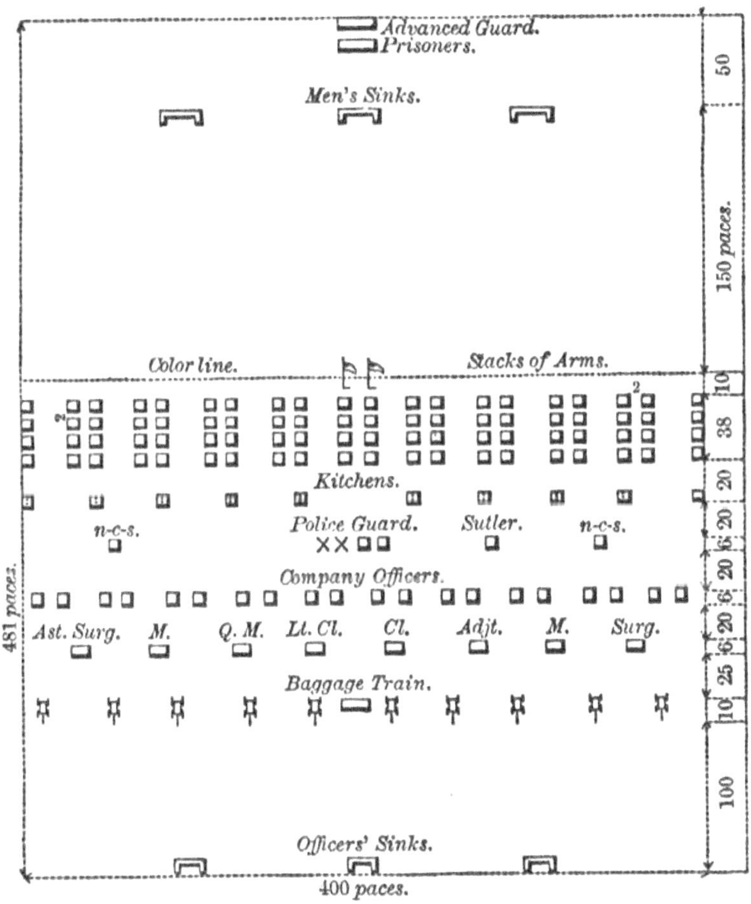

THE SANITARY CAMP

All the US Sanitary Commission returns were for inspections conducted at semipermanent Union army camps like the one described in army regulations. The inspectors did not accompany troops on campaign. Thus, the returns failed to take into account the many health challenges involved in one-night bivouacs, where the officers had little if any choice of a stopping place. In semipermanent camps, on the other hand, officers usually had the opportunity to select locations as well as time to make sure their men followed sanitary principles in arranging their living quarters.

For this type of semipermanent camp, the kind in which soldiers lived for the majority of their time in service, Civil War sanitarians had plenty of advice. Columbia College professor John Ordronaux recognized that stricter rules of hygiene were needed in semipermanent camps than in temporary bivouacs. He identified three main concerns: selecting dry ground, locating close to fresh water, and sheltering the men from persistent winds. Surgeon General Hammond went into more detail by noting how much moisture was retained by differing soil types. The worst was a sandy upper layer with clay beneath, which inhibited proper seepage and kept the surface damp. But gravel subsurface combined with a sandy top layer was good. Ground that was already exposed to air and sun was better than vegetated ground that had to be cleared for the camp. Regular maintenance was important. Hammond advised the men to sweep company streets every day, to air their tents by raising the walls and opening doors daily, and to expose their bedding to air and sun. For flooring inside the tents, he wanted them to use a layer of straw, which had to be replaced every week. Hammond also urged that beef-slaughtering areas should be located far from camp and offal should be burned. Commission official W. H. Van Buren echoed all these recommendations and added that the men should dig a small ditch at least eight inches deep around every tent to connect with deeper main drains along company streets.[4]

In general, army regulations paid attention to these prescriptions while instructing officers in how to select campsites. General-in-Chief Winfield Scott, while advising the governor of New York in how to establish camps of instruction, urged him to find a site with "a rolling surface or porous soil" that also was close to good sources of wood, water, and railroad or canal facilities. Numerous orders issued by various headquarters throughout the war reminded subordinates of basic considerations and urged them to follow the regulations already established. Moving the campsite to fresh

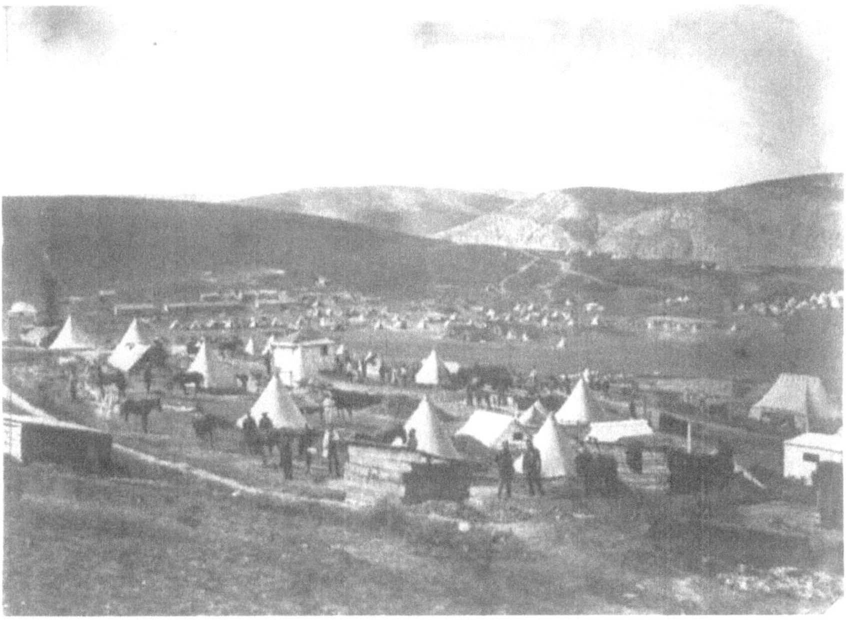

British Camp near Sebastopol. Identified as the camp of the Fifth Dragoon Guards, looking toward Kadikoi, this photograph by Roger Fenton depicts an army encampment as it was supposed to be arranged according to sanitarians. The mostly conical tents are separated by wide intervals for good air flow. There are several wooden huts as well. (Library of Congress, Manuscript Division, Fenton Crimean War Photographs, LC-USZC4-9178)

ground now and then was considered good policy. If natural drainage was poor, the only recourse was to dig ditches deeper and increase daily maintenance to keep them unclogged by silt or garbage.[5]

Many soldiers understood the necessities of a healthy campsite after a few months of experience. Maine artilleryman William B. Lapham noted that the three essentials were wood, water, and a type of soil that drained well. The troops often took personal interest in keeping the place clean and decorating it with cedar trees and bushes cut from nearby woods. The company streets of the Eighty-Fourth Illinois were swept so often they became "almost as hard as a brick pavement" during the long encampment following the Battle of Stones River (December 31, 1862–January 2, 1863). It was not uncommon that units had to clear a chosen campsite of vegetation, and at times they had to level off rough undulations of the ground to provide level surface areas for tents. How well their commander chose a campsite had a direct effect on the men's morale. "Bad camps and comfortless nights disgust more men with campaigning than battles, and kill more horses than marching," asserted Lt. Frederick Whittaker of the Sixth New York Cavalry. An officer who had peculiar ideas of his own about the proper campsite or arrangements tended to be disliked by the men. When Brig. Gen. Alfred T. A. Torbert commanded the First Cavalry Division in Maj. Gen. Philip H. Sheridan's Cavalry Corps, Army of the Potomac, he sometimes kept the men waiting for an hour and a half while staff officers searched for a campsite that could accommodate the entire division in one field. Often the place wound up being a plowed field that proved muddy and uncomfortable. The men were happier when Brig. Gen. Thomas C. Devin replaced Torbert and let them camp in a dispersed arrangement and often allowed them to settle in the woods, although camping among trees was frowned upon by Civil War sanitarians because it inhibited the flow of fresh air around and through the tents.[6]

CAMP ARRANGEMENTS

All regiments were supposed to arrange their camps according to the regulations, and the evidence suggests that most of them more or less did so. The degree to which they complied varied according to the type of man who commanded the unit. Some were sticklers and adhered very closely to the regulations, while others only approximated that standard by allowing variations on the formula. A minority of regimental commanders paid no attention to the regulations and allowed their men to pitch tents in any order they wished. If the camp was located in woods, regulations largely went out of the window because trees inhibited the orderly arrangement of tents and company streets. The Thirteenth New Hampshire arranged its camp at Falmouth soon after the Battle of Fredericksburg (December 13, 1862) to conform to the terrain, which was a slope draining into a brook. The tents were "mixed up, and angling in every direction, as the contour and drainage of the land demanded," wrote the regimental historian. "There can be on this camp ground neither order nor regularity."[7]

The regulations stipulated that only the privates live along company streets. A separate row of tents for noncommissioned officers, another row for company officers, and still another for the field and staff officers of the regiment were made perpendicular to the company streets. At least in the Seventy-Fifth New York, a fourth perpendicular line consisted of company kitchens. The regimental camp encompassed all members of the unit in a tight space of ground but in an orderly fashion that was designed not only

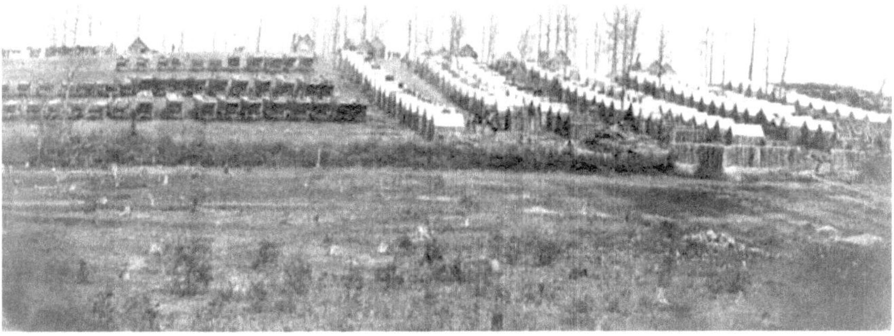

Winter Quarters. The Fiftieth New York Engineers constructed a model semipermanent camp near Rappahannock Station, Virginia, which was photographed in March 1864. The huts were uniformly built with tented roofs and exactly aligned along streets. The camp is laid out on a slope to facilitate water runoff, and there is plenty of open space around the huts for proper air circulation. Pontoons on wagons are parked to one side, larger huts for officers are on another side, and a stockade with a gate opening allows entry to the camp from along yet a third side. (Library of Congress, Prints & Photographs Division, LC-USZ62-76824)

to promote sanitary measures but also to maintain the tenuous but real distance between officers, noncommissioned officers, and privates. It was, in other words, a well-ordered social space in the military environment with important medical concerns underlying the order.[8]

Because they left a physical impression on the land, Civil War camps have become an object of study by historic archaeologists, although they often find relatively little in the way of material remains. Large and semipermanent camps, such as those constructed for enduring the winter months, tend to leave behind more physical evidence on the ground than smaller, regimental camps that existed only for a few weeks. If soldiers lived in huts built with foundations dug into the earth, the archaeologist can find and study the impressions. They often discover hearths and fireplaces dug into the earth, with their telltale campfire scorch marks. Places leveled for tents also leave their mark on the earth, and of course material objects turn up, such as personal possessions, military items, and the bones of domestic animals butchered and eaten in the camp. Archaeologists have confirmed through the material evidence that the regulations were more or less followed. For example, the Fourteenth Connecticut stayed in one camp at Milton's Mill near Brandy Station, Virginia, November 10–26, 1863. Here, five hundred men lived in an area of 108,000 square feet in a rough approximation to the army prescription, allowing each man on average 216 square feet of ground.[9]

CAMP CLEANLINESS

Following the army regulations for camp selection and layout established the foundation for a healthy environment for the living space. But the next step was for the men to take care of that space by keeping it clean of their garbage and draining the tent areas to reduce the accumulation of moisture. Work to promote good camp hygiene included regular inspections by the medical personnel, detailing men to police the grounds (even if that meant assigning cleaning duties as punishment for those who broke regulations), and changing campsites now and then to get away from the filth accumulated at old sites. It could also mean felling trees to let in more sunshine.[10]

Most soldiers came to appreciate that cleaning the site and keeping it dry were keys to a healthy camp. Whenever decorations appeared, such as small cedar trees replanted along company streets or arbors erected across those streets, that was a sign of unit pride in the appearance of its campsite. These additions always accompanied a high degree of cleanliness and orderly layout of the tents. Members of the Twelfth Indiana spared no labor in making their winter quarters a showcase at Scottsboro, Alabama, during the early months of 1864. Word of it spread, and men came from their own camps in the area to see it. Theodore R. Davis sketched the camp for an illustration in *Harper's Weekly.* The troops constructed a hut to serve as a guardhouse, built storerooms for quartermaster and commissary supplies, and erected a regimental chapel.[11]

But in contrast to the model camp of the Twelfth Indiana, many regimental camps were dirty and disorderly. In some cases, the troops simply shoveled the garbage into the middle of company streets and left it there to decay. Capt. Rufus D. Pettit allowed the men of his Battery B, First New York Light Artillery to plant their tents "just wherever suited the occupants to put them" and also paid little attention to camp police. Some camps, improperly located downslope, suffered from water runoff from higher ground where latrines, slop holes, and even dead horses and mules were located. If the officers did not compel their men to properly bury animals left nearby, the stench was "extremely unpleasant, if not really unhealthy." In the best of conditions, camp life could produce "noise, *mudd* and damp and discomfort" that only strict attention to cleanliness could avert. If a regiment accustomed to a clean camp had to move to a site recently vacated by one that had lower standards, the first order of the day was to clean up the area before settling in.[12]

THOSE RESPONSIBLE FOR CAMP CLEANLINESS

The evidence arising from soldier accounts and official army reports indicate a disturbing lack of uniformly clean camp procedures despite all the regulations, rules, and sanitary advice available to regimental commanders. So much depended on how conscientious those officers happened to be, how seriously they took their responsibility for the health of their men, and especially how ready they were to listen to and cooperate with the medical officers of their command. It is not that all regimental surgeons were good sanitarians; coming from civilian life just as did their regimental commanders, some were aware of sanitary principles and others were not. But another level of this problem lay in the fact that medical officers could only advise, not order, within the regiment. If his advice was ignored by the colonel, the surgeon had some leeway to improve conditions but could never thoroughly do so without the cooperation of the commander.

Alfred L. Castleman, one of the thirty-four inspectors whose returns are used here, provided a case study of tensions between the regimental surgeon and his commander during his yearlong tenure as surgeon of the Fifth Wisconsin. On the way to war, the regiment arrived at Harrisburg, Pennsylvania, on July 27, 1861, to find Camp Curtin filthy and the weather "intensely hot." Castleman took responsibility "to visit every tent twice a day, to see that they were thoroughly cleaned, and that the sides of the tent were raised so as freely to admit a current of air." He made the men strike their tents and move them a few feet every week to occupy fresh ground. Col. Amasa Cobb, a politician who later ran for Congress while still serving in the regiment, "was positively ignorant of the fact that we had a hospital on the ground," Castleman sarcastically wrote, even though it occupied three tents filled with sick men within fifty feet of his quarters. "I was now receiving but little support in my efforts for their health and comfort." Cobb tried to reduce Castleman's personnel, claiming he had too many staff members, but the doctor only had three nurses and two cooks for one hundred sick troops. When the colonel confronted the surgeon on this issue, Castleman

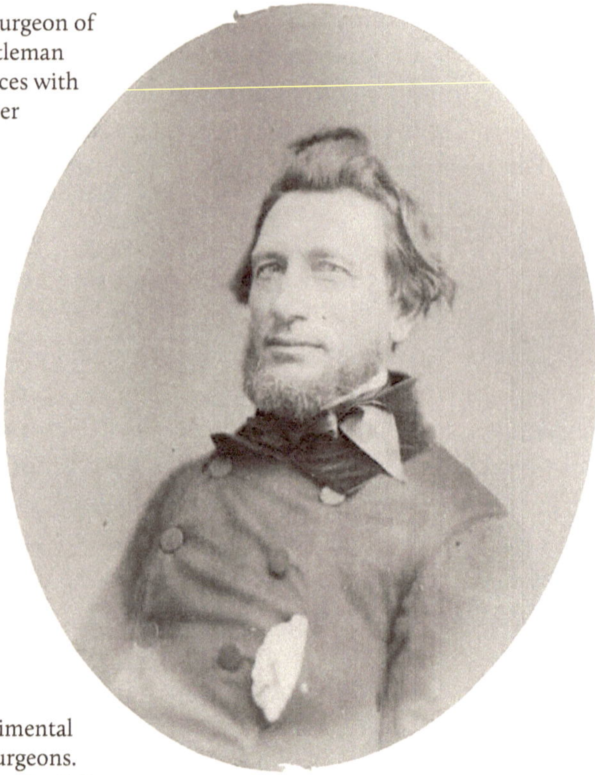

Alfred L. Castleman. As surgeon of the Fifth Wisconsin, Castleman wrote about his experiences with his regimental commander concerning a serious difference of opinion about exactly where the line between their respective responsibilities for the health of the men lay. Both men fought each other for months before they left the regiment—Castleman resigned and became a US Sanitary Commission camp inspector, while Cobb was elected to Congress. Their tussle reflected a persistent problem with preventive healthcare in the Union army: an imprecise delegation of authority between regimental commanders and their surgeons. This photograph was taken by Fuller and Johnson of Dane County, Wisconsin, in 1856. (Image 27916, Wisconsin Historical Society)

agreed to reduce his personnel only if responsibility for taking care of the sick was given to someone else, which forced Cobb to back off.[13]

"The jealousy existing in the military towards the medical department of the army astounds me," wrote Castleman. Commanders claimed that surgeons had no authority "except through them," and medical officers were incited to take up the other extreme view, claiming to be "the only officers in the army who are really independent of command." This bitter argument was unnecessary, to say the least, but fortunately it did not occur in all regiments. But in the Fifth Wisconsin, the quarrel hounded Castleman for the duration of his tenure in the regiment and greatly impeded his ability to care for the men. When the regiment moved to a different location, Cobb chose the new campsite without consulting Castleman and laid it out with tents far too close to each other. After some wrangling, the doctor obtained permission to rearrange everything. But Cobb had "interfered much with my sanitary orders," Castleman complained, "particularly those in reference to ventilation."[14]

Things came to a head in early November 1861 when Cobb overheard Castleman give orders to some men for cleaning the camp and ventilating the tents. The colonel ordered the men not to obey Castleman, irritated that the surgeon had not received his permission to order anyone to do anything. That was the last straw. Castleman decided to let Cobb handle all sanitary matters afterward and confined his duties to the regimental hospital. According to the doctor, the results became evident in only three weeks, as the sick list soared from 39 to 160. Gov. Alexander Randall happened to visit the Fifth Wisconsin on November 29, so Castleman pleaded his case and

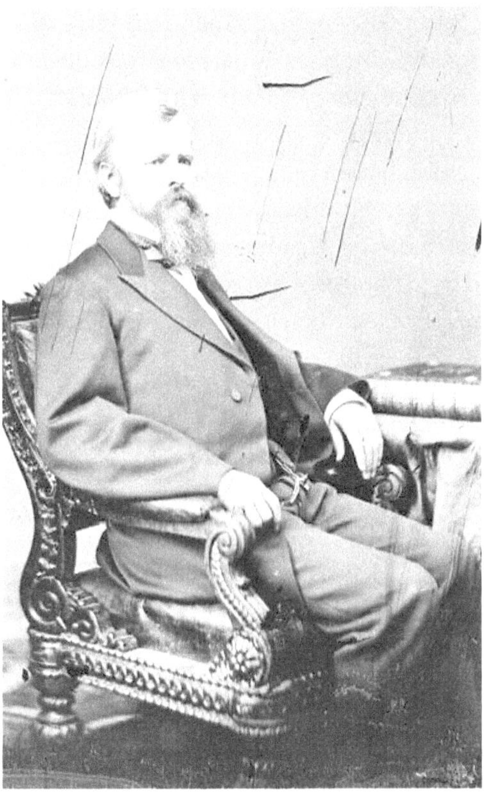

Amasa Cobb. As colonel of the Fifth Wisconsin, Cobb adopted a strident, even aggressive, attitude toward Castleman. He tried to minutely control all aspects of his position as regimental commander, refusing even to allow Castleman to order the men to clean up their quarters without his approval. Cooperation between colonel and surgeon later served the interests of the men far better than this kind of turf fighting. This photograph depicts Cobb as a congressman in Washington, DC, after his election to a House seat as a Republican in 1862 and his resignation from the army. Born in Illinois in 1823 but moving to Wisconsin with his family a few years later, Cobb engaged in lead mining and practiced law as well as serving in the Mexican War, in the state senate, as adjutant general of Wisconsin, and as speaker of the state assembly by 1861. (Local Identifier 111-B-3115, Mathew Brady Photographs of Civil War Era Personalities and Scenes, RG 111, Records of the Office of the Chief Signal Officer, 1860–1985, NARA)

convinced him to intervene. The next day Cobb rescinded his November 9 regimental order not to obey Castleman and "entrusted to the Surgeon of the regiment" all the "sanitary regulations of the camp." According to the triumphant surgeon, within six days he reduced the sick list to about 50 men. Another 75–100 men complained of poor health but were not really sick in his view, suffering only from colds, chafed feet, and other minor troubles.[15]

Castleman shared his experience by writing a book about his service in the Army of the Potomac, laying out the problems of sanitary care that stemmed from the lack of clarity about the power of surgeons to act within the regimental organization. His story also demonstrates that much of that problem stemmed from personal difficulties. Cobb was adamant about controlling everything within the regiment, while Castleman asserted the surgeon's right to be fully responsible for the men's healthcare. This overlapping of authority applied literally to every regiment in the Union army, but it did not always produce the bitter friction that it did in the Fifth Wisconsin. If a regiment's commander and surgeon were willing to cooperate rather than contest authority, the lack of clarity did not harm anyone.

Castleman documented another interesting strain in his book. On December 21, 1861, some other surgeons appealed to him to support their criticism of the Sanitary Commission. There seemed to be "almost universal prejudice" against the organization, although Castleman did not detail exactly why those surgeons disliked it. Obviously, he agreed with them since he consented to write a newspaper article criticizing the commission, but duties involved with the Battle of Dranesville (December 20, 1861) the day before diverted him from the task. In the end, he never got back to that assignment. But by April 1862, Castleman was happy that he had never written the article because his opinion of the commission had greatly improved. The organization had provided medical supplies when needed, and several months later its support following the terrible Battle of Antietam sealed Castleman's devotion to the commission. He had been "near battles, at battles, [and] in battles" before, "but never till today was I *through* a battle," he wrote on September 17, 1862. Castleman worked from dawn until 11 P.M. caring for the wounded and was forever grateful to receive twenty pounds of chloroform from the Sanitary Commission to help his efforts.[16]

On December 22, 1862, Castleman submitted his resignation as surgeon of the Fifth Wisconsin. Cobb approved and sent it up the chain of command. Three days later Cobb himself resigned as colonel of the regiment to accept a seat in the House of Representatives from Wisconsin. "I am worn out by the labor of the last year and a half," Castleman wrote in his diary.

He needed to "rest for a time," although he left the regiment with some regrets, "for I have grown to love it, both individually and in mass." A few weeks later Castleman became an associate of the Sanitary Commission, concentrating his camp inspection duties with the army in Middle Tennessee in 1863. He included an appendix to his book praising the commission as having "an inestimable power in the relief of the sick and wounded," both in the Army of the Potomac during the first year and a half of the war and in the Army of the Cumberland in 1863.[17]

Castleman represents a bridge between the experienced regimental surgeon and the camp inspector of the Sanitary Commission, for he did well in both jobs. Nothing better illustrates the fundamental significance of camp situation than the fact that so much information on it is available from army sources, soldier accounts, and other official documents. In other words, the commission could exert a bit less influence on the improvement of camp situation than on other subject areas of its inspection program precisely because the subject already had a hefty presence in army culture.

THE SANITARY COMMISSION AND CAMP SITUATION

Sanitary Commission inspectors had very high standards of cleanliness and often were appalled at the squalid conditions they found in volunteer regimental camps, especially early in the war. They had far less patience with substandard camp hygiene than the army personnel who largely agreed with them about the need for some level of hygienic care. Medical officers in the field tended to be more lenient than the commission workers in their efforts to enforce sanitary measures.

Frederick Law Olmsted and Elisha Harris looked at the camps of twenty regiments in the area around Washington, DC, by July 9, 1861, and found camp police almost nonexistent. Bits of discarded food littered the floors of tents, around the tents, and even along company streets, with flies alighting on them. Olmsted and Harris often detected a musty smell inside the sleeping quarters. The tents were too close to each other, none had a full drainage system, and all had very poor ventilation. Many men slept directly on the ground without any protective layer between their bodies and the moist earth. Their report stunned commission executives and was a key document leading to the creation of the camp inspection program.[18]

But that initial assessment by Olmsted and Harris was not typical of the reports that soon followed. Those first volunteer regiments were thrown together quickly and rushed to the field with little time for preparation or observance of sanitary rules. As the war lengthened and the process of mobilization became more regular, one can see a wider variety of sanitary conditions in Union army camps. They ranged from those that warmly pleased the sanitarians to those that continued to appall them, with the majority falling somewhere between those extremes.

When Union forces occupied Ship Island, located a few miles off the Gulf coast of Mississippi, late in 1861, the troops carefully established their camps on this nearly barren sand island, which lay but a few feet above the water level. "A most vigorous inspection each week detected any lurking filth," reported commission agent George W. Avery. In Virginia Dr. Franklin B. Hough happened to catch the Thirty-First New York just when it was changing its camp from a muddy location to a better spot and clearing off the brush. As he approached, Hough heard the sound of axes and saw columns of smoke as the men burned the vegetation, the smell of "green wood, oak & cypress, [and] sassafras" permeated the air. The colonel rode about directing everything, and Hough gave him many bits of advice about how to lay out the camp.[19]

One could find plenty of regimental officers who knew what they were doing when it came to camp situation. In many cases intelligent commanders had to battle unusual environmental conditions. The Twentieth Indiana took the field in August 1861 with good ideas. Its first camp at Cockeysville, Maryland, was well selected, "gravelly and dry, with a good elevation," and the commander made sure the grounds were well policed and the men had good straw to sleep on. Even so, Surg. Orpheus Everts reported a sick list amounting to 8 percent of the troops. The regiment moved in late September to the newly occupied Hatteras Island off the coast of North Carolina, where it endured terrible storms that washed out its camp at high tide. The men took shelter in Fort Clark even as the sea tore away part of the parapet. In early November the Twentieth moved to Fortress Monroe and took up a campsite in a wheat field on land twelve feet above high tide. The ground was primarily clay, so Everts made sure the men thoroughly ditched around their tents and graded the company streets for better drainage. Working along the coast, commission inspector Marvin M. Marsh thought that the coastal environment was such that a higher degree of attention to camp drainage was necessary to maintain a proper health regime.[20]

FIFTEENTH CORPS MEDICAL INSPECTION REPORTS

Aside from the many inspection reports of camp situation filed by Sanitary Commission agents, the medical inspectors appointed in the Fifteenth Corps from 1863 on provided another insight into the environmental conditions of semipermanent camps. A survey of many of their monthly inspection reports gives us a clue to how well the regiments of that corps fared. In April 1863 those troops were living along the Mississippi River bottomland near Vicksburg in environmental conditions that were far from ideal. The report for the week ending April 12 included 297 evaluations of a variety of subject areas, all related to camp situation. Of that number, 97 (32.6 percent) rated good, 81 (27.3 percent) rated fair, and 119 (40.1 percent) rated bad. The results were not at all flattering, mainly because bottomland was far from ideal for situating a camp. But later in September, when the corps was settled on high ground in semipermanent camps near the Big Black River east of Vicksburg, conditions were much better. Of 229 evaluations, 165 (72 percent) were good, 48 (21 percent) were fair, and only 16 (7 percent) were bad.[21]

Surg. E. O. F. Roler, who acted as medical inspector of the Second Division and later for the Fifteenth Corps, generally praised the camp situation in September 1863. It was "exceedingly favorable," with the sick list low and consisting mostly of intermittent fever and diarrhea at levels that were commonly expected even of well-ordered camps. Roler did find too much stable manure, camp rubbish, decaying vegetable matter, and animal offal near the camp of the Eighth Missouri and ordered the refuse removed.[22]

The Fifteenth Corps soon left its camps at the Big Black River and moved to East Tennessee that fall. After the Battle of Chattanooga (November 23–25, 1863), it entered winter camps in northern Alabama, where the men once again had a chance to fix up their situation. By now, Surg. John M. Woodworth handled the medical-inspection duties, and he offered considerable praise. Especially when located on level land, extensive drainage ditching took care of excess water. Woodworth particularly praised the camp of the Twenty-Fifth Iowa. "Grounds and qrs. are very clean, and the camp ornamented with evergreens: the men are neat and clean in their persons and clothing." Jumping forward nearly a year, after completing the March to the Sea, Fifteenth Corps regiments continued to receive favorable reports for good order and cleanliness in December 1864. But reports filed in June 1865, when the corps was located outside Louisville, Kentucky, indicated that the camps tended to be too crowded and too shaded. They were situated too often among the trees, and not enough sunlight penetrated to the tent areas. "The narrow space between the tents is used as a receptacle for bits of food etc., and does not admit of being policed."[23]

Reports from the Fifteenth Corps on camp situation show that many factors influenced the environmental conditions. The swamps of the Louisiana bottomland near Vicksburg offered the worst environment and it showed in the elevated bad ratings. The high ground along the west side of the Big Black River in Mississippi made it easier for the regiments to achieve higher good ratings, and the men were generally able to maintain them at other locations with favorable environments. A likely reason for the crowding at Louisville in June 1865 was the need to get the camps under some shade for protection from the scorching summer sun, but that violated a cardinal rule of sanitary science. Moreover, it is possible that officers and men by then were much more interested in going home than in their camp situation.

SANITARY COMMISSION CAMP INSPECTION RETURNS

The Sanitary Commission program of camp inspection began much earlier than did the Fifteenth Corps inspections and extended across the entire Union army; it therefore yielded a different perspective on camp siting. Commission executives approved the inclusion of twenty-three questions concerning this subject area on their best standard form, No. 19a, divided into two major categories, "Character of Camp Site" (thirteen questions) and "Arrangement and Condition of Camp" (ten questions). These questions included the need to identify who selected the site; whether it had been occupied previously, and if so, when it had been evacuated; whether military or sanitary factors guided the site selection; if it was on a hill top or a slope; the amount of shading and shelter from wind; proximity of wood and water; and a division of topsoil type into sandy, loose gravel, loose or firm loam, or clay. The same questions that applied to topsoil also applied to subsoil. Further questions related to how well the camp arrangement conformed to army regulations, how far apart were the tents, and whether artificial drainage was systematic and complete. The drainage ditches were also of interest—their depth and width, whether they were straight or angled, and how well they were kept clear of rubbish. Finally, special attention was paid to whether the areas immediately around the tents and the company streets were kept clear of garbage. The questions were written so the inspector could simply write yes or no in response, but he always had the opportunity to supplement that answer with comments.

The camp situation of the regiments varied pretty widely across the spectrum, as should be expected. From the better ones we descend into the middle range, where good aspects of the twenty-three questions concerning camp situation coexisted with bad aspects. These drew from inspectors a mix of comments as they detailed for the regimental commander and the commission what they saw as defects in camp arrangement. The overall results for the 280 camp inspection returns were 39.6 percent good, 41.5 percent fair, and 18.9 percent bad. The fact that fewer than one-fifth of the units were rated as bad implies that, in general, camp situation passed most inspections. But it is also important to examine how the inspectors evaluated the subareas under this topic.

One can read dozens of positive comments and see many of the questions answered "yes" in the 280 returns. But inspectors did answer "no" to some questions, which offers other insights. Inspectors praised selections that planted a regiment on good sloping ground, on the proper soil, and with an eye toward protecting the site from strong winds while still keeping a good circulation of air. Camp cleanliness drew praise wherever it could be found, while the near presence of stagnant water was criticized. If the drains were wide and deep enough (usually six inches to one foot), straight, and connected to a system that encompassed the entire camp, that also pleased the inspector. But many soldiers tended to view these channels as a convenient dump for garbage, which blocked the free flow of rainwater, which was understandably criticized by the inspectors. Company streets also had to be kept clean, and inspectors were pleased if the men "turnpiked" them, which meant grading the street with a ridge in the middle to drain rainwater off into gutters along the side. The width of company streets ranged from five to twenty feet; inspectors preferred wider streets. In a few cases there were no company streets, with the men allowed to place their tents anywhere they wished, and this was criticized. In a handful of other regiments, company streets were paved with stones or cedar poles, and gutters were covered in places for the men to more easily cross them. Such efforts were highly praised.[24]

Wide variation existed in the results on the details of camp arrangements. The distance between tents in a regimental camp only rarely conformed to army regulations of two paces. One can find distances anywhere from four inches to eighteen feet in the returns, with only about half a dozen returns indicating that the distance came close to regulations. Moreover, the entire regimental camp at times occupied only "half the proper area," as with the Second New Jersey, or two-thirds of the area specified by regulations, as with the Thirty-Second New York.[25]

Creating drains around the tents was an obvious advantage in dealing with rainwater. Of 232 returns that specifically mention this topic, inspectors rated 102 (43.9 percent) as good, 62 (26.7 percent) as fair, and 68 (29.4 percent) as bad. For the bad ratings, the biggest problem was that ditches dug around the tents often were not connected with those alongside the company streets to create a full system of drainage for the camp. Another problem was that these drains often were not kept clear of camp garbage or silt from runoff and thus became clogged and useless.

Inspectors also considered whether the campground was conducive to natural drainage—in other words, if the slope and soil conditions took away rainwater or allowed it to percolate down, reducing the need for artificial drainage in the form of ditches. Of the 77 returns that specifically mentioned this topic, 33.8 percent rated good, 40.3 percent rated fair, and 25.9 percent rated bad. For the bad ratings, it is possible that officers responsible for locating the camp might have paid less attention to this issue than was warranted or that they had only limited choices in camp location. But the worse the natural drainage, the more important it was to have a complete and clean system of ditches.

The most complete system of drains to appear in the returns was located at Camp Parapet near Carrollton, Louisiana, north of New Orleans. The camp lay on completely flat land lower than the adjacent Mississippi River and was protected by a levee. It had a ditch three feet wide and three feet deep entirely around its perimeter. Although the Confederates had initially established the camp before the fall of New Orleans, the Federals improved its drainage system. Its streets were fifteen paces wide, and the tents were from one to two paces apart. Tent sites were raised by carting in earth and shells to raise the ground level.[26]

Inspectors took notice of whether a regiment kept the areas around its tents clear of camp garbage, especially food scraps. Of 225 returns that specifically mention this issue, 79 (35.2 percent) rated good, 116 (51.5 percent) rated fair, and 30 (13.3 percent) rated bad. Thus, only a few regiments did poorly in this subarea. Company streets fared even better than tent areas, with 45.7 percent good, 41.4 percent fair, and 12.9 percent bad among the 232 returns that specifically mention this topic.

Sometimes inspectors wrote with unusual admiration for a regiment's site selection. "This camp is very pleasantly situated [two miles north of Falmouth] on a side hill facing a little to the north of west," F. U. Johnston wrote of the Seventeenth Maine in February 1863. "The level land slopes sufficiently to drain the ground completely." Johnston was equally pleased with the camp of the Seventy-Second Pennsylvania three-quarters of a mile northwest of Falmouth. "This regt is located on the spur of a hill running towards the east falling with a gentle slope to the valley below and also on either side into a valley, so that there is natural drainage in three directions." Inspector W. M. Chamberlain focused on the nature of the soil while visiting the camp of the Fourth New York Heavy Artillery near Alexandria, Virginia, in March 1862. He found the regiment divided into not one but four camps, and all were "well located for Sanitary interests upon lofty and dry sites with a soil of loam and gravel and subsoil of gravel, well situated for drainage." For his part, Alexander McDonald wrote with the highest praise of the 119th Pennsylvania in March 1863. "The camp is excellently located on the south side of a hill, well laid out, kept in perfect order & is in all respects a model camp."[27]

In some cases the inspector recognized that unusual environmental conditions militated against selecting an ideal site. Regiments stationed on the Atlantic and Gulf coasts as well as those along the lower Mississippi River often found themselves near salt water, marshes, or swamps. The men therefore lived on very sandy soil and endured hot, often windless weather conditions. The Seventh Vermont was stationed on Santa Rosa Island near Fort Pickens on the northwest coast of Florida. The island was "a mere tongue of white sand shining" in everyone's eyes, wrote Dr. Edward A. Crane. It was "entirely destitute of vegetation" on the west end, where the Vermonters were camped on ground "but a few feet" above sea level, and "thoroughly exposed" to the Gulf sea environment. Similar conditions were endured by the Thirty-Eighth Iowa while camped along the Rio Grande in Texas. The land there was arid, vegetation scanty, and the temperature unbearably hot. Even up the Mississippi River as far as Bird's Point, on the Missouri side nearly opposite Cairo, Illinois, the presence of swampy land restricted available campsites so that it was impossible to position regiments far enough away from stagnant water to satisfy sanitary inspectors. Even near Washington, DC, and Portsmouth, Virginia, with their low-lying topography, one could find quite a few swamps.[28]

Camp cleanliness was possible even in poor environmental conditions, but the officers and men had to take that idea seriously. At times regimental commanders offered excuses for the dirty state of their camps. The Ninth New York Heavy Artillery stayed on ground recently occupied by another regiment and not cleaned up before they moved in. Plus, huts were being built for the artillerymen. The colonel used this as an excuse, claiming there was no point in cleaning up the camp as it would be vacated soon, even though inspector T. B. Smith noticed a "great amount of sickness" and was sure it was made worse by "the emanations from the filth surrounding" the men. Crane found a similar situation with the Twenty-Fourth Connecticut at Baton Rouge, Louisiana. It had moved into its camp six days before he visited, and Crane found the site still unorganized and unclean. In fact, he could not coax enough information from regimental officers as to why these conditions prevailed so as to completely fill out his return.[29]

Even within a single regiment, camp inspectors found variations between companies that at times were startling. William F. Swalm toured the camp of the Twenty-Sixth Wisconsin in March 1863, noting that two or three company streets were "very cleanly, and in one the drainage is very good." But in the rest he rated both the streets and the drains as poor or only moderately clean. That was a clear sign of laxness on the part of the regimental commander and commendable attention to camp sanitation on the part of only a few company officers. F. U. Johnston ascribed ethnic differences to the fact that the camp of the Sixty-Ninth Pennsylvania exhibited "but little regard to camp streets," with tents and huts placed randomly and too close together. The place also lacked a proper drainage system. "The regt is composed almost entirely of Irishmen officers and all—so that neatness that is evident generally where Americans control is not here visible."[30]

When they found especially bad camp situations, the inspectors were not shy about reporting them. "This is the most miserable camp I have yet visited," Johnston wrote of the Ninth New Hampshire in January 1863. It vividly exhibited "the effect of neglect of officers and the ill effects of Idleness on the men." The regiment camped among trees on top of a hill, and after eight weeks the men had cut down everything in sight but had not yet constructed winter huts. They dug pits and stretched their tents over them, living partly underground, and put these ill-advised habitations too close together. The company streets were "hardly recognizable," and nearly all the tent pits had standing water. No wonder the troops seemed "badly demoralized." Few camps were as bad as this, but many failed to meet proper standards. The most common defect was poor or even nonexistent camp policing, which resulted in far too much "decaying matter about *within* and *between* the tents," as Robert Collyer wrote of Castleman's Fifth Wisconsin in

August 1861. Robert Jones referred to the "great ignorance" of how to run an army camp on the part of regimental officers in the Thirty-Sixth New York. While many inspectors immediately connected the rising sick list with a foul camp, others admitted that they also saw camps with poor sanitation but surprisingly little sickness among the men. Robert Jones expressed this dilemma. He found the Fortieth New York camped on a "humid site" and with "prevailing filth," which he assumed was "enough to account for the disease now existing and to produce much worse." Two months later, in September 1861, he once again inspected the regiment. This time it occupied a different spot, but Jones still found the place a "dirty camp with a general disregard of the laws of health." Even so, the inspector could not account for the fact that the regiment had "a remarkably Short Sick-list" at this second site.[31]

When an inspector found problems, all he could do was to suggest remedies. Collyer advised that a stagnant pond and "a nasty ditch" near the Fifth Wisconsin be drained. Both would "breed mischief if not seen to at once" because of the "broad, sludgy, green" conditions on their surface. If tents were too close, the obvious suggestion was to move them a bit. If drains were inadequate, details should work to improve them. Often the inspectors' suggestions related to relatively small matters that could elevate a camp from a good one to a model example for others. But at other times their suggestions related to fundamental issues designed to correct very serious defects. Inspectors took into account, however, extenuating circumstances. If a regiment intended to occupy a camp only a few days, it could be forgiven if the men did not fuss with housekeeping chores.[32]

Inspectors did not systematically revisit regiments that had bad camps to see if their suggestions for improvement took effect, although there were a handful of cases of this happening. For example, in addition to Robert Jones's two visits to the Fortieth New York, Dr. George A. Blake revisited that regiment a month after his first inspection to find some real improvement in its camp situation. A company of the Fortieth New York that had previously settled in a ravine and suffered greatly from typhoid fever had been moved to a hillside, with "reports [of] improvement of its general health." Blake also found that the horses were picketed farther from camp and that "decidedly odorous heaps of manure," which had been located too close to the regimental hospital during his first visit, had been moved much farther away. The "general appearance of the men and of the camp is vastly better than when first inspected." Blake did not explicitly take credit for these improvements, perhaps because he honestly knew that they could have resulted from trial and error on the part of the regimental officers.[33]

In terms of camp cleanliness, some Sanitary Commission inspectors found the gold standard. Godfrey Aigner exuded admiration when he identified the camp of the Twelfth Illinois as the best he had yet seen in the early months of the war due to its "attention to military hygiene." It was "a model regiment. Its camp is beyond comparison the best regulated and cleanest," which "furnishes altogether a splendid illustration of the beneficent results which follow a strict adherence to sanitary rules by the commanding officer and his staff on the government of their men." That was high praise indeed from a physician with wide experience and a discerning eye. The things that drew the most praise included adherence to army regulations, cleanliness of tent areas and company streets, deep and clean drains and graded streets, and the clean and neat appearance of the men's clothing. Jesse W. Page was impressed that Col. Silas P. Richmond of the Third Massachusetts, a state militia organization called up for nine months' service in the middle of the war, created "a permanent police of 20 men detailed daily with a sergeant, and reporting for duty" to Surg. Alfred A. Stocker to keep the camp clean.[34]

Inspectors also were impressed by the extras that cropped up in a few regimental camps, things that went beyond army regulations and sanitary principles but added to the appearance of the place and the spirits of the men. Bernard J. Bettelheim noted that two Kentucky regiments near Murfreesboro, Tennessee, constructed "beautiful & still more useful Corduroy Roads" to make it easier to move about camp. The Ninth Indiana and 110th Illinois did better by constructing a footpath and a wagon road, laying down a gravel pavement on them. Bettelheim gave credit to brigade leader William B. Hazen for the graveled path and road and noted that the great amount of surface rocks in the area facilitated such work. Several inspectors praised regiments for taking the time and effort to decorate their camps with arches made of evergreen boughs and small cedar trees replanted near the tents. Such an arrangement gave the camp "a wonderful aspect," in Bettelheim's words.[35]

Sanitary Commission agents fully understood that the quality of personnel made all the difference. That applied not only to the colonel and the surgeon but also to the rank and file. If the unit had a healthy mix of professional men among the privates, one could expect better of its camp. "The men are mostly mechanics," Julius Nichols reported of the Thirteenth Massachusetts Battery, "and indeed appear enabled to turn their hands to almost any thing." They created a variety of camp furniture, "chairs, desks, or bed steads, of peculiar manufacture," to make themselves and their officers more comfortable. The men also were "in first rate spirits." When a call for mechanics to do some work at nearby Fortress Monroe was issued, more than fifty of the ninety battery members reported they could do the job. When Nichols inspected the camp of a battalion belonging to the Third Pennsylvania Heavy Artillery, he was impressed by the pride taken in their camp by the men. It was spotless, and he also credited the attention of senior Capt. George K. Bowen, a civil engineer before the war. "I find him much given to order and regularity and he has his men in very good condition both as regards their health and drill." But Nichols also noted that the battalion contained "very many men of good Education and many I found had left good business prospects at home for this service." He also wondered if they were in part motivated by the news that they would constitute the permanent garrison of Fortress Monroe and wanted to prove that they were worthy of the good quarters they expected to inhabit there.[36]

There were several upbeat reports filed by camp inspectors throughout the war. In this first subject area on the standard form, a topic already much discussed within the US Army culture of healthcare, promoters of sanitary principles found their work aided more often than retarded by the military system. They highly praised the volunteer officers who did well. When George G. Edgerly inspected the camp of the Tenth Regiment, Corps d'Afrique at Port Hudson, Louisiana, in October 1863, he was mightily impressed. "The neatest and best regulated camp we have ever seen," he wrote of the Tenth, which later was designated the Eighty-Second US Colored Troops. Edgerly credited this to Lt. Col. L. S. Jalosky, who apparently was a "nephew of Louis Kossuth and formerly Capt under Garibaldi in Italy." Jalosky's men were "always cheerful."[37]

If one relied solely on personal accounts to gauge camp situation, it would be easy to come to quick but not necessarily accurate assessments. With hundreds of thousands of volunteers in the field filling thousands of semipermanent camps, personal accounts fail to offer a broad-spectrum picture of the whole. Systematic examination and reporting, as with the Fifteenth Corps medical inspection reports and the US Sanitary Commission returns, are the only way to get close to a broad coverage of this significant topic. The commission returns are more numerous and far more extensive in their coverage of different aspects of camp situation than are the Fifteenth Corps reports. Those commission returns offer a complicated answer to the question of how well semipermanent camps were situated as far as sanitary principles were concerned. But then, complicated answers are more valuable than simple answers for understanding complicated questions.

Union army camps were neither uniformly dirty nor uniformly clean. Moreover, the camp inspection returns illuminated the many varied aspects that went into proper selection of sites for semipermanent camps in the Civil War. It was not just a question of whether they were dirty; it was a question of how well a camp was situated to take advantage of the best environmental influences to promote the health of a mass of soldiers living in close contact with each other. The need for plenty of fresh air; ground sufficiently drained of rainwater; the ready accessibility of good, potable water; and proper spacing of tents were as important as keeping the grounds free of trash.

3

Shelter

Whereas the subject area of camp situation focused on the link between the regimental encampment and the natural and built environment, the second subject area, shelter, focused more tightly on the immediate protection of soldiers against the elements. Military housing involved barracks, which were purpose-built large buildings to house numbers of men; tents, which constituted temporary and portable housing; and huts, small structures made from scratch with readily available material near the campsite. Barracks were permanent or at least meant to last for the duration of the war, constructed by the military system, and always located well to the rear. Tents also were made or procured by the military system, and they became a symbol of the war experience; the phrase "tented field" often was used to denote life in the army. Huts were the only one of the three shelter types made by the men themselves from whatever they could find and to no standard, authorized plan in contrast to barracks and tents. Huts were a feature of winter quarters and thus meant to last several months. For the average Union soldier, living under a tent or in a hut was the most common experience, with far less chance of living in a barracks even for a short while.

Many sources deal with this subject, which was so important to the average soldier. Personal accounts, Fifteenth Corps medical inspection reports, and official documents all testify to the soldier's need to find something that would keep the rain off in wet weather and give him the chance to sleep warmly in cold seasons. Army regulations paid quite a bit of attention to the sheltering of the troops, and the supply system worked hard to provide proper tents for them.

PRECEDENTS

A recent historical experience with military shelter, the Sebastopol Campaign of the Crimean War, was a foreshadowing of the early experience of the Civil War. English soldiers often were housed in common bell tents at the start of the campaign. These shelters were more than 13 feet in diameter and 10 feet tall, with 512 cubic feet of air inside for the fifteen men expected to live in them. With only 34 cubic feet of air per man, they also had very poor ventilation. The troops tended to pitch these tents too close to each other, according to one English military surgeon. As the siege continued, soldiers were placed in huts that were made along two standard types approved by the army. The Portsmouth Hut, 15 by 27 feet interior dimensions, was 6 feet tall to the eaves and 12 feet to the ridge. It contained 3,645 cubic feet of air for twenty-five men, about 146 cubic feet per man. The Chester Hut, introduced later, was bigger, but both types had thin walls and, some believed, poor ventilation.[1]

The French army initially used a large tent with two poles and a top shaped like a roof but found it inadequate for the Crimean weather. An especially fierce storm played havoc with them in November 1854. The army then switched to a conical tent with a single pole, sending enough to the theater of war to accommodate 280,000 men, not counting officers. The shelters were manufactured mostly in Toulon and Marseilles, but some were made in England.[2]

Other European armies varied in the way they sheltered their troops. The Russians relied heavily on barracks with bunks and straw mattresses, preferring a large square tent with a pyramidal roof to accommodate fifteen men in the field. The Prussians dispensed with tents on campaign, relying instead on housing the troops in civilian quarters or bivouacking without cover. In the Sardinian service, there was a mix of conical and French-style shelter tents, the latter designed for use by only two men.[3]

In the Civil War, Union soldiers utilized all these types of shelter over the course of time.[4] They found that every type had its advantages and drawbacks as far as comfort and convenience were concerned. Sanitarians had much to say about which type was better and which was worse for health, even though the US Army had relatively little to say about these sanitary matters.

SANITARY PRINCIPLES CONCERNING SHELTER

"Good air is more essential than good food," wrote John Ordronaux. "A human being consumes about 18 pints of it per minute, or nearly two hogsheads and a half per hour." Ventilation of living space was therefore of prime importance. Every man needed at least 108 cubic feet of air, which amounted to 6 by 6 by 3 feet of air space, "with a renewal of 40 cubic feet per hour." Physicians were divided as to whether this could be better accomplished in tents or huts. Dr. Robert Jackson, the inspector general of army hospitals in the British service, favored huts but Ordronaux preferred tents. Jackson noted, however, that the tent had to have walls that could be raised for ventilation and a trench dug around it for drainage. They had to have intervals of at least 4 feet between the tent stakes to avoid crowding. The men should be told to open the door and raise the walls for ventilation when possible and sleep on an india-rubber blanket to protect themselves from the damp earth. The tents needed to be aired daily and moved a few feet twice every week. The problem was that the crowding of bodies in a small, enclosed space with moisture arising from the earth produced bad air inside the tent. It also polluted the ground and produced a disease environment inside the shelter. Ordronaux advised moving the entire camp to fresh ground every three months. "Long after a camp has been broken up, a faint, sickly animal smell reveals the place of its site, and shows the continuing presence of deleterious emanations from the soil."[5]

Ordronaux disliked barracks, but he probably was heavily influenced by reports from England that depicted army barracks as grossly overcrowded and extremely unhealthy living environments. He advised that if used, barracks should be located away from swamps, slaughterhouses, cemeteries, and narrow streets. The site should get plenty of sunlight and air, with the building facing northeast and southwest. It should be no more than two stories high and hold no more than fourteen men per room. Ordronaux prescribed at least 400 cubic feet of air per man, with an influx of 20 cubic feet of fresh air per minute. This meant opening windows and doors a lot. To keep the interior space clean, the men should scrub the floors once a week and whitewash the walls and ceilings twice a year. They should sleep on iron bedsteads supporting straw pallets. Urinals or "night buckets" made of tarred canvas should be made available, with latrines located in a separate building, the latter disinfected with ashes twice a week.[6]

Surgeon General Hammond conducted an experiment concerning clean air in military living spaces. He closed a room of 1,280 cubic feet of air and slept in it overnight. In the morning he found the carbonic-acid level inside had risen to more than twice the normal rate, but after letting fresh air pass through the room for three hours, it had reduced to the normal level. He saw this as proof that army shelter had to incorporate the influx of fresh air on a regular basis to avoid unhealthy environments and concluded that the tent was far superior to barracks or huts for this purpose. Especially for the care of the sick and wounded, tents were superior. They should be made of cotton duck rather than linen or hemp. Under no circumstances did Hammond allow for the men to dig an excavation to live in, which would only increase the moisture problem inherent in living in close contact with the ground.[7]

In practice the Union army followed these prescriptions for tent living in a sporadic way. There is evidence that some volunteer regiments followed the regulations and changed tent sites now and then. They often dug drainage ditches around each tent because the benefits were obvious. Many soldiers who neglected this essential feature of camp sanitation soon found their living quarters underwater. Fewer regiments took care to find straw or pine boughs to make a foundation for sleeping on the ground. A few dug excavations in which to live, but that was not common because the problems involved were obvious—a hole that filled with mud and water after a rain.[8]

TENT TYPES

The volunteers used a variety of tents during their Civil War service. One of the two more common types was the Sibley, designed for about a dozen men. Some sort of conical or bell tent had been in use by the British Army since at least 1810, and American militia units picked it up by the 1840s. In the United States, Henry H. Sibley, a graduate of the US Military Academy, patented improvements on the basic concept to create the tent named after him. Some observers assumed he was inspired by the Native American wigwam in his design, but of course the same conical shape was prevalent in both English and French military tents long before his time. Franklin B. Hough thought the Sibley was taller and wider than the French bell tent used in the Crimean War, with a bigger opening for better ventilation. The center pole rested on an iron tripod so that it could be raised and lowered to let in air at the bottom. A circular opening at the top one foot in diameter could be closed or opened to promote air circulation. This also allowed for a small camp stove to be placed under the tripod, with a smokestack

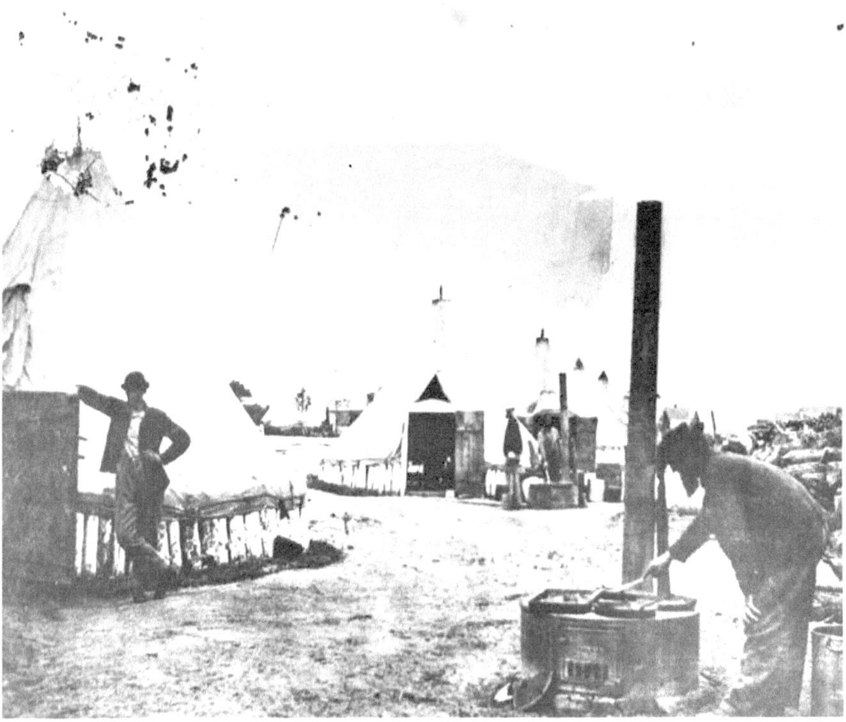

Sibley Tents on Stockades. The ubiquitous Sibleys, the favored among many conical tents available in the 1860s, are here raised on stockades to increase their interior-height advantage. These even have wooden doors and door frames for entering and exiting. The stove upon which the man on the right is cooking was not issued by the government but instead was purchased from civilian vendors by the troops. Their utility for cooking in camp is obvious. (Library of Congress, Prints & Photographs Division, Civil War Photographs, LCDIG-ppmsca-33108)

sticking out through the top hole. At eighteen feet in diameter and twelve feet tall, the Sibley was a chore to handle. A communal living arrangement, it also demanded a communal effort to set up. It had to be transported in wagons, increasing the transportation requirements of a regiment.[9]

The Sibley tent was very widely utilized early in the war, although supplemented by a handful of other conical tents designed for several men that were very similar to it. But by midwar, the Sibley was largely replaced by the shelter tent, which was designed for only two men and was much more portable. At times one found the wedge tent in use. It consisted of two halves like the shelter tent but was much larger than the two-man affair, accommodating up to five soldiers. Officers and noncommissioned officers used a square wall tent, which had vertical sides and was more commodious than the conical or shelter tents. The largest, most commodious tent was referred to as the hospital tent. It had walls four and a half feet tall and was twelve feet high at the ridge. Made of heavier canvas than the other types, it could be opened at both ends and joined with others to make a long ward.[10]

Soldiers improvised their tent arrangements by building so-called stockades. This consisted of splitting posts in half and setting them upright and tightly together, with the split side toward the inside. Then they placed the tent on top of it to give themselves much more headroom. The stockade could also be constructed crib fashion using full logs notched at the corner joints. The crib design was faster and easier to make. Stockades appeared early in the war for the Sibley tent but became more popular later when the shelter tent was issued because the shelter design prevented the men from standing up inside. Stockades obviously were possible to construct only in a camp of some duration.[11]

LIVING IN TENTS AND HUTS

For bedding, the soldier was issued a woolen blanket and a rubber blanket, but some men found that this alone was not enough to prevent the cold, moist air emanating from the ground from affecting their health. They learned to cut tree boughs or collect pine straw, or their officers found and issued wheat straw to serve as a sort of mattress and comfortable foundation for their blankets. But there is plenty of evidence that many men did not bother with this and simply slept on one or both of their army blankets on the bare ground. Time and energy often dictated this. Every soldier had to decide if it was worthwhile to make a comfortable foundation. During the Siege of Vicksburg, however, it was obvious the Union army was planted for some time to come. Therefore, one saw many elaborate sleeping arrangements, including wild cane from the ravines used to make raised bedsteads a few inches off the ground.[12]

For heating their tents in a winter camp, there were several options. Early in the war, small sheet-iron stoves were manufactured and sold to troops in the field, but that does not seem to have been a very common item due to the cost. More often, the men improvised with available material. Franklin Hough found many such arrangements while inspecting regiments during the winter of 1861–62. These mostly consisted of small hearths with attached chimneys, but the material included everything from brick, stones, and mud to sod. "The thousands of acres of oak timber, cut down as a military necessity, allowed no limit to be placed upon the luxury, except that of transportation." Many tents were heated by digging a trench through the middle and covering it with flat stones. Then the occupants connected the trench to a chimney at the rear of the tent while building a fire in it at the front. The heat communicated along the trench, warming the stones, and the fumes exited through the chimney. This arrangement or something similar to it worked well.[13]

To a greater or lesser degree, the men spent time fabricating extra comforts in camp. They scrounged lumber to make seats and tables or erected brush arbors to shade themselves from the sun. Anything that increased the ease and comfort of camp life was usually allowed by the officers. In some units, such as the First Rhode Island Cavalry, this sort of thing was so often done that bugler George Sargent thought the regiment's camp looked "more like a band of travelling Gypsies than a military encampment." If regulation candles were in short supply, light could be improvised by making what John D. Billings called a slush lamp. This involved taking an empty sardine can and filling it with the leftover grease from the company kitchen. Then, by inserting a rag in a corner of the can to serve as a wick, one could suspend it from a ridgepole with wire that came from hay bales.[14]

In semipermanent camps, such as winter quarters, the tent arrangement could blend in with the hut arrangement. For example, stockade tents could be made higher and more elaborate so that really only the roof consisted of canvas; by that time, the soldier had what was really a canvas-roofed hut. That arrangement made perfect sense because the roof was the most complicated part of a field hut. If made of wood, it could easily leak and make life miserable for the occupants, but a canvas roof was more reliable.

A good winter hut involved much labor because it was a miniature log cabin. Rice C. Bull of the 123rd New York recalled that his regiment's first two weeks in the field were spent near Arlington, Virginia, in September 1862. Here he and the men "learned how to care for ourselves and how better to overcome the conditions we had to contend with." The experience prepared them for making good winter huts at Harpers Ferry, Virginia, in November. The men divided into squads of six, cut logs from nearby woods, and notched them at the end to construct a crib, with an opening for a doorway on one wall. They dug up clay to chink the cracks for insulation. The chimney had a base of stone, but the rest was made of small limbs

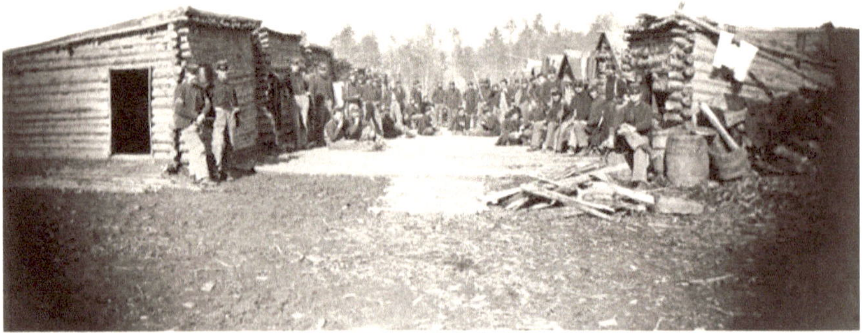

Huts Along a Company Street. These were very substantial huts created to house several men each. There is even a corduroyed street between the two rows. Laundered clothes are drying at several buildings. The caption to the image indicates these were former Confederate huts now used by Federal soldiers near Brandy Station, Virginia, close to the Orange and Alexandria Railroad. For another perspective on these huts, see the image "Slop Barrels" in chapter 5. (Library of Congress, Prints & Photographs Division, Civil War Photographs, LCDIG-ppmsca-32951)

heavily daubed with clay. The roof consisted of tents, and empty cracker boxes served as tables. Bull's squad chipped in to purchase a "small sheet iron stove which was a great luxury."[15]

Huts were a communal form of living, and given latitude, most groups roughly built theirs in similar ways. But some men preferred wooden roofs, and if boards were readily available, they could build them. The Thirteenth New Hampshire, demonstrating an obvious familiarity with woodworking, stripped off the bark of yellow-pine logs and piled it up to press and dry out over a few days. It was "a capital roofing material" that also could be used to make cabin walls. "Half the houses are papered with Harpers, and other pictorial papers, and maps and pictures of all sorts, tacked on all over the inside of walls and roofs," wrote the regiment's historian. The officers occupied larger huts; the smallest of them measured ten by sixteen feet, with two glass windows and a brick chimney.[16]

As with civilian homes, soldiers tended to accumulate little comforts in winter quarters that they did not need once active campaigning resumed in the spring. Even items that could be useful in the future had to be discarded. "All clothing that you could possibly do without," recalled cavalryman George Sargent, "all extra cooking utensils, blankets, and rations had to be left behind in order to make the load for your horse as light as possible."[17]

Some regiments lived in barracks for short periods of time. Billings reported that barracks were typically designed for only one company and were long, one-storied structures "not unlike a bowling alley in proportions." The entrance was at one end, and a walkway ran through the center. The bunks usually were placed one above another on both sides. When the 117th New York assembled at its first rendezvous at Camp Huntington in Rome, New York, Hermon Clarke found barracks living "pretty tough," with three or four men sharing a bunk only five by six feet. "And of all the noises you ever heard, the loudest and meanest are heard here from dark until 10 or 11 o'clock." Straw mattresses typically constituted the bedding. With tents, the shelter could easily be opened to let in fresh air and sunlight, but not so with barracks. That is why Col. Franklin S. Nickerson ordered the troops of his Fourteenth Maine out of their barracks at New Orleans on every good day to air themselves and their belongings. While empty on June 11, 1862, the barracks were to be thoroughly cleaned. Two days later Nickerson issued a stern circular compelling all company commanders to personally oversee this process. "Some have done nobly: others have entirely neglected my previous order."[18]

On rare occasions volunteer regiments lived in civilian houses, usually abandoned by the owner. This was a common way to house soldiers in Europe, but it had negative connotations dating from the period before the American Revolution and was strongly frowned upon during the Civil War. The Eighth Illinois Cavalry, however, put up in citizen houses while staying a while at Alexandria, Virginia early in its service. The companies were scattered about in residences on different streets in town and in two churches.[19]

"A soldier has a great many houses to live in," thought Clement Abner Boughton of the Twelfth Wisconsin. Judging from their personal accounts, very many men were interested in huts, especially those constituting a winter camp. They filled their letters, diaries, and memoirs with minute descriptions of these makeshift cabins. "At home it would be called a good pigsty," wrote Sargent, "but out here it is a palace." In the winter camp of the Eighty-First Ohio at Corinth, Mississippi, the men gave names to their huts. "Alhambra, Burnett House, Wild Cat Den, Possum Rest, Red Pepper Cabin, Robbers Roost, Bully Boys, [and] Cripple's Home" were some remembered by Edwin Witherby Brown, who admitted there were other names that "would not bear repeating." The general arrangement of these huts usually was left to chance, but on occasion unit commanders issued plans for the little community. Capt. Jacob Roemer of Battery L, Second New York Light Artillery thought his winter quarters at Lenoir Station near Knoxville, Tennessee "had more the appearance of a permanent village than a temporary camp." The next winter Roemer not only laid out the general arrangement of his battery camp but also specified for his men exactly how big each hut should be.[20]

SOLDIER REACTION TO TENTS

One would think that living in a hut or a barracks would have been the preferred mode of sheltering in the Civil War, but that was not so. Most Civil War sanitarians agreed that tents were preferable as military housing because of their portability, the natural limit on the number of men they could accommodate (especially the shelter tent), and the freedom to rearrange them to better conform to sanitary standards. They were the ideal housing for soldiers even if they wore out relatively fast under the heavy conditions of field use. Overwhelmingly, soldiers preferred to live in tents, or at least in some combination of tent and hut. Even for a winter encampment, Brig. Gen. Alpheus S. Williams thought that tent living was best.[21]

Sibley tents generally were well liked by Union soldiers. They could raise the walls for air circulation and often stockade them to create more head room for the fifteen to twenty men in each one. While usually free to choose their tent mates, Capt. Frederick W. Alexander detailed each gun detachment to occupy one Sibley tent to promote unit cohesion in his Baltimore Battery. Wooden floors typically were placed in the tents, and some had bunks. Many believed the Sibley tent was the best military housing available. Commission inspector Lewis H. Steiner certainly agreed with that assessment, arguing that huts had too little ventilation and light in comparison with the Sibleys.[22]

But quite a few soldiers recorded significant problems with the Sibley tent. It was "large and comfortable" but at the same time "hard to manage and heavy to transport," wrote Robert B. Stewart of the Fifteenth Ohio. If the wagon train failed to keep pace with the regiment, the troops were stuck without shelter for the night. Other men complained of the constricted space inside. When closed up, the Sibley became a hot house of humanity. "To enter one of them of a rainy morning from the outer air," wrote John Billings, "and encounter the night's accumulation of nauseating exhalations from the bodies of twelve men (differing widely in their

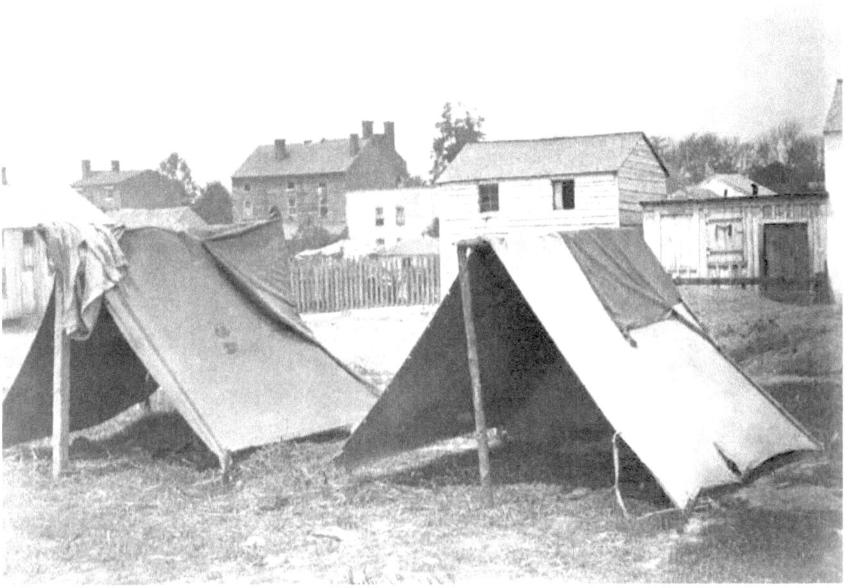

The A Tent. These two examples of a simple tent of the Civil War were photographed by Andrew J. Russell on July 6, 1865. The A tent had no wall, thus it was not easy to enclose the occupants either on the sides or the open ends, but it was tall enough to allow for some standing up and movement inside. In this case, the occupants have acquired more canvas to construct a back wall for themselves. The A tent, often called a wedge tent for obvious reasons, was widely used by enlisted men in semipermanent camps. (Library of Congress, Prints & Photographs Division, LCDIG-ppmsca-13670)

habits of personal cleanliness) was an experience which no old soldier has ever been known to recall with any great enthusiasm." Moreover, if the men stretched the canvas too tightly, rain tended to shrink it and loosen the pegs that attached the conical tent to the ground. The next gust of wind blew it over.[23]

The Sibley was ill-suited for an active campaign because of its bulky nature. It was relegated to semipermanent camps by the midpoint of the war, when the shelter tent offered a good alternative for active campaigning. By that time, quite a few soldiers had become active haters of the Sibley. Louis A. Simmons of the Eighty-Fourth Illinois characterized the tent as "murderous, and totally unfit for white men to live in." Members of the First Wisconsin Battery were delighted to tear them up so the Confederates could not use them when its division evacuated Cumberland Gap and retreated to Ohio in September 1862.[24]

The wedge tent, or A tent, was a viable alternative to the Sibley. It also afforded communal living arrangements but on a smaller scale—only four

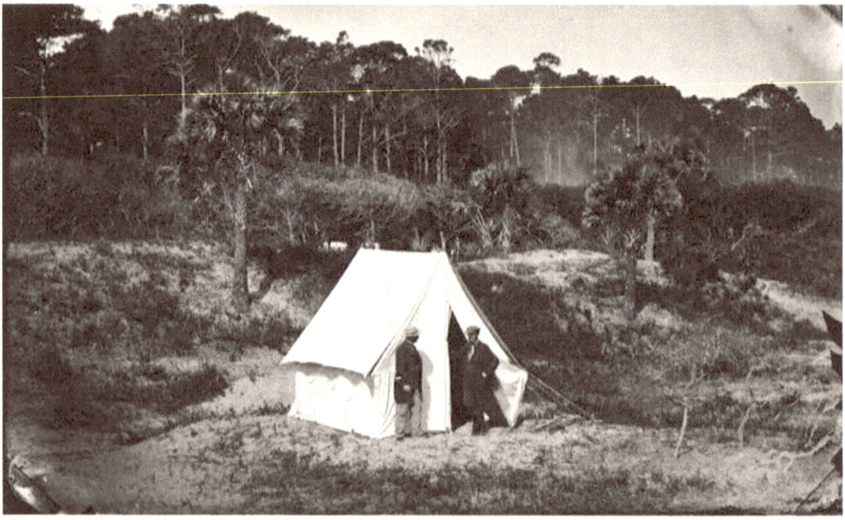

The Wall Tent. Taken by Haas and Peale on Morris Island, South Carolina, in July or August 1863, this image shows the advantages of the spacious wall tent compared to the A tent. The wall raised the A-frame of the tent high enough so that one could easily stand up and walk inside. Typically, officers were allowed wall tents rather than enlisted men. (Library of Congress, Prints & Photographs Division, Civil War Photographs, LCDIG-cwpb-04761)

to six men per tent. It consisted of two large pieces of canvas erected in an inverted "V" and really was little more than sleeping quarters for them. The canvas pieces were six feet long and supported by two poles six feet tall. Placed on a stockade, it provided more interior room for the occupants. This type of tent had a long history in the European military experience and was widely used by state governments and the Federal government during 1861 and 1862. But it also required wagon transportation and thus tended to be more suited for semipermanent camps than active campaigning. Wall tents, with much more head room, were reserved for the use of officers.[25]

The solution to providing cover for troops on active campaign came at midwar with the introduction of the shelter tent. With each soldier carrying a small piece of canvas, it was designed so that two pieces could be connected to form a small version of the wedge tent. Thus, it cut down a lot on field transportation and was quick and easy to set up and take down. The shelter tent also was handy in a winter camp because it could serve as the roof for a wooden hut. They initially were not popular with the men but soon became their standard living quarters for the last half of the war, facilitating more rapid movement during long campaigns. Although small, the shelter tent became a tool of war that covered thousands of tired men more often than any other type of tent.

It was not an American invention. Thomas Robert Bugeaud, marshal of France and governor-general of Algeria, developed the concept as a way to impart a higher level of mobility among his French troops when suppressing native uprisings. Those highly mobile movements took place mostly in 1841–42 and were keys to the French success over Algerian freedom movements. "Our troops became movable and nomadic, like the Arabs whom they pursue," wrote Jean-Baptiste Louis Baudens, who praised the shelter tent for its use by French troops in the Crimean War. It was a small piece of linen 5.5 feet by 5 feet in dimension with buttons and buttonholes so they could be attached to other pieces. Each man carried one piece and clubbed with five other men to assemble a tent barely large enough for all to sleep in. The French soon replaced the buttons with eyelets so the pieces could be attached with rope instead of buttons. A Belgian army surgeon named L. Heureux modified this idea by using rubber cloth and arranging the piece so it could be used not only like the French shelter tent but also as a poncho for the individual soldier to protect himself in rainy weather.[26]

The American army adopted the French shelter tent and changed it only slightly by enlarging the piece to six feet square because American men tended to be taller than French men. It also used canvas instead of linen for the sections and instructed that only two men rather than six should join their pieces. The result was the most famous tent of the Civil War.[27]

The key to the shelter tent was mobility. The Union army simply was overburdened with materiel and had to lighten its load. It began to use the shelter tent as early as June 1862 and within a few months the new shelter spread throughout the Union army. Two stakes supporting a ridge pole was all that was needed to complete it. The shelter tent had both buttons and buttonholes that were combined with rope and eyelets. Wherever introduced, there was initial resistance to the new sheltering system. It offered little comfort and had to be carried by the troops. And at about four feet tall at the ridgepole, one certainly could not stand up inside it.[28]

In some regiments the tents were met with almost universal contempt. Tall men had to scrunch their bodies even while lying in them and the canvas did not seem capable of repelling heavy rain. Soldiers began to protest by likening themselves to dogs in a pen. Those of John Beatty's brigade in the Army of the Cumberland erected various signs to show their displeasure: "Pups for Sale," "Rat Terriers," "Bull Pups Here," "Doghole No. 1," and "Sons of Bitches Within." One day army commander William S. Rosecrans rode through Beatty's camp and was greeted with barking from the troops, on their hands and knees, who stuck their heads out of the shelter tents to give him an impression of what they thought about the new mode of living. The general found it amusing and promised them better accommodations.[29]

But Rosecrans could not follow through with that promise because the shelter tent was here to stay. The army officially required it for the rank and file, reserving wall tents for the use of officers, in General Orders No. 160, dated October 18, 1862. That order more generally outlined new regulations to reduce the field transportation of all units entering field service. The War Department later dealt with resistance to shelter-tent use by issuing General Orders No. 189, dated May 2, 1864, in which the authorities made it clear that if soldiers refused to accept the shelter tent, they would be issued no tents of any kind.[30]

Usually, the initial resistance to the shelter tent gave way to acceptance as the men got used to it. According to Louis Simmons, the men of the Eighty-Fourth Illinois soon came to realize that they could make themselves reasonably comfortable in them, and "within a month all were perfectly satisfied." For others, acceptance came on the first rainy night during a campaign when realizing how quickly and easily they could assemble their shelter without having to wait for the wagon train. But a certain percentage of Union soldiers persisted in criticizing the shelter tent even as they relied on it. A common complaint was that the canvas did not repel heavy rain. "The water goes through them just like a sieve," wrote Sylvester Strong of the Twentieth Wisconsin. The canvas filtered the rainwater and dispersed it into "a nasty mist" inside the tent, wrote Alpheus Williams regarding the "miss-named 'shelter tents'" used by his division. If the rain persisted, this mist soon turned into a series of big water drops pelting the occupants "like a leaking roof," noted Rice Bull. Some men learned that they could lessen the leaking by wiping the inside of the canvas with a cloth. "As soldiers we had to get used to anything," remembered Bull, "and we soon became used to the little tents and were thankful to have them."[31]

Despite general orders, other tents were not phased out so quickly in favor of the shelter tent. Many units in Rosecrans's army continued to use Sibleys during the early months of 1863 while in winter quarters at Murfreesboro, giving them up only when setting out on the Tullahoma Campaign in late June. But the desire for bigger tents persisted even beyond the midpoint of the war. Quartermaster General Montgomery C. Meigs complained that his department continued to receive requisitions for Sibleys as late as April 1864. He pointed out that the army did not even make them anymore. Many of the units requesting bigger tents were in William T. Sherman's Military Division of the Mississippi, so Meigs lectured Sherman on this point. He noted that the Army of the Potomac had entirely shifted to shelter tents for its rank and file with no bother, and he also argued that these tents were not only more convenient but healthier for the men.[32]

Although the most famous tent of the Civil War, the shelter was really only one of several types commonly used. The Federal government procured a wide variety of tents through a mixed process of relying on eight major contractors combined with its own efforts to purchase the raw material and make them. The Quartermaster Department was responsible for this, expending a total of $30 million on tents during the Civil War. They were made with a material called "duck," a name given to the cotton canvas used to make sails for ships. A prodigious number of tents were provided the Union army during the course of the war. For a force that totaled close to 3 million men, the Quartermaster Department obtained 50,884 Sibley or some other type of conical tent; 44,688 hospital tents; 103,998 wall tents; 526,474 wedge tents, and 4,546,436 shelter tents. In fact shelter tents made up 86.2 percent of the total 5,272,480 tents used by the Union army during the Civil War. With 790,000 shelter tents on hand at war's end, the Federal government gave them to various groups over the years such as veteran reunions, to be recycled into book covers, and to shelter flood victims as well as Jewish refugees from Russia.[33]

Even though the shelter tent was the most heavily used shelter of the Civil War, it was supplemented by many other types. During the last half of the war, many officers tried to impose uniformity in tent usage. Those orders tended to be issued by headquarters in areas where little active campaigning took place and thus applied to semipermanent camps rather than to bivouacs. In the Department of the South, those orders included a mandate to provide arbors over every tent for shade; installing wooden floors or bunks to raise the sleeping soldier from the ground; and striking tents, airing bedding and clothes, and cleaning bunks and floors at least three times a week. Officers were ordered to inspect the tents of their men every night to ensure they were properly ventilated. Conscientious surgeons, such as Burt G. Wilder of the Fifty-Fifth Massachusetts, fulfilled these orders almost to the letter.[34]

But sanitary routines were unevenly applied to tent life across the whole army. Lt. Willoughby Babcock noted that in his Seventy-Fifth New York, the men struck tents once every two weeks while in camp near Baltimore during October 1861. They also tipped up the wooden floors only to find

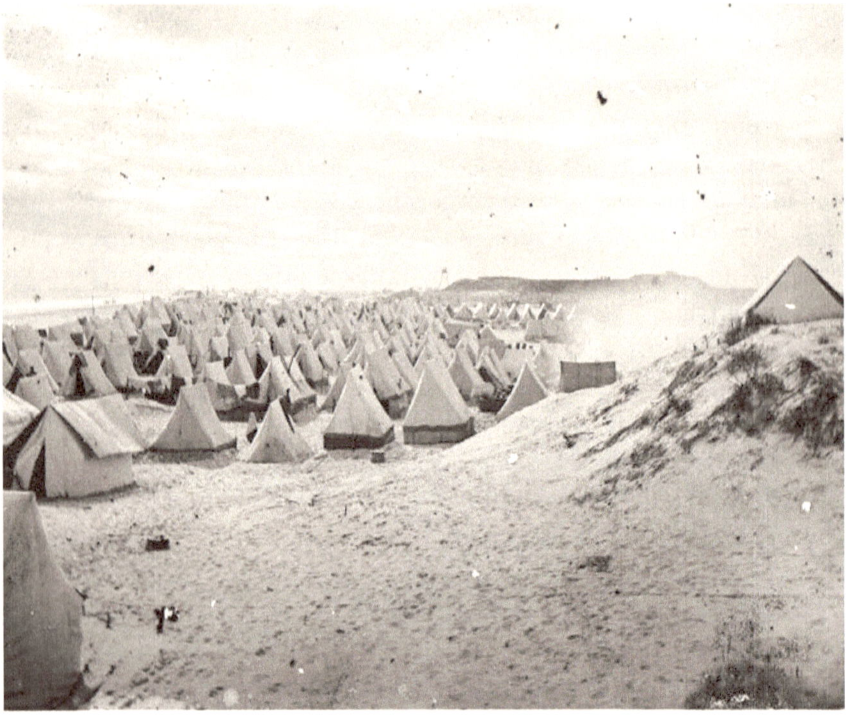

The Tented Field. This photograph by Samuel A. Cooley depicts a Union regiment camping on Morris Island, South Carolina, near the entrance to Charleston Harbor. It gives a good idea of the snug quarters, tents tightly positioned close to each other, that was typical of Federal semipermanent camps during the Civil War. These are A tents raised on stockades. Note the ocean on the left and the sand dunes on the right, which means the view is toward the south. (Library of Congress, Prints & Photographs Division, Civil War Photographs, LCDIG-cwpb-03363)

that rats had burrowed under them during the past two weeks. They leveled the ground again and aired everything. This was all done in unison, with officers giving orders and the drummer tapping out signals so that "down goes the whole camp in an instant." A number of other units, including Dr. Alfred Castleman's Fifth Wisconsin, the Twentieth Indiana, and Brig. Gen. John J. Peck's brigade, routinely struck tents and cleaned up the ground, at least early in the war. Orders to continue doing so appeared at the midpoint of the conflict, which reflected a constant need to reinforce this basic sanitary principle.[35]

Rice Bull remembered the first time he lived in a "tented field" after joining the 123rd New York in the fall of 1862. The tents were brand new and "looked white and attractive."[36] That was unusual. Most soldiers remembered tents that had become muddy, sunbeaten, and soaked with heavy rain and that wore out quickly in the field.

FIFTEENTH CORPS MEDICAL INSPECTION REPORTS

Reports by the medical inspectors of the Fifteenth Corps reinforce the conclusion that tents wore out quickly. In the first report filed, for early April 1863, when the regiments were camped on the soggy Louisiana bottomland near Vicksburg, the comments were not complimentary. The inspector regularly noted not only that there was a variety of tents (the shelter had not yet supplanted the other types) but also that most were "in bad condition." For the Sixth Missouri, they were "worthless, being full of holes and quite rotten." The inspector found that in the Eighty-Third Indiana, up to sixteen men crowded into each bell tent and from eleven to twenty-one in every Sibley tent. Only Battery E, First Illinois Light Artillery managed to keep its tents "in admirable order." By September 1863, when the corps rested in camps near the Big Black River, its situation had improved a lot. Still, there was a bizarre variety of tent types. Shelters were rarely mentioned by the medical inspector, but at least most of the wedges and the few Sibleys were in good shape. Only in a few units, such as the Fourth Iowa and Ninth Iowa, were the tents "worthless for wet weather." In fact, despite the real improvement in tent covering, the corps still presented a notable difference in the quality of its field shelter from unit to unit. That variety ranged from excellent tents well set up to boarded huts and old tents torn and leaking. The most common problem was failure to protect the occupants from rain, the cause of which was tents having worn out and officers having not yet replaced them.[37]

During February and March 1864, when the Fifteenth Corps wintered in northern Alabama, the most common shelter was the wedge tent along with huts. The medical inspector noted that many men slept directly on the ground without any foundation between their blankets and the earth. Sanitary conditions varied widely from regiment to regiment, with some quite clean and others absolutely filthy. Even the Eighteenth Wisconsin, which stayed in the courthouse at Huntsville, had poorly ventilated and overcrowded sleeping quarters; the men also cooked and ate in their quarters, making them quite dirty. The medical inspector blamed these conditions for a sharp rise in sickness in that regiment at the same time that illness was decreasing in all others of the division. Some regiments in the corps stockaded their tents, a few were still using conical tents, and some used a wide variety of tent types plus log cabins. In the artillery units the men tended to live better; equivalent in size to an infantry company, the battery was easier to superintend by its officers.[38]

The surprising discovery is the fact that the shelter tent had not yet replaced the Sibley or the wedge for rank-and-file living by early 1864, despite strict orders from Washington that only shelter tents were to be issued. How and why that happened is not explained in the readily available documents. Another major point is that, over and above the type of tent used, Fifteenth Corps medical inspection reports clearly show that officer supervision of camp sanitation was very uneven. About a third of the regiments had very poor ratings, while the rest ranged from roughly average to superior. One has to conclude that the Fifteenth Corps lagged behind most other large formations in the Union army in terms of switching to shelter tents and maintaining good camp sanitation over the long term.

SANITARY COMMISSION CAMP INSPECTION RETURNS

US Sanitary Commission camp inspection returns do not offer such a concentrated view of one large formation of the Union army over time as do the Fifteenth Corps records. They are more episodic, constituting something like snapshots of individual regiments rather than whole corps. But those snapshots are revealing, nevertheless, and cover many more regiments than do the Fifteenth Corps medical inspection reports.

The best of the five versions of the inspection-return form included five questions relating to shelter, but one question had four additional subquestions. The commission wanted to know what type of tent was used, how many men lived in each one, and whether officers supervised proper ventilation during the night. Whether and how often the tents were struck for thorough cleaning also was of interest. In addition, four questions related to the proper spacing of tents to reduce overcrowding, but they were included in the segment of the form that dealt with camp situation. The form also had eleven questions in the camp-situation section that related to the drainage system and four that related to the cleanliness of areas immediately around the tents.

Commission inspectors saw all types of shelter (tents, huts, and barracks) in the semipermanent camps of the Union army. But they reported more heavily on tents than any other kind of shelter. A wide variety of tent types was in use across the board. The most common were conical tents, 36.4 percent of the kind named in the returns. While the Sibley was the conical tent most often noted, eleven other conical tents were mentioned as well: Bell, Haskell's Folding Tent, Eldridge, Butler, Yale, York, Warner, Cincinnati, Fremont, Portland, and a French conical tent. The next-most-often-noted tent type was the wedge, at 32.2 percent of the mentions. Three other types—shelter at 9.4 percent, A at 5.1 percent, and wall at 3.4 percent—were relatively uncommon. Regiments with a mix of different tent types represented 13.5 percent of the 258 returns that included specific mention of this. It may come as a surprise that the shelter tent rated so few mentions, but one must keep in mind that the camp inspection returns were weighted toward the first one-third to one-half of the war, a time period when conical tents still dominated the semipermanent camps and before the shelter became standard issue. When it was mentioned, the shelter tent often was used as a roof for a hut in winter quarters.

The camp inspection returns also indicate that huts and barracks were less widely used in Union army semipermanent camps than one might expect. They are mentioned in only 26 returns, which, added to the 258 returns in which tents are mentioned, makes a total of 284. That number is higher than the 280 returns examined because in some regiments both huts and tents were used simultaneously. But of the 284 total, huts appear only in 9.2 percent of the references.

While sanitarians generally preferred that soldiers live in tents than in barracks, they also prescribed several features to enhance the healthy advantages of living under canvas. They deplored, for example, the tendency of many soldiers to dig a pit and stretch their tent over it. This was mentioned in only half a dozen returns and therefore does not seem to have been a widespread practice. Sanitarians also strongly advocated a wooden floor for the tent, and this was mentioned as existing in seventy returns. It was important to strike the tent on a regular basis to air the ground under it, and this practice was performed in sixty-six, or 37.1 percent, of the units inspected. That meant that in 62.9 percent of the regiments for which this practice was mentioned, striking did not occur at all or so irregularly as to amount to no striking.

For some regiments, there was a practical reason for not striking tents. In more than a few units, the canvas was so old and worn out that officers were afraid they would fall apart if struck. "The tents are the most wretched worn out mildewed rotten concerns," wrote William M. Chamberlain about the Eighth New York. In other regiments tents were not struck because cold weather made it uncomfortable to do so.[39]

One thing the commission agents found when attempting to answer the questions relating to shelter was a strong tendency for tents to be placed too close together. There was little trouble in lining them up along company streets but frequent trouble in planting them too close to each other. James Gall found that the tents of the Second North Carolina (US) were "back to back & touching each other" near Portsmouth, Virginia, in September 1863. This fully blocked air circulation and created "an accumulation of refuse matter of all kinds between the tents." Improper drainage was another common problem. In many regiments the men simply did not understand how important a deep and wide ditch could be, especially on flat land, and the result was flooded tents and huts. Henry Oliver found that the huts of the Fourth New York Battery had dirt banked up against the lower walls, which allowed moisture to soak through the crevices and create a damp environment inside. He saw one hut with a drainage ditch literally dug right through its middle to lead water to the door.[40]

But commission inspectors also admired many regimental arrangements, citing them as fulfilling army regulations and sanitary principles alike. E. J. Dunning carefully looked at the camp of the Twentieth New York and found the men "better prepared to make themselves comfortable than any I have yet seen." Their tents were properly arranged, the area around them thoroughly drained, and the quarters embellished with benches and tables. Many had wooden racks for the storage of arms and equipment as well as wooden floors for comfort. These troops had made their camp their home. "Passing along the streets men are seen in the tents plying their trades of shoe making and tailoring, while those moving around the quarters exhibit a cheerfulness and alacrity that are not always perceptible among our volunteers."[41]

Quite a few regiments had beds raised above the ground in their tents, typically about twelve to eighteen inches. In the Eighth Maine wooden floors were removed daily and the ground was raked, a precaution that helped keep out rodents. In the Second North Carolina (US), two-thirds of the tents had raised bunks, indicating a lack of uniform practice in the regiment. But Gall found that most of the tents were clean whether bunked or not. The men also were "quiet, respectful & orderly," and kept their weapons and equipment in good shape. He also found that most bunks in the

First US Colored Troops were raised above the ground, but even those that rested on the surface had boards or poles between them and the soil.[42]

Bedding material varied from regiment to regiment. Some used sacks filled with straw, called bed ticks, while others simply collected material from the area—including hay, leaves, and tree boughs—and spread it on the ground. Members of the Zouave d'Afrique, a unit of white soldiers who served as the bodyguard for Nathaniel P. Banks, took the time to interweave grass and thatch into a matting to sleep on. The regulars in Battery D, Fifth US Artillery slept on "fir twigs spread on the ground to the depth of 2 to 8 inches," wrote Dr. Edward A. Crane, who found it "a very excellent kind of bedding, fresh and clean in its appearance, in this camp it is removed and replaced every week."[43]

Commission inspectors recorded a long list of good and bad regimental habits. When Robert Jones visited the Fortieth New York early in the war, he found the tents, inhabited by five to seven men each, were a mess. Food remains, dropped clothing, and many other items lay about inside and outside. The tents were too close, and many were completely closed even in good weather. While some had straw or leaves as bedding, none had any wooden floors, so most men were "greatly exposed to the dampness of the earth." While some tents had trenches around them, all the ditches were too shallow and none connected to the main drain along the company street.[44]

But the most persistent problem lay in air circulation. This was what Surg. James P. Prince of the Twenty-Second Massachusetts and later of the Thirty-Sixth Massachusetts believed right after the war. Not a commission inspector but a physician who obviously understood and agreed with sanitary principles, Prince argued that this was the "crowning fault of the medical administration" early in the conflict. "The men were allowed to shut themselves up in their tents and cabins very much as they pleased, in ignorance of the danger of poisoning themselves with foul air of their own production." They became susceptible to typhoid and intestinal fevers "from the crowd poisoning and of pneumonia from the sudden transition from these sweating dens to the cold air of winter as they came out for roll call and other purposes."[45]

Overall, the mixed record of tent setup persisted throughout the war. This was inevitable in an army of amateurs, despite the heavy level of field experience they accumulated. Many regimental commanders and even a certain percentage of regimental surgeons failed to take proper ventilation seriously and did not think they needed to force the men to pitch their tents farther apart from each other. And yet it did not help the cause of camp sanitation when inspectors admitted ruefully that some companies that neglected sanitary principles happened to be among the healthiest in the regiment.[46] That was not common, but one certainly can find such reports in the returns.

Another common result of the inspections was to document how often regiments had to put up with worn-out tents and a variety of them as well, despite the effort to streamline the army to shelter tents. James Gall found that members of the Fourth US Colored Troops were living in "old worn out Sibley tents," which had been condemned by another regiment and reissued by a stingy quartermaster, late in 1863. "They are ragged & leaky & dirty & very much over crowded, from 13 to 20 men sleeping in each tent." He advised the colonel and surgeon either to build stockades and raise bunks or to construct wooden huts as an alternative.[47]

A cluster of camp inspection returns filed by Bernard Jean Bettelheim also demonstrated how varied and poor the tent coverage of many regiments could be even at the war's midpoint. He visited several units in the Army of the Cumberland in their winter quarters near Murfreesboro early in 1863 and heard numerous complaints about the army's effort to streamline field transportation by reducing the number of tents issued. Sibleys were still being used by the Fifty-Seventh Indiana, although they were very leaky. Surg. G. W. Phillips of the Seventy-Fifth Illinois blamed "the bad condition of his tents" for the rise of sickness in the ranks.[48]

Another cluster of returns, filed by George G. Edgerly after visiting regiments that garrisoned Port Hudson in October 1863, documented not only bad tents but also bad living habits among the troops. The Eleventh Regiment Corps d'Afrique possessed tents that were "very old and poor many of them badly torn, and afford but a poor protection in time of a heavy rain." Those in the camp of the Third Regiment Corps d'Afrique were so worn that they failed to keep out the rain during a storm, and Edgerly found standing water inside nearly every one he inspected. It was not just the Black regiments that received bad tents. The Sixth Michigan also had to endure equally poor shelters. Its colonel and surgeon told Edgerly that they had tried repeatedly to acquire new tents but without success. Those in the camp of the Second Vermont Battery were "nearly worthless, being old, rotten, and ragged."[49]

Only a handful of the 280 returns examined here related to a regiment quartered in barracks. Generally, those returns indicated that the buildings were properly planned and constructed along sanitary principles. Only one company usually occupied each building. Inspectors looked at air circulation, sunlight, and cubic feet of space. Quarters for officers and noncommissioned officers were always separated to some degree from those of the privates. The kitchen usually was in a separate structure. Gordon Winslow praised the barracks occupied by the Fifth New York at Federal Hill near Washington, DC, in January 1862. The buildings, which had clapboard sides and shingle roofs, were relatively spacious, and a piazza linked several of them into a group. Officers made sure the men aired their bunks daily and neatly folded blankets at the head when not in use. "The Hygeine, as perfect as competent inspection & care can render it," was approved by Winslow.[50]

Barracks were seldom mentioned in the camp inspection returns because so few regiments had the opportunity to occupy them. But despite Winslow's glowing praise, the available information does not support the idea that barracks were better housing for soldiers than tents or huts. The Fourth Iowa occupied a hastily erected barracks at Rolla, Missouri, during the winter of 1861–62. It consisted of five buildings, each forty-four by one hundred feet, and housed two companies. The walls were nine feet tall and the ridge twenty feet above the floor. While no complaints were lodged about these structures, those at Benton Barracks just south of St. Louis were a different matter. This was a permanent army post that processed thousands of soldiers during the war, but its accommodations were worse than the temporary barracks at Rolla. They were "greatly overcrowded," wrote Henry W. Warriner, with two companies in each room. That meant that up to 170 men crowded into a space thirty-two feet wide, sixty-two feet long, and twelve feet high. "The rooms are unlighted usually except through the 'breathing' holes that is by day," but the ventilation was too limited for the number of men occupying each room. "*More Holes* or *fewer Men* required," he wrote.[51]

When he inspected barracks for the commission, Robert Ware found less than perfect conditions at Camp Butler near Newport News, Virginia in February 1862. The Seventh New York occupied barracks with insufficient light and inadequate means of ventilation, which were common faults of military buildings in the minds of sanitarians. But after joining the Forty-Fourth Massachusetts as surgeon, Ware encountered a much worse situation. Fever broke out in the regiment because its barracks were located too close to a swamp in occupied North Carolina. Latrines were located too close to the buildings, too, and the latter were shoddily made of green pine lumber with too little air space for each man. "We are having our first experience of severe sickness here in the shape of congestive fever, of which three men have died within ten days, several others being very sick," Ware told a correspondent. "One man died in twelve hours from the time of attack. It is more savage than anything I ever saw, except some cases of scarlet fever in children." By late February 1863, nineteen men came down with a serious fever, and a dozen of them died. An autopsy revealed inflammation in the membranes of the brain and spinal cord. This was identified as cerebrospinal meningitis, similar to what had been called an outbreak of spotted fever in Massachusetts from 1807 to 1816. Ware issued quinine as a prophylactic, and the regiment had to change its location before the problem disappeared. Sanitary principles had not been observed originally, and the relatively closed environment of the barracks interior had intensified the problem, with disastrous results for the men affected by the fever.[52]

One would think that buildings were better military housing than tents, but that notion has to be modified in light of the affliction that struck the Forty-Fourth Massachusetts. It was even more important to plan and construct barracks along sanitary principles than it was to organize a tent city because they were essentially permanent whereas tents could easily be put up, taken down, and replaced or relocated as needed. Tents housed far fewer men per unit and, as long as they were arranged properly, limited the spread of diseases compared to barracks.

Huts shared more of the advantages of tents than the disadvantages of barracks. They also housed only small numbers of men per unit and were faster and easier to construct but not easy to take down and move. A "small hut" used by the Sixty-Ninth Pennsylvania was eight by ten by twelve feet in dimension, according to inspector F. U. Johnston. Commission inspectors found hutted communities to be fairly well constructed along sanitary lines, but a major problem they reported was the persistence of cellars in many of them. This was, of course, an important point as far as most sanitarians were concerned, but Ware had to admit that the First Minnesota, which was "living in 'cellars' more than any regiment I have visited," did not seem to suffer from it. The men had open fireplaces "of some sort" to warm their huts, and those fires helped dry out the interior. In contrast, Alex McDonald found huts occupied by the 147th New York in March 1863 to be "so much excavated as not to be easily drained & are consequently damp after every severe storm."[53]

It was very rare for inspectors to find regiments quartered in civilian buildings, and when they did the record was mixed. Henry Oliver carefully looked through the quarters of the Eighth Illinois Cavalry in Alexandria, Virginia, early in 1862 and recorded a seriously high rate of sickness. One company occupied the basement of a church, another roomed in a machine shop, and many used houses that had been abandoned by secessionists. Crowded ten men to a room and scattered in numerous buildings, the sick list rose from 30 in October 1861 to 342 in November, 396 in December, and 455 in January 1862. This rise had started even before the regiment had reached Alexandria on January 24, but it sharply increased after its men began taking up quarters in civilian structures. Still, Oliver could not pinpoint exactly why these civilian quarters seemed to increase sickness.[54]

Julius Nichols also could not explain why the Nineteenth Wisconsin, quartered in civilian structures in Norfolk, Virginia in March 1863, did not fare better. He noted that in many ways its residence in a city provided the men with "good warm houses, with comfortable stoves, and fire places, with the advantages of City Markets." In these ways, the Wisconsin men fared better than their comrades living in "tents in the wilderness." But Nichols also noted the widespread occurrence of pulmonary diseases among the Nineteenth, "while the 148th NY in tents, near a damp swamp and exposed to all bad weather have not a single case!"[55]

The only possible way to explain the peculiar disadvantage of living in civilian houses is that they were not designed for the accommodation of soldiers. Instead of ten men to a room, the entire building was meant to be occupied by a family large or small and with the care of a fulltime housekeeper and cook, whether in the form of a mother or a female servant. Most of the sanitary rules concerning overcrowding, proper air space, and ventilation were ignored whenever a regiment took up residency in the civilian buildings of a town or even in the isolated civilian structures of a farm or plantation.

Specially constructed military barracks were much better than civilian houses because they could, if the planner and builder paid attention to sanitary rules, eliminate many of the problems associated with private residences. But even here, if the design and construction did not take sanitary principles into account, barracks could be more dangerous than safe, as vividly demonstrated by the experience of Ware's Forty-Fourth Massachusetts. Although constructed with very little oversight, huts typically provided better housing than barracks because, again, they were designed for small groups of men. That is why sanitarians at times allowed that huts were acceptable for housing soldiers in the field.

Ironically, considering the many problems with housing described in this chapter, when one looks at the statistical results of the Sanitary Commission inspection returns, the topic of shelter comes out looking quite good. The good ratings amounted to 50.0 percent, the fair to 45.4 percent, and the bad to only 4.6 percent. Shelter was one of the handful of topics that most officers and surgeons recognized as of high importance in soldier welfare, even if they could not always do something about the problems associated with it.

When Union soldiers moved to the "tented field," they more often than not literally did live in tents. Those canvas homes came in a variety of shapes and sizes, but the one that they became most familiar with, the shelter tent, represented the state of the art in soldier housing. The French had developed the first individual-tent shelter system in world history, and Civil War soldiers employed the concept in a huge way in their conflict. Despite its discomforts, it was the best way to shelter men in the field because of its mix of utility in covering the soldier and portability to reduce wagon transportation, thus increasing army mobility. With relatively little use of barracks and civilian houses, the Union army was largely a tented force, and the millions of canvas units produced and issued testify to that fact. This aided the health of the soldier more than threatened it because the tent was the most flexible form of soldier housing, adjustable to meet standards of air flow and lowered occupancy. The typical Civil War hut also had many of the tent's advantages in these ways and thus was acceptable in light of the era's sanitary principles. Being a tent dweller, for the most part, helped Union soldiers survive the war.

4

Clothing and Personal Cleanliness

While camp situation and shelter dealt with protecting soldiers from the elements, Civil War sanitarians focused their efforts more familiarly when examining the soldier's clothing and his personal habits of cleanliness. Both subject areas were intimately connected with his body, directing his attention to personal care and appearance in a way that likely was a new idea for many Union soldiers, who were not used to examining their clothing or thinking of their personal cleanliness from the standpoint of health and military effectiveness.

Preventive-healthcare advocates in the armies of other countries had also been considering the best types of clothing material, how well the items fitted the man, and the best colors for uniforms as far as reflecting or absorbing the sun's hot rays. In addition, the idea that a clean body encouraged health was by no means an invention of military sanitarians. An important cleanliness movement had been developing in Europe and the United States for many decades before the Civil War. Efforts to develop a proper uniform and compel soldiers to change their underwear and bathe regularly have to be seen within their proper contexts both in and out of the military sphere. Soldiers themselves had something to say about clothing and especially personal cleanliness, which need to be considered. The Sanitary Commission camp inspection returns offer us a diagnostic gauge to see how far these advanced concepts regarding clothing and clean bodies penetrated the ranks of the volunteer force. These regiments fared well in clothing, but in some ways they did poorly when it came to personal cleanliness.

CLOTHING

In the long view of military history, uniforms had been required for armies only for about two hundred years or so before the Civil War. They had always been governed by a mix of utilitarian concerns combined with attention to show and display. In large, well-established peacetime forces, such as dominated the military scene of Europe by the mid-nineteenth century, display tended to overshadow practical concerns; the latter really came to prominence only during major wars. Colorful, showy uniforms demonstrated the prestige of the government, enticed new recruits, and overawed the populace in times of internal unrest, even if they countered the health and effectiveness of soldiers in field service.

According to John Ordronaux, the concern about soldier clothing then current during the Civil War began with French military operations against Algerian rebels in the 1830s and 1840s. French officials began to question the utility of their standard uniforms and tried to modify them to improve agility. "Everything *heavy* and *constraining,* or *impeding* in any way the free movement of any muscle in either arm or leg, neck, shoulder, or back, was discarded," Ordronaux wrote. "Loose pantaloons, and jackets, small collars, or none, light kepis instead of heavy shakos, shoes in the place of boots, lighter rifles and muskets, took the place of the former heavy arms and accoutrements."[1]

The extreme result of this French reevaluation of soldier clothing was the famous Zouave uniform, which combined concerns for agility and display in one suit. With its baggy trousers, short jacket, modest collar, and fezlike head covering, it solved many of the problems concerning health and agility. With its colorful, even gaudy, appearance, it was the most showy military clothing in world history. A handful of Union regiments in the Civil War adopted the Zouave uniform, but most of them were required to switch to regulation dress after a few months.[2]

The Union army's uniform had been crafted with an eye toward utilitarianism and economy rather than display. It avoided most of the problems identified by sanitarians but not all. There was no high, stiff collar, but no unusually loose pantaloons either. For head covering, the standard was a kepi, but hats were allowed. The uniform was made with wool, about which sanitarians argued, but they could not mount much in the way of a strong argument about most aspects of the uniform, even though they could not enthusiastically praise it. Cost was a huge factor in this; with close to 3 million men to clothe, the Federal government considered the economics more than the sanitarian aspects of the army's uniform.

Government-issued clothes would become worn out in field service. Each man therefore received a clothing allowance of forty-two dollars a year, which was more than the cost of the initial full issue. If replacement costs totaled more than forty-two dollars in one year, the overage was deducted from his pay. If he used less than that amount, he received the balance in cash. If the quartermaster could certify that clothing was lost in action, it was not counted against a man's allowance. The official issue covered the soldier from head to foot, inner and outer garments, and included two shirts, two pairs of underwear, two pairs of stockings, and two blankets (woolen and rubber).[3]

Ordronaux favored woolens for both under and outer garments, including socks, as best for warmth and lightness. William A. Hammond agreed, citing wool's ability to trap air particles and retain body heat. It was the best fabric for cold weather. But he warned that woolen clothing must be kept clean, as it retained skin exhalations more than other fabrics. The surgeon general differed from Ordronaux, however, in advocating cotton for underclothing, at least during winter months. Cotton was the most commonly used fabric derived from the vegetable world. Linen made from flax was better for underclothing in the summer because it absorbed perspiration well. Hammond favored a white cotton or linen jacket and trousers of the same make for the summer. All clothing should be loose fitting, especially on the limbs, chest, and abdomen.[4]

The color of the uniform had definite advantages and disadvantages. Ordronaux cited statistics indicating that for every twelve soldiers wearing red who were hit in battle, only seven wearing green and five wearing gray became casualties. While darker, muted colors were safer in combat, they also absorbed the sun's rays and made the soldier hot in summer weather. Brighter colors such as white, red, and orange were too easy to see in the field. Hammond believed that the colors adopted by the Union army, sky-blue trousers and darker blue for the upper garments, were ideal for field service.[5]

For covering the head, Hammond favored straw hats for summer and woolen hats for winter. The forage cap in use by the army met his approval. The term *forage cap* referred generically to an undress working cap used in a variety of forms by various armies. In the United States the Model 1858 type became the most common form of cap gear in the Union army. It had a visor to provide shade for the eyes and a waterproof covering. In contrast, the felt hat was heavy and provided, in Hammond's opinion, no advantage over the forage cap. European shakoes with helmet string were horrible, as they confined the man's neck in a straightjacket. Hammond also condemned the leather stock and cravat, but these European influences had never taken permanent hold in the American army.[6]

Federal authorities issued headgear in the form of two broad types. The Quartermaster Department gave 1,068,849 hats and 1,124,773 caps to the troops during the fiscal year that ended June 30, 1864. Straw hats were rare, but the Department of the South mandated their issue for men enduring the heat of summer along the South Carolina coast in 1863. Early in the war a craze for the Havelock as a protection against the summer sun could be seen. This was a linen flap extending from the back of the forage cap to protect the back of the neck. It had been used by Sir Henry Havelock's troops in quelling the Indian uprising of 1857, and many Union soldiers wore it during the summer months of 1861 in Virginia. But even though Ordronaux liked it, the item never caught on anywhere else in the war zone and soon disappeared, even in the East. William T. Sherman called it "a useless contrivance" while preferring felt or straw hats. The Sanitary Commission suggested the best way to deal with summer heat was to wear a silk handkerchief in the crown of the hat, but it is doubtful most soldiers could do so.[7]

When it came to footwear, everyone agreed that shoes were better than boots for infantrymen. Hammond focused a lot on the size of the sole, noting that it had to be wide enough to fully support the foot. He also warned that frequent marching could elongate the foot up to half an inch, so the sole size had to take this enlargement into account or the result would be callouses and ingrown toenails. He favored hard upper leathers for ankle support.[8]

The poncho was useful in wet weather. Made of unbleached muslin that was coated with vulcanized india rubber, it was a rectangle sixty inches wide and seventy-two inches long, with an opening in the center through which one passed his head. It was based on the Spanish American woolen poncho.[9]

All sanitarians agreed that changing one's clothes for sleep at night promoted good health. W. H. Van Buren recommended the men sleep in their underwear and shirts. "Sleeping in the clothes is never so refreshing, and is absolutely unhealthy," he wrote. In fact, Ordronaux urged a soldier to strip completely for sleeping now and then because "his body receives the benefit of an air-bath, and both his day and night garments have an opportunity to be aired." This also prolonged the life of the clothing. Some army officers supported the idea that soldiers ought to undress at least their outer garments for sleep, but this was by no means a universal concern in the Union force. Most men did not use separate clothing for sleeping as they had done at home, but would take off their coat, boots, and vest. "Some, however, stripped to their flannels," remembered John D. Billings. "There were a few in each regiment who never took off anything, night or day, unless compelled to." Even officers found it hard to follow good principles in the field. Sherman admitted he had not undressed at all for almost two months during the Vicksburg operation in the summer of 1863. "I have slept in my clothes ready to jump to the saddle" at a moment's notice.[10]

SANITARY COMMISSION CAMP INSPECTION RETURNS

The Fifteenth Corps medical inspection reports did not pay substantial attention to the troops' clothing and therefore cannot be used to gain insight into this subject area. But the Sanitary Commission camp-inspection-return form included twenty-four questions relating to the bedding and clothing of soldiers. Commission officials wanted to know if the men slept on any foundation, such as a wooden floor, straw, hay, or leaves, and whether they simply slept on the bare ground with nothing more than a blanket between them and the earth. Most troops did use a foundation of some sort, especially as it was easier to find material while in a semipermanent camp. One of the twenty-four questions asked if the men changed their clothing for the night, and the answer overall was decidedly in the negative: The overwhelming majority of troops slept in the same clothing they wore during the day. The other questions related to whether the men had been issued the standard clothing and what condition the items were in, with the answers mixed. Most of the regiments had the items, but the quantity and quality varied widely. For example, many units had only one issued blanket per man instead of the standard two blankets, and the quality of these often was poor. The questions regarding blankets even distinguished between regular-army-issued items and other, privately owned blankets, and the inspectors did find some of the latter in use by the troops. Most men, however, had the regulation trousers, jackets, and overcoats in pretty fair condition. When a regiment did not have enough clothing, or if its items were in terrible condition, the fault usually lay in the kinks inherent in the supply system. Officers had to file requisitions, which went up the chain of command until reaching the appropriate quartermaster in a major depot on home territory before the items could be shipped, and delays could be expected.

Early in the war the Federal government was aided by state governments in supplying new volunteer regiments. E. J. Dunning found that the Twentieth New York had good jackets, trousers, two shirts, two pairs of stockings, two pairs of underwear, an overcoat, and woolen and india-rubber blankets, all supplied by the State of New York. The men purchased their own caps. The only poor items were the shoes, also provided by the state, and the men were waiting for replacements supplied by the central government. The Fifteenth New York Engineers also benefited from the Empire State's tendency to send regiments into the field fully supplied with state-issued clothing. In a handful of regiments, the men used items of clothing donated by concerned citizens back home. For example, Surg. R. W. Hazlett of the Second Virginia (US), later redesignated the Second West Virginia, encouraged his friends to send four boxes of mittens and other cold-weather clothing for the men to endure their first winter in the army.[11]

While states like New York were exceptionally good at providing the initial outlay for their volunteer regiments, this process did result in some confusion. Vermont, New York, Indiana, Rhode Island, and Wisconsin issued gray clothing to some regiments in the early months of the war because that was the color of each state's militia uniform. In fact, the Second Rhode Island went to the field wearing gray trousers and blue flannel blouses, mixing what soon became the standard colors of the opposing sides in the Civil War. In contrast, the Thirty-Sixth New York entered the field with full US Army regulation clothing that combined dark-blue top with light-blue trousers in good woolen cloth. But the regiment's blankets were flimsy, "most of them . . . already worn out," after only four days in camp near Washington, DC. Robert Jones further reported, "there are hardly ten left to each company." In fact, along with overcoats, Civil War soldiers had more difficulty securing good blankets than any other item in the clothing allowance. Blankets tended to receive a lot of wear and tear, forcing the supply system to repeatedly send replacements. The other problem was poor quality, which often really meant they were too light and thin. A blanket weighing at least two and a half pounds was minimally necessary for a soldier in the field.[12]

Even after nearly a year in service, the Third Regiment, Corps d'Afrique still had never been issued rubber blankets or knapsacks. Of 752 men in the Ninth Connecticut, 250 had only one shirt, 70 had none, and 250 had no overcoat. The overcoats given the Seventy-First Pennsylvania were "miserable things of a brownish color," reported Robert Ware. Other regiments put up with inadequate overcoats made of felt or saltinet, consisting of "a light, spongy fabric which you can look through." It was not unusual for inspectors to find regiments overdue for new issues of various items. The men of the Fourth US Colored Troops suffered with "poor" clothing, and "their shoes are worn out," as James Gall put it in November 1863.[13]

In terms of headgear, the majority of camp inspection returns are silent, which seems to indicate that there were few problems with that item of the standard clothing. One of the few exceptions related to the Fortieth New York in the summer of 1861. Some of the men had procured Havelocks on their own. But these troops complained about them because they kept the back of their necks too hot. Havelocks quickly went out of fashion, as the men preferred fatigue hats made of felt, the brims of which they could button up for better air circulation. "These are said to be particularly comfortable and serviceable," reported Jones. Footwear generally was acceptable, although no returns indicate that the men were fully satisfied with their army shoes, which were not particularly comfortable. Soldiers often complained that the standard sizes poorly matched their feet.[14]

While most regiments were clothed according to army regulations, several swayed from that standard. As indicated earlier, a handful of units adopted Zouave clothing. Maj. Gen. Nathaniel Banks had a company called the Zouaves d'Afrique that served as his bodyguard early in the war. Consisting of white men and aping the famous French Zouaves of Algerian fame, they wore red trousers and blue coats. The Fifth New York also wore Zouave clothing consisting of red pants, blue coats with red trim, and red caps with white trim. A bit more common than these gaudy outfits were a number of regiments that, for some unexplained reason, wore black trousers instead of the sky-blue regulation pants. The First and Second US Sharpshooters, on the other hand, had every reason for wearing green coats. Specially raised directly by the Federal government, they were supposed to serve as roving snipers and specialized skirmishers, taking advantage of natural cover on the battlefield. But there was no explanation why the First US Sharpshooters wore light-blue pants and the Second US Sharpshooters wore dark-blue trousers.[15]

The camp inspection returns overwhelmingly proved that very few soldiers changed their clothing for sleeping at night. Of the 280 returns, only 25, or 8.9 percent, indicated that either some or all of the men in a given regiment changed for the night. The standard issue did not include special clothes for sleeping.[16]

M. P. Buel was so impressed by the clothing of the First Nebraska that he effused in his report, "all new & excellent, the best furnished of any Regt. I have seen East or West." One would think that these men took pride in their appearance, a question the commission asked on the standard return. But overall the answers to that question indicated a decided lack of pride in the appearance of their army clothes. More often than not the men were not impressed by the uniform. "Not as a personal thing," Lewis H. Steiner wrote of this question when he visited the Third New York Heavy Artillery, while other inspectors just bluntly wrote that the men had no pride of any kind in their uniform. Bernard J. Bettelheim got to the heart of the question when he noted that the men of the Fifty-Seventh Indiana took pride in their army clothes only "when new & well fitting." So for them, it was not just the relative drabness of the uniform, which was designed more for utility than show, but how well the procurement process provided quality clothing items that fit the men. There was nothing the quartermasters could do about the normal wear and tear on clothing in the field, so the average Union soldier had to put up with torn, dirty garments far more often than he could take delight in a new suit.[17]

The Sanitary Commission inspection return included no questions relating to the design and fabric of clothing items and only one question relating to color. In short, most of the concerns expressed by sanitarians about constricting clothes or whether the enemy could readily see a particular color of uniform seem not to have concerned Frederick Law Olmsted when he drew up the inspection-return form. The apparent reason for this omission must be that the standard army uniform did not violate any of these principles, in his view. There was no high, stiff color; no gaudy colors; and no particularly tight fit, while the standard wool fabric was not viewed as a major concern. Army clothing generally passed muster, and the commission focused instead on whether the items were well made and issued properly.

When evaluating the overall results of this subject area in the 280 returns, clothing came off with a pretty good score. A total of 47.5 percent of the returns rated clothing as good, 42.2 percent as fair, and only 10.3 percent as bad. Providing clothes for its soldiers was one of the high-profile requirements of the Quartermaster Department. It devoted a bureau within its organizational structure exclusively to the complicated process of purchasing and making the numerous items on the clothing list.

PERSONAL CLEANLINESS

With the subject area of bodily cleanliness, the commission got up close and personal with Union soldiers. In this, the inspectors inquired about selected habits concerning the care of the body. Mostly, they were interested in how often inner clothing was washed and changed; how often outer garments were dusted; how often the men bathed, washed their faces, and combed their hair; and whether they suffered from body lice. As with all other subject areas, the inspectors asked these questions of the surgeons and regimental or company officers, but they were supposed to include their own observations as well. Of course, there were serious limitations on how far any unit officer could go in examining his men's personal habits, and the inspector had even less opportunity to personally observe these things. But the results, limited as they were, reveal quite a bit about how Union soldiers took care of themselves.

THE CIVILIAN WAR ON DIRT

This concern for military hygiene dovetailed with a social and cultural movement progressing toward a heightened awareness of body care and health that had been developing for decades before the firing on Fort Sumter. With slow beginnings about the middle of the eighteenth century, reformers had been urging Americans to see the body as an important link in their health. They portrayed the skin as a purifier of waste products that needed to be kept free of dirt; washing should not just be a process of pouring water over the skin but should include scrubbing the body. Even then, most Americans typically did not use soap when they began to scrub. According to historians who focus on the history of personal cleanliness, soap was not commonly used in body care until the 1850s and 1860s, at least in middle-class households. Advice books stressed that "a daily wash of face, hands, and arms with soap was necessary to remove perspiration, oil, and dust." Soap had always been used when washing clothes, but by the 1880s, it was widely marketed in convenient ways for both bathing and laundry purposes. Before the Civil War, most Americans had accepted the fact that laundry day should occur weekly rather than remain a "seasonal event" and that underwear should be changed or washed frequently. Cultural and social issues reinforced health concerns by positing cleanliness as a distinguishing feature between higher and lower classes, representing not only hygienic awareness but also civic responsibility.[18]

Those interested in military hygiene fully agreed with the health precepts of the cleanliness movement that ran current through North American and European societies. Edward Thornhill Luscombe, senior surgeon of the Thirty-Fourth Regiment of Foot during the Peninsular War, pointed out that officers bore an enormous responsibility for the personal cleanliness of the soldier. He advised them to inspect the troops weekly by requiring the men to remove their shoes, stockings, and jackets and to roll up their shirt sleeves. This limited inspection of the body was all that could be allowed, but Luscombe felt it was sufficient to gauge the personal habits of the men. Indicating that the Europeans were ahead of the Americans, he also urged that lots of soap be issued to the troops. In the United States, John C. Warren, emeritus professor of anatomy and surgery at Harvard University, recommended cold-water showers or baths as early as 1830. Such washing would purify the skin and serve as a tonic. But, while urging the use of a sponge, Warren made no mention of soap.[19]

AMERICAN SANITARIANS ON MILITARY HYGIENE

The Civil War was the first conflict in American history that drew concentrated attention from sanitarians to the topic of personal cleanliness for soldiers. Ordronaux went pretty far in this regard, advocating a sort of basic training for all Union army recruits in which they would be taught habits of cleanliness. A morning wash of face, neck, arms, and feet with cold water and a report by their officers on each man's state of cleanliness at roll call would be part of this training. A more thorough cleansing of the body every week, with proper air circulation of the sleeping arrangements as well, would complete this basic training in military hygiene. It may be needless to say that this was not done; Ordronaux was decades ahead of his time. During the entirety of a soldier's army service, Ordronaux wanted him to continue this regimen of weekly bathing and washing of clothes. He also at least mentioned the use of soap.[20]

Hammond regretted that the army did not pay more attention to soldier bathing. It was important to open up skin pores and to stimulate energy that promoted health. Bathing tubs were provided for patients in general hospitals, but no special provisions for bathing were arranged in barracks and semipermanent camps. Each soldier had to fend for himself or do without a bath. In this regard, European armies were far ahead of the Americans. According to Hammond, the British had only recently switched from providing nothing to arranging for a bathhouse in all barracks similar to the arrangement previously fashioned by the French army, which included a dressing chamber and a shower bath that could accommodate 350 men daily.[21]

The US Army, in its own fashion, was alive to the principles of military hygiene. A handful of army officers wrote books spelling out these ideas and urging soldiers to take them seriously. "Personal cleanliness acts like a charm against all disease," wrote Daniel Butterfield, a graduate of the US

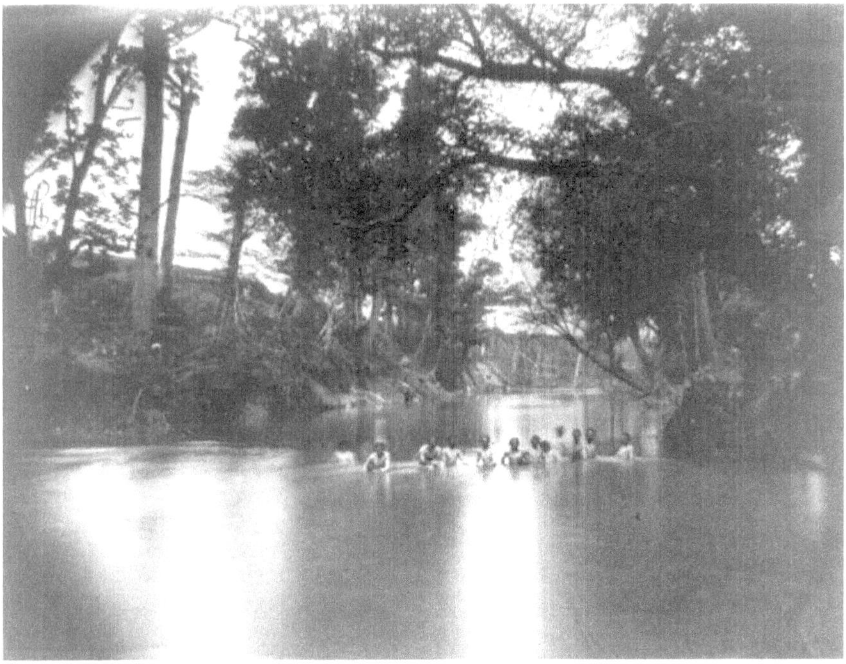

Bathing. Union soldiers are shown bathing in the North Anna River near the ruined bridge of the Richmond, Fredericksburg, and Potomac Railroad, which is in the background. This photograph was exposed by Timothy O'Sullivan in May 1864. (Library of Congress, Prints & Photographs Division, Civil War Photographs, LC-USZ62-91075)

Military Academy who rose to the rank of major general in the volunteer force. He advocated washing underwear every week and cutting hair every month so that it never grew more than one and a half inches long. Butterfield also urged a thorough cold-water washing of the scalp every morning and cutting the toenails and fingernails closely. Maj. James A. Congdon of the Twelfth Pennsylvania Cavalry wrote a book about the mounted service in which he drew attention to military hygiene. Congdon urged every trooper to keep two combs, one coarse and the other fine; a toothbrush; a sponge; soap; and two towels for his personal care. He went further than most in advising men to wash their face, neck, and hands as well as brush their teeth and comb their hair every morning. A bath twice instead of once a week rounded out the Congdon personal care system.[22]

Of course, officials of the US Sanitary Commission fully supported all efforts to teach Union soldiers how to fight dirt. W. H. Van Buren urged a thorough bath every week along with laundering of underclothing weekly. He stressed the importance of washing the feet every day and applying ointments to rid the body of lice. "The hair and beard should be closely cropped," he advised.[23]

PROBLEMS WITH ARMY HYGIENE

But as soon as the war broke out, it became apparent that actual conditions in the camps led men to often ignore the sage advice of sanitarians and army officers alike. Gov. John A. Andrew sent Samuel Gridley Howe, a physician, abolitionist, and veteran of the Greek War of Independence (1821–29), to look into the health of Massachusetts soldiers around Washington, DC, in May 1861. "There is more need of a health officer than of a chaplain," Howe wrote, "but the United States knows no such officer." He was astonished at the scarcity of soap in the army camps and the lack of provision for regular washing of clothes, making the extreme statement that laundresses were more needed at the time than nurses.[24]

Howe was realistic about the limitations of imposing sanitary principles in the camps. "It is difficult, if not impossible, to enforce perfect personal cleanliness among the soldiers beyond that of the head and hands. The rest must depend upon the individual habits and inclinations." The problem of body lice was "next to impossible" to solve, and even the more advanced European armies had not come up with a solution. "The *ova* of the insects seem to be omnipresent," and if the men wear the same clothes "unwashed or imperfectly washed in cold water, for several successive weeks, and when they are huddled closely together at night, the lice are sure to appear." The men initially reacted with horror at a lice infestation, but then "like other soldiers they will finally submit to what at home would be disgusting and insufferable."[25]

The problem of laundry facilities could be solved by hiring laundresses while in semipermanent camps, with each soldier paying fifty cents a month for their labor. Howe admitted it would be better to hire males for this service so they could accompany the regiment on campaign. He urged the issue of "a light, portable stove" to boil water and create a dry heat for washing and drying clothes while on the move. Hiring out laundry while in camp was feasible and (as we shall see) occurred in a minority of regiments, but providing for laundry services on the move was impracticable.[26]

In the scathing report filed by Olmsted arising from his tour of army camps in the summer of 1861, which sparked the camp inspection system, care of the body became a major concern. "In but few cases are the soldiers obliged to regard any rules of personal cleanliness. Their clothing is shamefully dirty, and they are often lousy." The uniform was "almost daily saturated with sweat and packed with dust."[27]

It is true that Olmsted saw the situation at its worst, looking at the first flush of volunteers who possessed far more enthusiasm than military sense, but the camp situation as it related to personal cleanliness improved a lot with the growing maturity of the volunteer army. Godfrey Aigner found that the twenty-three infantry regiments, one regiment and fifteen companies of cavalry, and ten batteries of artillery he inspected in the vicinity of Cairo, Illinois, during the fall of 1861 conducted routine washing of underclothing on a weekly basis. The men dusted their outer garments weekly rather than daily and bathed in warm water pretty often. Still, some degree of body-lice infestation occurred in every regiment. Aigner's biggest criticism was that officers in all units failed to thoroughly or consistently superintend their men's personal habits. Even so he concluded, "the volunteers keep their persons as clean as the generality of people in the localities they come from," a believable way to look at the issue, which highlighted the failure of the army to change civilian habits to meet the needs of military hygiene.[28]

The army actually tried to make men toe the line when it came to personal cleanliness. Regulations placed the burden of oversight on company commanders and, to a slightly less degree, on noncommissioned officers. "The utmost attention will be paid . . . to the cleanliness of their men, as to their persons," the army officially stated. "Where conveniences for bathing are to be had, the men should bathe once or twice a week. The feet to be washed at least twice a week. The hair *kept short,* and beard neatly trimmed." The army also required the troops to wash their hands and faces every day and to "brush or comb their heads." To promote this reasonable agenda, the Quartermaster Department issued a prodigious amount of underwear, more than 4.7 million pairs to an army of nearly one million men, during the fiscal year ending June 30, 1864.[29]

But getting the troops to obey these injunctions was another matter. Men were naturally "careless of cleanliness," thought William W. Belknap, commander of the Fifteenth Iowa, and needed supervision. A member of the Sixteenth Ohio made a similar comment in a letter published by the *Tuscarawas Advocate,* bluntly stating that "men in the army have to be watched like children at home, if they would be kept clean." John Billings more accurately differentiated between types of soldiers as he discussed the "wide difference in the habits of cleanliness" in the Tenth Massachusetts Battery. On one end of the spectrum were those as fastidious about washing their underclothing every week as they would have been at home.

On the other end were those who would do so only "under the severest pressure. It is disgusting to remember, even at this late day, how little care hundreds of the men bestowed on bodily cleanliness." Every unit had its share of troops who were "regardless of all rules of health."[30]

These general statements held a good deal of validity, but they need to be modified by the variations that are apparent in attitudes and practices concerning personal cleanliness. Commission inspector Marvin M. Marsh, for example, noticed a difference between the Army of the Potomac in Virginia and the troops stationed within Union-held enclaves along the South Carolina coast in the Department of the South. He visited the latter department in the summer of 1863, after its headquarters had issued specific orders for the men to bathe or wash at least twice a week and change their underclothing once a week. Yet the men in the department seemed to have less regard for personal cleanliness than those in Virginia. They complained of having poor water available along the coastal shelf where their camps were located, but Marsh believed the real problem was poor officer supervision. Over the course of two weeks, he saw only one man bathing in the sea, and although told by officers that the troops washed their hands and faces daily, he knew that this practice was "by no means universal in any regiment." At this same time similar orders supporting personal cleaning habits had been issued in the Army of the Potomac and were more carefully obeyed.[31]

Some officers tried their best to fulfill army directives about teaching their men how to maintain bodily cleanliness, but it was difficult to do. "I have the camp thoroughly cleaned every day and compel the men to be cleanly in the persons, believing filth to be the great originator of disease," wrote Col. William H. Raynor of the Fifty-Sixth Ohio in his diary. While Raynor seems never to have complained of the results, there is a tone of utter frustration in the orders issued by Col. Franklin S. Nickerson when trying to bring his Fourteenth Maine up to an acceptable standard of personal cleanliness. "Once more in the name of decency and humanity," he ordered company commanders to enforce regulations concerning "the washing of the persons" of their troops. "The condition of the men to day, notwithstanding my earnest appeals, is a disgrace to civilization." He threatened to dismiss officers incapable of improving the condition of their troops and reducing to the ranks any noncommissioned officer who did not set a good example for the men. "See that it be done not simply tell them to do it," Nickerson commanded.[32]

Underclothing tended to become the focus of personal cleanliness in the army, perhaps because it was the seat of so much filth and was the most private part of clothing. Officers could not truly inspect those items as they could the outer garments and had to trust the soldier to obey injunctions about caring for them. Lt. Frederick Whittaker of the Sixth New York Cavalry frankly admitted that most troopers did not wash their underclothing weekly; in fact, it was not unusual for them to do so only after several weeks had passed. In part, this was because the woolen underwear they used was not at all easy to wash and dry. Cotton or linen would have been better material, in his view. Moreover, the woolen fabric offered ample safe havens for body lice, again in contrast to cotton or linen. It probably was for this reason that inattention to underwear promoted body-lice infestation.[33]

The only recourse for prevention was frequent washing of underclothing because the army issued only one pair of drawers at a time to each man; he could not simply change and wash later. To do the job properly meant building a fire, boiling water, applying soap, and scrubbing "till every bone in our bodies ached," recalled George Sargent of the First Rhode Island Cavalry. The woolen fabric, resulting in thick and heavy underwear, rendered this job much harder than was necessary. "It took time to wash and dry so we had to know we would halt for at least a day before we could undertake the job," recalled Rice C. Bull. Regiments tended to set aside full days for laundry—for some it was Monday and others Saturday—during which everyone got the distasteful job out of the way. More often than not, the soldier did his own washing, but some relied on refugee slave women to wash their underwear and shirts for a small fee or gave it to an obliging member of their company, who also did it for a fee. The soldier further promoted his own health if he bathed regularly, but that process also was complicated in the field. Some of them performed the ritual conscientiously, but most did not. "I never left a Saturday night go by without having a bath and a change of underclothes," wrote Frederick W. Wild of Alexander's Baltimore Battery. While planted along the Union line at Petersburg, several regiments constructed bathhouses similar to those regularly set up in general hospitals. But this was an extremely unusual arrangement for units in the field, made possible only by the long, static nature of the Petersburg Campaign and the effect of good officer supervision.[34]

The most distressing result of inattention to bathing and washing underwear was the prevalence of body lice. Most men naturally dreaded an infestation both for the physical discomfort and the shame associated with it; still, lice were almost inevitable. Even vigorous attention to personal cleanliness did not necessarily eliminate the possibility of finding a louse on one's clothes, although it certainly reduced the chances. Lice lived in the soil until a warm body neared. They thrived among human populations that lived closely together without proper cleansing and clothes washing. Vermin have been a feature of army life forever because soldiers present an appropriate host population for them to thrive on. Living on the blood of the host, lice laid eggs along the seams of clothing. Worst of all, lice could carry the organism, a cross between a virus and a bacteria, that caused typhus fever. Thus, lice infestation was a problem far worse than discomfort and embarrassment. While excavating the mass grave of French army personnel near Vilnius, archaeologists discovered parts of five types of body lice that had carried this organism and estimated that one-third of Napoleon's soldiers carried infectious louse-transmitted diseases. Frequent washing of clothes in hot water reduced the risk of infestation, as did frequent washing of the body, but the only sure cure was mercurial ointment. This was "a capital germicide and insect exterminator" for body lice, wrote Charles Beneulyn Johnson, hospital steward of the 130th Illinois. Proper application along the seams of the shirt and trousers and even on the underclothing seemed to work more often than not.[35]

Keeping clean in the army, both for comfort and personal health, was no easy task. The military experience intensified physical closeness among soldiers, placing a premium on regular washing of clothes and body, while most men tended to think that other matters, such as drilling and weapons use, were more important elements of military life. The army itself, as represented by the officers and noncommissioned officers, bore a huge responsibility to teach them how important hygiene could be in their health and then to supervise their washing and bathing. The inspection reports indicate how well the military system carried out this vital responsibility.

FIFTEENTH CORPS MEDICAL INSPECTION REPORTS

The Fifteenth Corps medical inspectors paid attention to personal cleanliness but without devoting much time to it. The one thing that comes clearly through their reports is that cleanliness was closely tied to the environment. When the corps was struggling to exist along the muddy bottomlands of Louisiana during the early months of 1863, the men were absolutely filthy. A report for April 12 listed a total of eighteen regiments; nine of them, or exactly half, rated bad when it came to personal cleanliness, while only five, or 27.7 percent, rated good. But while staying on high ground near the Big Black River in September, medical inspectors rated seventeen of nineteen regiments as good when it came to personal cleanliness. In March 1865, at the end of the difficult march through the Carolinas, First Division commander Charles R. Woods complained that his men were "not wearing the hair as ordered by regulations. Each enlisted man will be required to have his hair cut as prescribed." Soon after that, corps headquarters issued orders reminding company commanders that they were responsible for their men's cleanliness and that noncommissioned officers were supposed to "see that the men wash their hands and faces daily; that they comb and brush their heads; that their hair is kept short; [and] that those on duty are properly dressed." It is obvious that attention to personal cleanliness had to be reinforced from the ground up on a repeated basis during the course of the war. Most of the men never learned to do this on their own, and even many officers never learned to consistently apply the regulations they were told from the beginning of their army service it was their responsibility to enforce.[36]

SANITARY COMMISSION CAMP INSPECTION RETURNS

The Sanitary Commission inspection returns reveal a varied and complex picture of personal cleanliness in the Union army. Fourteen questions on Form No. 19a were devoted to aspects of personal cleanliness. The commission wanted to know how often the men washed their underclothing; did they dust their outer garments; did officers supervise these necessary tasks to see that they were done properly; did it appear that the cleaning regimen was effective; did the men bathe frequently and were they supervised; did each wash his head, neck, and feet daily; was evidence of neglect in personal cleanliness part of the regular inspection routine of the unit by its officers; did the men suffer from vermin infestation; and whether any effort was made to deal with the pests. The return, in other words, explored all the relevant aspects of personal cleanliness in a thorough way.

Overall, the results reflected a wide array of attention paid to personal hygiene. There were some regiments that shone brilliantly, but more units did poorly, and many others muddled through with mediocre results. One can readily find inspector's comments that frankly reported no systematic attempt to keep clean on anyone's part. That was true not only of the first wave of volunteer regiments at the start of the war but even of old regiments halfway through their war service. There was no distinction between races; white regiments joined Black regiments in scoring at different levels. Men in a number of units deployed mercurial ointment when the inevitable louse appeared, although Surg. Alonzo M. Morrison of the

Twenty-Third Kentucky told his assistant surgeon, William L. Hasbrouck, to sprinkle coal oil over the blankets and men's clothing to deter vermin "with decided advantage." But one could not expect total victory. "Do what you may you cannot keep soldiers clean from vermin," concluded Dr. W. C. Pace of the 110th Illinois, "even the Doctors have them."[37]

From the poor end of the spectrum to the better, the returns documented everything. Inspectors did not hesitate to praise when they thought it justified, and they found good hygienic regimens from the start to the end of the war in a few units. They occasionally encountered regimental bathhouses, good oversight by officers, and soldiers who actively sought ways to bathe even when it was not easy to do so. "The men are very cleanly. Once or twice a week they are marched to the river by companies and compelled to give themselves a thorough scrubbing," George G. Edgerly reported of the Tenth Regiment, Corps d'Afrique at Port Hudson.[38]

But the middle range of the spectrum is the most important because it represented more accurately the average Union regiment than either of the two extremes. The average can be broadly summarized. Most regiments had regulations in place instructing the men to wash their underclothing every week and to dust their outer garments either weekly or daily. They also had regulations for the men to daily wash their faces, heads, and necks but rarely their feet. Most also had some kind of officer supervision for enforcement, although in some units that assignment was given to noncommissioned officers. But most regiments did not perform officer supervision well, simply blending personal cleanliness into a general weekly inspection that included many other aspects of soldier life, such as how well the men maintained their weapons. Even among the better regiments, vermin was present to some degree.

The references to care of outer garments almost always referred to regular dusting, not washing. Inspectors mentioned this aspect in 187 returns, and in 176 (94.2 percent) of them they indicated that some regulations existed requiring the men to dust. For a couple of regiments, clothes brushes were purchased by means of the company fund, although that was extremely rare. In a few regiments the men were "expected" to dust without a formal requirement, and for 11 of the 187 regiments, there was no expectation or requirement of any kind on the matter.[39]

A similar situation prevailed when it came to washing underwear. Of 211 returns that mention this topic, 191 (90.5 percent) indicated that the men were officially required to wash weekly; only 20 (9.5 percent) had no such requirement. In a small number of units, the men were to wash daily, twice a week, or "as necessity requires." The army simply did not provide laundry facilities even in semipermanent camps. Hiring laundresses was an option only for a small number of regiments—four are mentioned in the commission returns as having the services of washerwomen. In the Sixth Wisconsin one man in each company washed the clothes of his comrades weekly. But most Union soldiers had to learn how to do their own washing under difficult conditions.[40]

Inspectors compiled quite a bit of information on bathing habits. The frequency depended a good deal on the season because cold weather put a damper even on soldiers who were willing to bathe frequently. Typically, regiments exercised a good bathing regimen in warm seasons and completely stopped bathing during the winter months. The men instead only washed their faces, hands, and necks in cold weather. But the lack of proper bathing facilities dampened the habit even in good weather. At times this was due to a shortage of water, but more often it was the lack of privacy. For most, the only choices for a bath were a nearby stream or an empty pork barrel serving as a bathtub. Even while staying at Benton Barracks outside St. Louis, the Fifty-Fifth Illinois had "no facilities" for bathing. Officers in a handful of regiments simply encouraged the men to bathe in their tents, using a sponge if available, but this method led to uneven results. Typically, even when a unit took bathing seriously, the men usually did it only once a week. In some regiments the troops had to be forced to the task. "Ordered to do so," Aigner noted of the Tenth Iowa. "Sergeants make the men do it."[41]

The presence of body lice seemed to be an indicator of how well a regiment observed the rules of personal cleanliness, although inspectors came to doubt that assumption. They also came to doubt whether they could ever know exactly at what level infestations occurred. A total of 267 inspection returns mentioned vermin; of that number 139 (52.1 percent) indicated no infestation at all. Another 106 (39.7 percent) indicated some degree of infestation, while another 15 (5.6 percent) indicated a rare occurrence, and 7 (2.6 percent) admitted a bad infestation. In other words, if we take these results at face value, a bit more than half the regiments were lice free, and almost half had some degree of infestation.

The problem was, however, that inspectors had to rely on what the surgeons and officers told them concerning this delicate topic. Many of them came to question that testimony. Robert Ware and William M. Chamberlain recorded officer assertions that no vermin existed in their regiments, but the two added a question mark next to that notation on the return.

Inspectors did not ask the rank and file, and of course they could not personally observe whether lice constituted a problem in the camp. One suspects that many officers covered up the truth and tried to make it appear that their men had no lice. But another aspect of this issue was that in some cases the surgeons and regimental officers simply did not know whether their soldiers had lice or not. "Capt. can't say," Ware noted of an officer in the Second Battalion, First Wisconsin Artillery. "Surgeon does not know[.] Some of the officers say yes to some little extent," Franklin B. Hough wrote of the First Connecticut Artillery. Chamberlain also noted that when asked this question, some officers replied "no complaint" was received from the men, so they assumed there were no lice in the regiment. In the end, the inspector rarely was satisfied with his opportunity for knowing the truth about pest infestations. "Could not learn definitely," Henry W. Warriner commented of a battalion of the First Nebraska Cavalry.[42]

It is very likely that well over half the regiments inspected had some degree of vermin infestation, although only a minority of them considered it a serious problem. Even in those with good hygienic practices, a handful of men outside the mainstream of personal habits suffered from body lice. Lax attention to personal hygiene could increase the level of infestation, but strict attention rarely eliminated the presence of lice from a regiment.

Army regulations strictly required short hair and beards that were combed daily. In some regiments this was attended to with acceptable results; in others the regulations were hardly acknowledged or openly ignored. As with everything else, it all depended on how seriously officers took the injunctions. In the Seventh New York Heavy Artillery, the men followed these rules "as far as possible," according to T. B. Smith. But in the Pioneer Corps of the Army of the Cumberland, the men "willingly" obeyed the regulations. Officers in the Fifteenth Maine were well aware of the regulations but chose not to enforce them. In the Forty-Fifth Massachusetts, however, officers strictly followed the rules.[43]

In many ways the most important information provided by the commission's camp inspection returns is how well officers enforced a wide variety of army policies concerning personal cleanliness. Among volunteer units, the officers generally came from the same class and community as the rank and file. As a result, many of them did not take sanitary principles any more seriously than did many of their men. Moreover, faced with a wide range of responsibilities, even well-meaning officers often placed personal hygiene low on their list of priorities. Seeing that their men were well drilled; had good, serviceable weapons; and were relatively well fed came first. Combing their hair and taking a bath came last.

A total of 170 returns specifically mentioned officer supervision of clothes care, washing underwear, and dusting outer garments. Of that number, 158 (92.9 percent) indicated that officers or noncommissioned officers supervised or inspected the men to see that it was done. But that is a very misleading statistic. For the overwhelming majority of those regiments, inspection merely meant that the company or regimental officer was supposed to include personal cleanliness as part of his overall weekly or monthly inspection of the troops. How well they did so was the big question. Typically, this inspection was a proforma affair in which the officer at best merely glanced about to see that the men were in reasonably good shape. He rarely if ever specifically focused on personal cleanliness unless someone was outrageously dirty.

A surprisingly high number of regiments assigned officers or noncommissioned officers to supervise the men's bathing, amounting to 52 percent. But there is every reason to question how closely this was done. It was, after all, a private affair, and no enlisted man would have welcomed an officer or a noncommissioned officer watching him do it. That is why 48 percent of the regiments openly admitted there was no officer supervision of bathing.

Inspectors were required not just to rely on what the regimental surgeon and commander told them but also to personally observe, as far as possible, all subject areas listed on the standard return form. Their opportunities for doing so were limited. If the men happened to be washing and drying their clothes when he visited, the inspector took this as a sign of healthy adherence to sanitary principles. But if their clothes seemed dirtier than usual, he came to the opposite conclusion.[44]

Personal cleanliness was one of the fifteen subject areas on the standard form in which officer supervision was unusually important. Gauging the answers to all fourteen questions relating to this topic, the good ratings were 28.9 percent of all 280 returns, while the fair ratings were 52.5 percent and the bad 18.6 percent.

In the end, commission inspectors could cluck their tongues at the many examples of poor hygiene they found in army camps. But they also recognized something else that was inexplicable. Some units with poor hygienic regimens seemed to enjoy acceptable or even good health. "The men do not look as cleanly as they ought," admitted Warriner of a battalion in the First Nebraska Cavalry. But he explained this apparent contradiction to sanitary theory by noting that they were "mostly miners and hardy enough to triumph over dreadfully *un* Sanitary conditions. So that on the whole they are in a very fair state of health."[45]

It was an uphill struggle to enlist Union soldiers in the war on dirt. Officer and private alike came directly from civilian lives in which, as members of a young male population, they were not necessarily attuned to principles of personal care that meshed well with army regulations or the ideas of prominent sanitarians. As temporary soldiers, they generally learned to mostly accept that regimen and the principles that undergirded regulations about washing clothes, bathing, and combing their hair. But that is about all that can be said of their record of personal cleanliness.

5

Slops and Sinks

There was general agreement that disposing of waste products in semipermanent camps was a necessity. The army already was keen on ridding the living and working areas of anything offensive to sight or smell and that posed a health hazard to the troops. For their part, Civil War sanitarians paid much less attention to this issue, probably because it was so obvious that waste needed to be syphoned out of the camp through some system of disposal. Thus, there is very little theoretical literature about waste disposal. But the camp inspectors paid a good deal of attention to the topic and included it in their returns in order to document how well the army was doing what it obviously needed to do.

The two concerns associated with waste disposal were slops and sinks. The first referred to the products of cooking and eating. Slops also included the waste associated with cattle butchering in the field, whatever waste came out of the cooking process such as grease and soured foods, and the table scraps left behind by the men after eating their meals. Sinks referred to human waste products: urine and excrement. The Civil War–era military jargon referred to the facilities designed to handle these as "sinks" rather than "latrines." In both cases of slops and sinks, regimental officers were expected to set up systems to handle the waste in a sanitary manner. These systems were quite simple but not always effective.

SLOPS

One can find several readily available army-issued documents about the handling of kitchen and food refuse. Army of the Potomac headquarters mandated by midpoint of the war that a hole should be dug near every company kitchen in a semipermanent camp into which "all the refuse matter" should be piled. When the matter reached a point two feet from the top, the hole was to be filled in and a new one dug. Offal, blood, and dead animals were to be buried at least four feet deep, kitchen refuse three feet deep, and manure two feet deep. These specific instructions were worked out by Jonathan Letterman, chief medical officer of the Army of the Potomac. Similar orders from the same time can be found, for example, in the Department of the South in occupied South Carolina.[1]

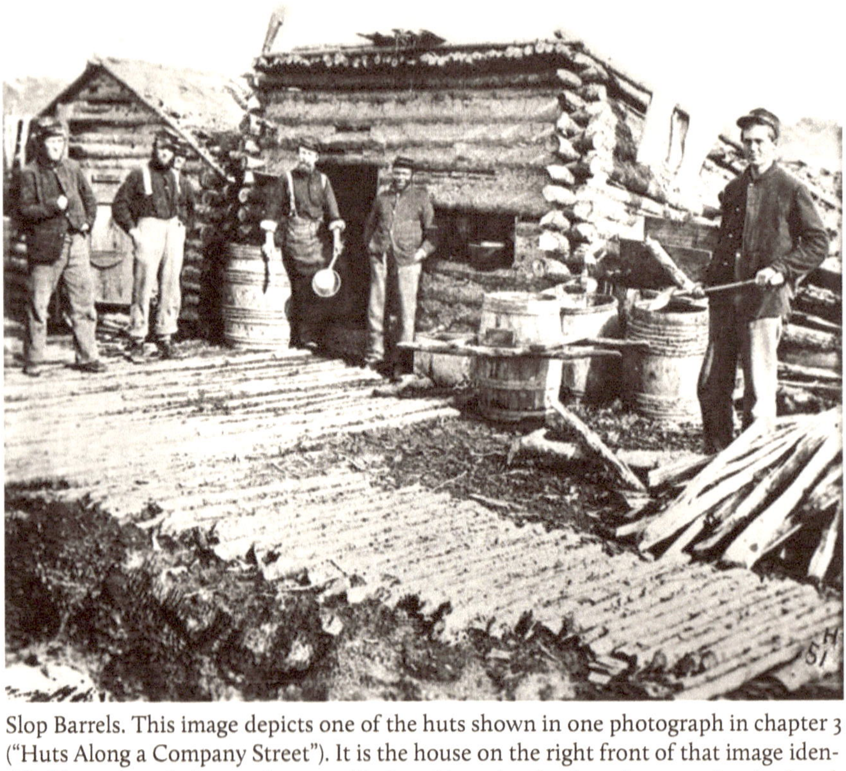

Slop Barrels. This image depicts one of the huts shown in one photograph in chapter 3 ("Huts Along a Company Street"). It is the house on the right front of that image identified by an inscription as the camp kitchen. Note the slop barrels conveniently placed for the disposal of kitchen waste and food bits. One of the barrels is fixed with handles to be readily carried by two men for emptying elsewhere. (Library of Congress, Prints & Photographs Division, Civil War Photographs, LCDIG-ppmsca-33110)

Such orders filtered down the chain of command and had their effect according to how conscientious lower-level commanders happened to be. In the First Brigade, Third Division, Fifth Corps, Army of the Potomac, the issue was taken seriously. An order issued late in July 1864 required holes to be dug at least one hundred feet from the camps. It further specified a hole's dimensions as six to eight feet deep, four feet wide, and six feet long. Each regiment was to collect its slops in barrels or boxes and empty them twice a day in these holes from 5 to 6 A.M. and from 6 to 7 P.M. The brigade commander required that this order be read to every company so that each and every enlisted man as well as all officers would be informed.[2]

FIFTEENTH CORPS MEDICAL INSPECTION REPORTS

The big question with slops as well as with all other army orders was how well they were obeyed. Personal accounts cannot be counted on to offer a consistent or widespread answer to that question. We must rely on the results of inspections to find out if the men and their officers thought it important to dispose of their waste.

Fifteenth Corps medical inspectors found extremely lax conditions in several veteran regiments that had been in service for two years. "'Slop holes' are dug in midst of camp," wrote Surg. Edward O. F. Roler in September 1863, "and are full of debris." Five months later his successor found "meat and other articles of food scattered indiscriminately about camp" when he inspected the Fifteenth Michigan at Scottsboro, Alabama. "Mens qrs. very dirty. No inspection of camp or quarters made by the officers." Even in June 1865, just before muster out after their war service, "joints of meat and other decaying substances are thrown out near the quarters, and the stench is readily noticed," reported Surg. John M. Woodworth about several Fifteenth Corps regiments.[3]

SANITARY COMMISSION CAMP INSPECTION RETURNS

The Sanitary Commission standard camp inspection form devoted nine questions to the subject of slops. These started with a quick visual survey by the inspector to detect the presence of food scraps in the tent areas, in the drains, and on company streets. Questioning regimental officers, the inspector was then supposed to find out if the unit had a systematic process for disposing of camp waste and report whether odors of decay could be smelled. The form included three questions concerning regimental animals—horses, mules, and beef cattle. How many animals each regiment had, how far from camp they were kept, and whether the dung was removed daily were the matters of chief concern.

From the 280 returns used in this study, inspectors reported that only forty-two units had no systematic method of waste disposal. They did not add much in the way of explanation, and one assumes regimental commanders simply let their men do as they wished in this matter. Ironically, there was no hard connection between especially dirty camps and units reported as having no waste-disposal system, indicating that when left to their own volition, most of the troops understood the importance of keeping the camp relatively clean of food waste. On the other hand, considering the fact that 238 out of 280 unit reports indicated some degree of system imposed on the unit by its commander to handle this daily chore is a positive sign of how well sanitary awareness had infiltrated the minds of volunteer officers.

Inspectors found a range of conditions in these camps concerning the disposal of waste. "No special plans for slops & refuse which are scattered about the camp," Robert Jones wrote of the Fortieth New York early in the war, after it had been in camp near Washington, DC, for a full week. A number of regiments did not bother to dig holes, but the men simply disposed of collected food waste by throwing it on the ground just outside the camp's confines. In many other regiments the waste was thrown into any natural depression that was handy so as to avoid the trouble of digging a hole. For Battery B, First New York Light Artillery, that was a small stream that ran through the camp. For the First Connecticut Artillery, it was a nearby ravine, and for the Twelfth Connecticut, it was the Mississippi River.[4]

The artificial drains dug around tents and along company streets also became handy dumping places for kitchen waste. "An open sewer or trench leads from the cooking places along the rear of the company quarters which is used as a garbage sink, and a terrible nuisance," E. J. Dunning commented of the Twentieth New York camp. Edward A. Crane found "bones fragments of food bottles slops and all unclean things" filling a main drainage ditch along the edge of the 128th New York camp north of New Orleans. One might bend the rules if winter weather made it difficult to collect and properly dispose of garbage, as the regimental officers of Battery G, First New York Light Artillery told Henry Oliver. But a more discerning view of excuses could be adopted, as William M. Chamberlain did of Battery A, First New York Light Artillery when he judged that its officers and men displayed "a careless [want] of cleanliness" after he saw "Slop & food Scraps all about" their camp.[5]

Inspectors found relatively few regimental camps suffering from foul odors. Only 14 of the 280 returns contained comments on bad smells. Most of these were due to animal dung and rotting food. When George L. Andrews visited the Fifth Wisconsin, he smelled "sour beans & bread," which was no compliment for the unit's company cooks. W. M. Prentice saw plenty of food scraps and smelled unpleasant odors in the camp of the Second Tennessee (US), even though the regimental officers insisted that they had a systematic method of waste disposal. While only 14 returns mention bad smells, several others reported no odors, although the inspector inserted a note of caution. The weather happened to be quite cold during these visits, and the inspectors found little to praise in the unit's camp police. They predicted that the arrival of pleasant temperatures in spring would likely bring out the odors suppressed by cold weather.[6]

But camp inspectors also found much that was good about waste disposal when they visited some regiments. The most common way to dispose of camp refuse was to use tubs or empty barrels to collect it and then dump the contents well away from camp. A handful of regiments made arrangements with local farmers to take the refuse away, either selling it or giving it away to be used as swill for hogs. Some units burned the refuse or took the trouble to cart it half a mile from camp for disposal.[7]

A few regiments arranged an elaborate method of taking care of kitchen slops while spending six months in semipermanent camps near Murfreesboro, Tennessee, early in 1863. Alfred L. Castleman described it as digging a large hole six feet wide and deep for each company, then covering most of it with wood, brush, and dirt. An opening just large enough for a barrel was left in the middle and covered with a lid. Most of the time these slop-disposal setups were completely closed to prevent gases from escaping. Arranged in a line, they had "rather an ornamental appearance" compared to the "unsightly & filthy pits usually left open." Castleman saw this arrangement in the camp of the Forty-Second Indiana. Bernard J. Bettelheim saw something similar when he visited the Thirtieth Indiana and Seventy-Ninth Illinois, calling them "barrel-kitchen-sinks." A few regiments in the East, such as the Third Massachusetts and First US Colored Troops, also made such arrangements, which were termed "kitchen cesspools" by some camp inspectors. These Eastern cesspools appeared in 1863, at the same time that they appeared in the West.[8]

The simplicity of the idea—that to promote health one needed to get rid of kitchen refuse and keep the campgrounds clean of food scraps—was so apparent that slops achieved a relatively high rating in the camp inspection returns. Overall, the good ratings amounted to 57.8 percent, while 22.1 percent were rated as fair, and 20.1 percent were rated as bad. One could argue that given the obvious benefits of waste disposal, it is a bit surprising that only slightly more than half the regiments inspected achieved a good rating. No matter how obvious the need, no matter how energetic the officer enforcement, sanitary efforts always smashed into the rock of general indifference on the part of many privates and their noncommissioned-officer colleagues. Left to their own devices, a surprisingly high percentage of them seem to have been quite willing to live in filth.

SINKS

The situation was a bit worse, ironically, when it came to disposing of human excrement, a topic that should have elicited even more concern and concentrated effort than slops. But the problem of placing latrines where they could be convenient but not offend the sensibilities or harm the men's health tended to be more difficult for Civil War soldiers to solve than one might have expected. The army had already established pretty good guidelines for this, specifying how far from camp to dig pits and outlining the daily regimen for maintenance of those holes. The problem was that officers and men alike tended not to follow those sound regulations, and a surprising number of regiments did not even bother to dig pits at all, forcing officers and men alike to find a convenient tree near camp. Far too often when it came to setting priorities among the many things that a Civil War regiment had to take care of, sinks tended to be placed pretty far down the list.

"One of the fondest recolections [*sic*] of a Soldier and the last to be forgotten is the path from his tent to the SINK," recalled Amos York of the Eighth Indiana after the war. Col. Alfred Gibbs, a graduate of the US Military Academy and veteran of the Mexican War and of battles with Apaches before the Civil War, commented to Surg. Benjamin T. Kneeland of the 130th New York that the smell of the latrine was an inescapable part of army life. He called it "the patriotic odor, and it would stay by us as long as we were sufficiently patriotic to remain in the army." But Kneeland managed to reduce the smell, if not eliminate it, by having men apply an inch of fresh dirt over the top of the latrine contents every day. Kneeland pointed out that this process was mentioned in Deuteronomy 23:13, which reads, "Outside the camp you shall have a place set aside where you shall go." The following verse adds, "You shall keep a trowel in your equipment and, when you go outside to relieve yourself, you shall dig a hole with it and then cover up your excrement."[9]

The best way to get rid of human waste was to set up a water-based system for its disposal. The Romans had engineered such a system with their communal latrines that incorporated two constant flows of water: one to carry away the waste and the other to clean oneself. This system was made available to civilians in large cities as well as to the garrisons of permanent posts. It was not possible, however, for armies on the move or in semipermanent camps to set up such an elaborate system, which also had to be located near a reliable source of water. For the majority of instances, a simple pit or trench had to suffice. This was how the allied forces provided easement for the troops in the operations against Sebastopol during the Crimean War. The men applied dirt or lime on a regular basis, but the holes were too big, which exposed a lot of the raw contents to the atmosphere. One could barely smell it during cold weather, but it became obnoxious in warm temperatures, leading the men to dig narrower trenches instead. European armies generally relied on trenches that, in the Prussian cavalry service, were thirty feet long and three feet deep when the troops were in the field. They generally called for a fresh covering of dirt and the application of some sort of disinfectant every day and digging new pits on a regular basis.[10]

SANITARIANS ON HOW TO DEAL WITH HUMAN WASTE

Civil War sanitarians offered clear and simple advice about disposing of human waste in army camps. When in barracks, it was best to have a system connected with an underground sewer regularly inspected by the medical officer of the post. So that the men did not have to go to the latrines at night, a urinal should be set up in each dormitory for their use. In field camps toilet facilities were arranged from scratch by digging long, deep, and narrow trenches a certain distance and downwind from the camp. Surgeon General Hammond cautioned officers never to place the sink near a source of water. Some degree of privacy was included as well, which could be accomplished by digging the hole near bushes or cutting brush to erect a screen. The sink needed a sitting rail for the convenience of users, while a separate sink should be dug to accommodate the patients of the regimental hospital. Every day a layer of fresh dirt should be thrown on the contents of all sinks, dousing them with disinfectants twice a week to complete the sanitary regimen. Cheap disinfectants included chloride and sulphate of lime (gypsum) in powder form, sulphate of iron (green copperas) in solution form, and sulfuric- and muriatic-acid gas. But the easiest was simply to spread lime or campfire ashes over it. A urinal could be fashioned from a bucket with a cover and large enough to serve twenty men. Soldiers had to be instructed to use the bucket even in daytime because urinating on the ground near the tents caused the soil to become "foul and offensive," as John Ordronaux pointed out.[11]

THE ARMY ON HOW TO DEAL WITH HUMAN WASTE

Unlike slops, the topic of sinks drew a good deal of attention from the army and from officers charged with the oversight of camps. Regulations established the location for latrines as 150 paces "in front of the color line," with separate facilities for officers on the opposite side of the camp and 100 paces from the tents. Sinks for the men could, if more convenient, be placed on other sides of the camp but never on the same side as the officers' sinks. Regulations mandated bushes for privacy and a layer of fresh dirt over the contents "occasionally."[12] They did not specify the number of sinks required per regiment.

Many military commands in the field issued orders regulating sinks largely along these lines. In the short-lived Army of Kentucky, headquartered at Louisville in September 1862, the medical director issued a set of instructions specifying that two sinks should be dug for every company's contingent of enlisted men, with two additional sinks for all the regimental officers and a separate one for hospital use. The officers' sinks "should always be distant from those for the men." Each should be from four to six feet deep, 160 paces from the nearest tent, and "as narrow as they can well be dug." The enlisted men needed a total of seventy-five feet of trench and the officers twelve feet. Regular inspection could ensure that no odor emanated farther than 20 paces from the pit. It was important for each regiment to issue orders requiring the men to use the facilities and punish those who disobeyed. When nearly full, up to eighteen inches from the top, new holes had to be dug. The medical director gave specific instructions about the critical area at the edge of the latrine trench. Officers should see that boards, poles, or fence rails were placed along the edge to serve as footholds because urine tended to fall there rather than in the pit. Subsequent users could largely avoid standing in urine-soaked soil if such a wooden pavement were added. The all-important sitting rail had to be secure and yet overhang the edge of the sink for obvious reasons. Its posts were placed overhanging the edge, supporting a rail not more than

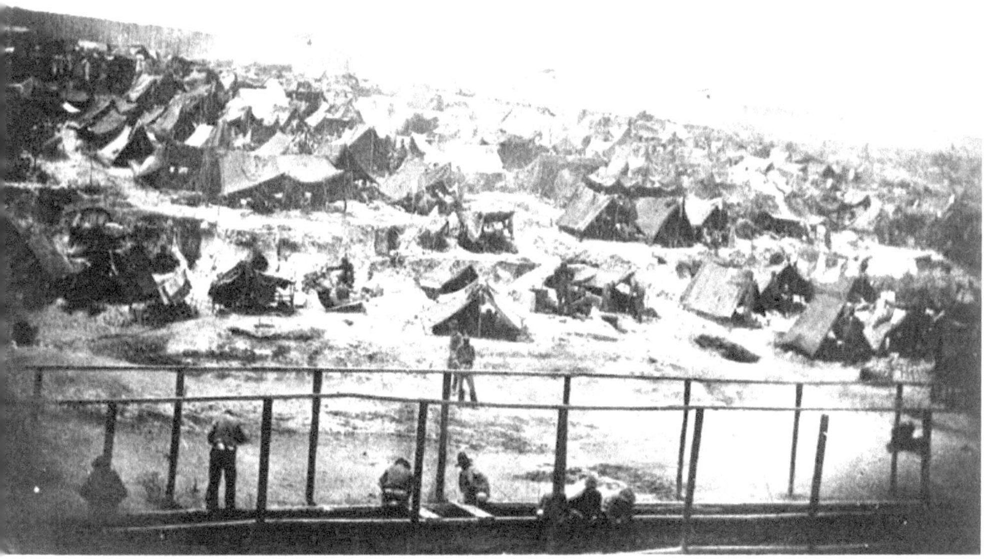

Sink at Andersonville. This is the only known photograph of a Civil War sink. It was taken on August 17, 1864, with a southward view across the prison compound. The Confederates held over 31,000 Union prisoners of war here by the late summer of 1864. This was not a typical sink, which was supposed to be at least partially shielded from public view by brush or trees, and it seems to have been supplied with a stouter sitting pole than was typical. (Library of Congress, Prints & Photographs Division, Civil War Photographs, LCDIG-ppmsca-33767)

fourteen inches high. Stakes had to be placed "at frequent intervals" under the rail for added strength. Medical inspectors did not need to remind the men what would happen if the rail broke while they were sitting on it.[13]

The medical inspector of the Army of Kentucky expounded on the basic problem of sink design. A wider trench helped promote decomposition of excrement by exposing more of it to light and air flow, but the wider the trench, the more foul odor came out of it. Those odors led to health problems such as camp diarrhea and typhus, or so people and many health professionals of the era believed, as part of the general miasma theory of disease inception. That was why they emphasized regularly applying disinfectants. "The health of the men is more concerned in the management of the sinks than in any other one particular incident to camp life," concluded the Army of Kentucky medical director.[14]

To some degree, all other Union commands issued orders for the management of human waste in camps, and they largely resembled the details endorsed by the Army of Kentucky. In the Army of the Potomac, the sinks were to be dug eight feet deep, with six inches of fresh soil added over the contents every day. Old holes were to be replaced with new sinks when the excrement reached within three feet of the surface. In the Department of the South, several sinks on different sides of a camp were to be dug, so only those on the downwind side on any given day could be used. The number of sinks per regiment and the distance from camp varied, but the need for effective supervision was universal. The object—keeping campgrounds clean of urine and excrement—was imperative.[15]

SANITARY COMMISSION COMMENTS ON WASTE DISPOSAL

How well did the army do in keeping itself clean of its own human waste? At least at the beginning, and according to Frederick Law Olmsted, it utterly failed. Inspecting twenty fresh volunteer regiments in the Washington, DC, area in ten days while accompanied by Dr. Elisha Hunt, Olmsted found that most of the sinks did not even have a sitting rail. "The edges are filthy," and awful stenches arose because no fresh dirt was leveled on the contents. The holes often were placed too close to the tents, and no effort was made to compel the troops to use them. Some men were "made sick to vomiting" by it, Olmsted contended. Samuel Gridley Howe found little better when he inspected Massachusetts volunteers assembled in camps near Boston. The worst problem was the lack of supervision provided by officers, which led to filthy conditions. Howe found only one sink that had some screening, but even it "was in a most neglected and filthy condition." He recognized that the distance from camp was very important. Too far, and the men would be disinclined to use the sinks, especially at night; but too near, and they would pose an offense to the noses and a threat to the health of the troops.[16]

It is not surprising that waste disposal should suffer among these first volunteer regiments, but for some the situation did improve with time. A. N. Read found a strange mix among the volunteer regiments at Camp Nevin in Kentucky when he visited in November 1861. At the Sixth Indiana's grounds everything was rosy, with sinks on the leeward side of the camp, deep in a patch of woods, and a nice walkway cut through the trees connecting them with the living quarters. But at the camp of another regiment, the identity of which was omitted in the published commission report that incorporated Read's finding, the situation was the opposite. A sink was located near the head of a small stream that collected surface drainage and was the only source of water for the camp. In addition, some men had a habit of not using the sink but depositing their excrement on the ground within the watershed of this stream. Perhaps they wanted privacy by being away from others using the sink and did not realize they were in the watershed. But this was such a bad set up that even the enlisted men complained until the regimental commander ordered the sinks relocated.[17]

Godfrey Aigner inspected twenty-three infantry regiments, one regiment and fifteen companies of cavalry, and ten batteries of artillery at Cairo, about 19,000 men, by November 1861. He concluded that the greatest problem was making all the troops use the sinks rather than easing themselves wherever they pleased. In only three or four regiments did the officers take this problem seriously and instruct camp guards to arrest anyone caught creating a "nuisance" inside or outside the camp. But Aigner only had to survey the grounds of the other regimental camps to see the "gross neglect of camp police," which gave "many a regiment, otherwise well reputed, a bad odor." He noted another persistent problem with camp sanitation—lax concern about disposing of animal waste. Every infantry regiment had a certain number of horses for the officers and more than that number of mules for drawing wagons. And, of course, cavalry and artillery regiments had even more horses and mules. Aigner found that most regiments kept these animals too near the men's tents and failed to properly dispose of the manure. "The daily removal of their dung is a myth dreamed of only by the authors of the army regulations and the Sanitary Commission Inspectors," he wrote with delightful sarcasm.[18]

There can be no doubt that, given time, some regiments learned how to properly handle human and animal waste. Maj. Gen. David S. Stanley recalled in his memoirs that the toughening campaign against Island No. 10 and the advance on Corinth, Mississippi, in the spring of 1862 "were opportunities to school our officers in the care of men. I did my best to learn." He specifically meant the need to construct good sinks and to see that the troops obtained their water before animals muddied up nearby streams for their own purposes.[19]

FIFTEENTH CORPS MEDICAL INSPECTION REPORTS

It is equally clear that progress in waste disposal was far from universal throughout the Union army. Fifteenth Corps medical inspectors found generally mixed results from efforts by regimental officers to dispose of human waste. When the corps was ensconced on the Louisiana bottomlands during the early months of 1863, the situation was at its worst. Of sixteen regiments inspected during the week ending April 12, eight of them were listed as having bad waste-disposal routines, and only four were rated as good, with the other four rated as fair. This situation improved dramatically by September 1863, when the corps camped along the Big Black River. Sixteen regiments achieved a good rating, only two received a fair grade, and only one was reported as bad. The poor ones suffered because sinks were dug too near the tents and not policed properly, a common fault of many regiments across the Union army. But it is interesting that this common problem never went away completely. Even in June 1865, some Fifteenth Corps regiments continued to neglect the more basic policing procedures. While the First Brigade of the Second Division did this job well, the division's other two brigades failed, "and as a consequence the men use the ground round about the camp." Even after four years of war, some small-unit officers still did not take waste disposal seriously.[20]

SANITARY COMMISSION CAMP INSPECTION RETURNS

The Sanitary Commission inspectors provided a wider view of this topic when they addressed the sixteen questions covering the disposal of human and animal waste in camps included on their forms. The commission wanted to know if the men urinated in camp and whether that occurred during the day or night, how far the sinks were located from sleeping areas, and whether the hole was properly dug and provided with a sitting rail and screens. Did the men apply fresh dirt and disinfectants regularly? Did the regiment have standing orders to use the facilities, and were those orders obeyed and enforced? Did officers have separate facilities or share those of the men? Finally, were horses and mules stabled at an appropriate distance from the camp, and was dung removed daily? These questions covered the subject area very well.

One can easily find pointed criticism of any given regiment's waste-disposal process in these camp inspection returns. "Men & officers ease themselves in the night behind woods & bushes," Robert Jones wrote of the Fortieth New York in September 1861. Robert Ware found that human excrement "occupys [*sic*] whole surface of the wood in rear of camp" when he visited the Seventy-Second Pennsylvania three months later. For the most part, when inspectors found widespread use of trees and bushes, it was because the regimental commanders had failed to have any sinks dug at all. In fact, a surprising percentage of returns indicated this problem. A total of 23, or 8.2 percent of the 280 returns used in this study, reported that regimental officers had not ordered any facilities to be created. At times the officers made excuses: they were waiting for lumber to construct nice sheds or the men were too busy with other duties (even though, as with the Fourth Maine Battery, the unit had remained in camp for a week). Others simply made no attempt to explain to the inspector why their troops were allowed to "look out for themselves as they please," as with Battery A, First New York Light Artillery. One can assume that many soldiers preferred to relieve themselves on their own hook rather than use a communal space. The brush, if any, only screened them from people around the camp, not from other men who were using the sink. In addition, there were cases where the unit had sinks, but the men continued to go where they pleased. In some instances it was because the sinks were poorly maintained and became very offensive. For example, in the Twenty-Fourth Missouri, the latrine had no sitting rail or screen and no fresh dirt or disinfectant, thus the men preferred to "go beyond sinks in the woods."[21]

Camp inspectors were supposed to personally observe conditions, but when it came to disposing of human waste, they all too easily saw and smelled the problems. While visiting the Fortieth New York, Robert Jones was forcibly struck by the pervading stench of excrement across the camp. He was convinced it caused the widespread diarrhea that affected the regiment at the time: "I myself was immediately disturbed in stomach and bowels by the disgusting odor." When visiting the Fifth Wisconsin, Robert Collyer happened to see two men "voiding" close to the tents "on the bare ground." Read had no difficulty seeing that the Eighteenth Ohio camp was in bad shape, with "the sinks unendurable the ground covered with the excrement of the men And all the waste running into a small surface stream from which the men obtained their water." Apparently, this was the regiment (mentioned earlier) that the commission officials decided not to name when they published portions of Read's damning report about the drainage of excrement-loaded ground into the water supply.[22]

These instances represented the worst results of camp inspections regarding the disposal of human waste. The inspectors found many other instances where attempts to ameliorate conditions had succeeded to a limited extent. Attention to urination really was largely separate from sinks because the men strongly tended to relieve themselves of this waste product wherever it was convenient rather than walking to the latrines. That is why the commission wanted to know if they urinated within camp limits, especially at night when it was inconvenient to walk to the sinks. The results on this issue were middling. Of 119 returns that specifically addressed it, 64 (53.7 percent) indicated that the men urinated in camp either at night or both day and night. Another 25 indicated that they did so sometimes, and on 30 other returns the inspectors noted that the men *probably* urinated in camp. On 77 of the 119 returns, regimental officers insisted that no urination in camp took place, or they at least stated that it was "not allowed" or that "no evidence" of it had surfaced. One can readily believe that urination in camp took place in far more than 53.7 percent of the visited units, with many regimental commanders and surgeons unwilling to admit it or unaware of it happening.[23]

Moreover, inspectors made their own comments on this issue. Their remarks tended to indicate that they did not always trust the testimony of unit officials as to whether the men relieved themselves of waste water in camp. "All soldiers do in all regiments," Henry Oliver cynically commented about Battery B, First New York Light Artillery. Based on his experience, George L. Andrews was sure that in cavalry and artillery units, the men tended to urinate "among the horses" so as not to be caught relieving themselves in camp. Other inspectors noted that the soldiers of some regiments had at least limited scruples. When provided with empty barrels, those of the Eleventh New York Battery and Twelfth New York Battery were pleased to use them within the limits of camp. The members of two battalions belonging to the First Wisconsin Artillery, which manned the Water Battery at Fortress Monroe, refrained from urinating in their camps but did not hesitate to relieve themselves in many parts of the fort itself.[24]

Another aspect of this topic with middling levels of success was in placing the sinks. Army regulations mandated that those of the men should be 150 paces and those of the officers 100 paces from the tents. Inspectors found a wide variance in this regard. Enlisted men's facilities were anywhere from ten yards to 1,000 feet from their living quarters. In most cases the officers did use separate facilities that were set apart from those of the men. But in 44 (17.1 percent) of the 257 returns that specifically mentioned this subject, the officers shared the same sinks as their troops; of course, for those regiments that had no sinks at all, the officers were automatically placed on the same level as their troops. Army regulations did not specify how many sinks were required per unit, so the number varied a good deal in actual practice. In some regiments each company had a separate sink, while in others there were only three sinks for the entire regiment, placed on three different sides of the camp.[25]

Making sure the sinks were properly provided with necessary adjuncts and were regularly policed tended to be a big problem. It obviously was important to have a good structure to sit on while relieving oneself over a hole. In 127 of the 139 returns that specifically mentioned this issue, there actually was a suitable railing; it is difficult to understand why a dozen regiments did not have any rails at all. Screens for privacy were provided in a majority of cases—117 of the 151 returns that specifically mentioned them, or 77.5 percent. But in nearly a quarter of these regiments, no attempt was made to provide privacy for the men. Screens usually consisted of bushes that happened to be growing between the sinks and the camp, but in some cases shrubs and tree limbs were cut and placed for this purpose. The Fifth Wisconsin provided good screens for newly dug latrines in one camp, but then six weeks later the regiment moved a short distance to the other side of the sinks. The men did not bother to move the screens, however, exposing their easing place to the full view of the new campsite.[26]

Regiments did very poorly in applying a layer of dirt on the excrement in these sinks and utterly failed to apply disinfectants. Of a total 174 returns that specifically mention this issue, only 11 (6.3 percent) indicated that fresh dirt was placed daily, 74 (42.5 percent) indicated it was placed occasionally, and 89 (52.2 percent) indicated no attention paid at all to this preventive measure. It was the most important thing that could be done to reduce the odor and shield the sink users from the noxious effects of an open sewer, yet officers and men far too often saw it as a choice rather than a necessary sanitary measure. No wonder they paid even less attention to applying disinfectants. Of 153 returns that specifically mentioned this topic, 137 (89.5 percent) indicated that the men did not bother to apply anything. Only 16 returns, 10.5 percent, indicated they applied something, usually on an occasional basis.

Officers were supposed to make sure that basic waste-disposal policies set by the army were followed. The majority of returns, 119 (76.6 percent) of the 155 that specifically mention this issue, indicate that the regiments had regulations in place concerning the proper way to dispose of human waste. That was all well and good, but it also means that almost one-fourth of regimental commanders did not think it necessary to establish regulations in their commands. Moreover, when one breaks down the evidence among these 119 returns, in 71 (60 percent) of them the unit commander claimed that the men fully obeyed the regulations, 26 (22 percent) asserted that they generally obeyed, and 21 (18 percent) could only say that the men *apparently* obeyed. That is not a sterling record of compliance by the troops or enforcement by the officers, especially when one had a right to question whether the 60 percent were telling the truth about full compliance.

Among those returns that exhibited frankness on the part of officers, one can see details of this problem. When local inspection of sinks took place, it usually was done by the officer of the day or by the surgeon. In cases where officers shared the same facilities as the men, they could take a quick personal survey of conditions when they were using the sinks. In one case the brigade commander "ordered all the men of his brigade to go to the sinks regularly each morning," but no word on compliance or enforcement was mentioned. In another, lone case the Nineteenth Indiana employed a "special police" squad to enforce regimental rules to use only the sinks and not spread "nuisances" around the campgrounds.[27]

Of course, the inspectors often found regiments with adequate disposal procedures and a handful equipped with more than what the army and the sanitarians required. A few units were in positions to link flowing water with waste disposal. If they were camped close to the seashore, tidal action came into play. On Ship Island, a lonely place off the coast of Mississippi, the Ninth Connecticut and Twenty-Sixth Massachusetts established privies on the north beach so that high tide could wash everything away from those structures on a regular basis. The Fifteenth New York Engineers and Fiftieth New York Engineers constructed a similar arrangement while camped on the bank of the Potomac River near Washington, DC, where they could take advantage of some tidal action. The latter regiment's arrangement also included damming a stream flowing into the river so attendants could release a flow of water through the latrine and supplement the tidal action. It was possible for a regiment camped inland near a good stream to do the same, but that happened only rarely.[28]

A few other regiments also enjoyed special arrangements for human-waste disposal. These included "a movable house" for the First Connecticut Battery and the use of civilian privies by the Eighth Illinois Cavalry when it was quartered in the buildings of Alexandria, Virginia. But for the overwhelming majority of Union regiments, the only recourse was a trench, a sitting rail, a screen, and making sure the men used them. Inspectors were delighted to report good conditions when and where they found them. "Each company has its own sink," wrote William F. Swalm about the Twenty-Sixth Wisconsin, "and all are policed every morning."[29]

While the disposal of human waste in regimental camps was uneven, the disposal of animal waste was little better. The inspection returns included questions about this issue, and inspectors recorded varied answers. The Third Pennsylvania Cavalry had 1,033 men and 1,050 horses present for duty when Andrews visited its camp. Details removed the dung daily, while in other regiments it was removed weekly. In contrast, the Third New York Cavalry devoted little care to dung removal, and the Twelfth Missouri Infantry, along with other regiments, did not bother to dispose of manure at all. Officers in the Second Ohio Battery claimed the unit was "not long enough in one place to make it necessary."[30]

The overall conclusion, based on the results of the Sanitary Commission camp inspection returns, is that too little attention was paid to waste disposal in the Union army. Among the 280 returns, only 36.7 percent rated good in this subject area, 30.0 percent rated fair, and 33.3 percent rated bad. It is not easy to understand why volunteer officers and enlisted men took the need to separate themselves from excrement and urine so lightly. Admittedly, digging a hole in the ground and erecting a wooden railing constituted very basic toilet facilities, but primitive as they were, this arrangement could have been made workable if proper care and attention had been devoted to it.

It should have been relatively easy for all Union regiments to have instituted effective systems of waste disposal in their semipermanent camps, but that seemingly attainable goal was not properly met. A handful of them, according to the camp inspection returns, did so in fine style. But the majority of Union regiments attained only a middling level of camp sanitation in terms of not only human- but also animal-waste disposal. Far too many of them paid so little attention to the problem as to serve as examples of how not to keep their camps clean. Part of the trouble was that young men eager to participate in combat placed low priority on seemingly mundane issues associated with army life. One can understand that attitude. But the seeming indifference of so many of their officers is not so easy to understand. Most of them also tended to be young and were citizen-soldiers like the rank and file, but when they accepted their commissions, they also accepted the responsibility of conforming to army regulations, and in far too many instances they failed to do so. Civil War soldiers did not need to live so intimately with urine, excrement, and dung as they too often ended up doing.

6

Food and Cooking

If it is true that an army marches on its stomach, then the quality and quantity of military rations and how the men prepared them assumes a vital importance not only in effectiveness but also in soldier health. In their own ways both the officers of the US Army and the Civil War sanitarians were well aware of that importance, but they did not necessarily agree on the details of how to keep soldiers healthy through diet. In fact, there were many and varied opinions on the question of how food affected health in Civil War America, and most of those opinions found some degree of expression when it came to military food. Likewise, civilian cooking habits and the difficulties of setting up cooking facilities both in army camps and in the field influenced military cuisine. Selecting food, cooking it, and eating it, something civilians tended to take for granted, was never easy in the army.

FOOD

Soldiers did not have the freedom of choosing their diet items. The army ration was heavily institutionalized, starting with action by Congress. The military affairs committee of both houses had primary responsibility for studying what should be included in the army ration and then proposing their recommendations to the House and Senate separately so those bodies could compromise on a joint bill. This oversight, based largely on the fact that Congress was responsible for paying for the feeding of the army, extended down to the smallest detail. The ration listed exactly which food items were allowed and the amount to be issued per man. Congress increased the ration in quantity and added more items on August 3, 1861, building in some flexibility as far as choosing from several options. In other words, commissaries could favor one or two items over others in some categories depending on soldier taste. These guidelines gave maximum flexibility to the fresh beef that most soldiers seemed to favor, stipulating that it could be issued "as often as the commanding officer . . . shall require it, when practicable." The daily issue per man amounted to one and a quarter pounds of fresh beef. This new ration also allowed for the issue of tea as a substitute for coffee. Congress provided a relatively balanced diet theoretically, but the options given commissaries, who tended to be influenced by the men's preferences, could work against the concept that eating enough fresh vegetables and legumes was important.[1]

Many observers boasted that the Union army ration of August 3, 1861, was the most generous military diet in the world when it came to variety and quantity, and they seem to have been right. European armies tended to downplay meat and emphasize vegetables and soups more than did the Americans. The French army in the Crimean War heavily invested in processed foods, mostly desiccated vegetables. This involved drying a number of vegetables, then compressing them into cakes for easy transportation. Soldiers in the field learned the best way to soak and cook them. It was a success, and members of the Delafield Commission were much interested in this new way of feeding soldiers. Most European forces tended to require some degree of self-supply in their military forces. That means in camp and garrison, only selected items of the ration, such as bread, was issued, leaving the men to individually or through a company arrangement purchase whatever else on the ration list they wanted. In the Russian army that arrangement was called the "artel," a company-level fund to buy fresh vegetables and other items. A similar institution, the "company fund," existed in the prewar US Army and in the Union volunteer force during the conflict.[2]

The British Army came closer to the American establishment than did Continental forces. Britain also had a company-fund organization for when the troops were settled in semipermanent camps, but its commissaries issued all ration items to the troops when they were on campaign. When it came to food preferences, British soldiers agreed with Americans that fresh beef was the most important item on the list. Officials recognized by the late 1850s the importance of consuming some vegetables as well, both fresh and desiccated. Bread was a given; it seems to have been accepted as a necessary part of the ration of all armies in one way or another. The only question was whether it was offered hard in the form of a cracker or freshly baked. The latter was generally preferred but available only when the troops were in semipermanent camps. Hard bread's advantage was that it could be stored indefinitely and was easily transported.[3]

Civil War sanitarians never subscribed fully to the diet reforms that swept through the Northern states in the decades prior to the firing on Fort Sumter. They did not endorse vegetarianism or the Grahamite effort to switch to whole-grain foods. But they generally supported a balanced, varied, and sensible diet accompanied by moderation in quantity. Surgeon General Hammond recognized the trends in American dietary habits. "No people eat more than the inhabitants of the United States," he admitted. "A healthy adult American" needed forty ounces of food daily, two-thirds of it vegetable matter and one-third animal food, plus twenty fluid ounces of good water and eight to ten ounces of tea or coffee. Hammond found the British Army ration, which tended to be more generous than Continental issues, to be inferior to the US Army allowance. For example, the British soldier was allowed only twelve ounces of meat on home station and sixteen ounces on foreign station compared to the twenty ounces issued to American soldiers wherever they were located.[4]

The company fund could play an important role in giving the soldier more options for his diet. It operated through a combination of excess quantities of certain rations that were regularly issued and the ability of men and officers to use that surplus to their advantage. If, for example, a company received more flour for making bread than it needed or wanted, it could return the excess back to the commissary for credit in their company fund. The unit could then use that money to purchase more fresh vegetables than the commissary would issue. Credit also was added to the company fund if a unit failed to receive a part of its allotted ration due to active campaigning or hitches in the military supply system. But the company fund, which seemed to work well in Russia, never really flourished in the Union volunteer army. The main reasons were, as Godfrey Aigner put it, the "stupidity or laziness of captains & the wasteful habits of the men." While a few regiments took advantage of this option and regularly operated company funds, the majority did not.[5]

UNION SOLDIERS COMMENT ON THEIR FOOD

Based on a survey of personal accounts, it is clear that many Union soldiers were quite satisfied with the army ration both in terms of quality and quantity. Of course, they tended to fare better when in stationary camps near a good line of logistics than when actively moving through the countryside. How well balanced their daily diet tended to be depended on many factors even when not on the move, but there usually was some degree of variety to balance the regular issue of fresh beef. That could include anything from several different types of vegetables to just a regular issue of Irish potatoes. "There is no danger of our starving," reported Sylvester Bartow of the Twelfth Wisconsin Battery to his wife. In the best case scenario, regiments received what the Army of the Potomac was issued early in 1864 before the onset of the Overland Campaign. That consisted of an issue of fresh beef every three days, fresh bread every three and a half days, potatoes every four and a half days, and other varied vegetables every two and a half days. Soldiers cherished their issue of soft, fresh bread. It was baked in large government bakeries in large cities and shipped fresh to nearby regiments. In many cases, regimental officers purchased or built their own ovens for baking. When fresh bread was not available, soldiers learned to deal with the ubiquitous hardtack cracker.[6]

Attitudes toward meat eating permeated Civil War America and army food as well. In this regard, the United States was allied with European food habits, especially those of Great Britain, for meat eating had been democratized on the Continent by the middle of the nineteenth century. Before that time it had been largely a feature of upper-class life, but rising standards of living for working-class Europeans meant that a much wider cross-section of society could afford meat as well as fresh vegetables, sugar, and dairy products. While there was a feasible balance of food preferences on the Continent, residents of the British isles tended to overemphasize meat, as did those of the United States. Meat became "the grand symbol of their rising standard of living," as historian Vincent J. Knapp has written of most workers and peasants.[7]

"The fresh-meat ration was thoroughly appreciated by the men," recalled John D. Billings of the Tenth Massachusetts Battery. The army allowed each man twenty ounces of fresh beef every day, in contrast to only twelve ounces of pork or bacon, and encouraged commissaries to issue it as often as requested. Commanders and commissaries took that encouragement seriously and tended to feed the men's craving for this ration item. They maintained herds of beef cattle that accompanied the armies, and a few were slaughtered whenever needed. For hours after an issue, the atmosphere around army camps was permeated with the odor of frying, broiling, or boiling beef that whetted the appetites of most men. Salt beef was issued periodically, but the men overwhelming rejected it in favor of the fresh article.[8]

In practice, army commissaries overemphasized meat and underemphasized all other items on the ration list. No other foods were as seriously undervalued as fresh vegetables and fruit. A general order issued by the Adjutant General's Office in July 1864, after three years of army eating, allowed that "when deemed necessary, fresh vegetables, dried fruit, molasses, pickles, or any other proper food may be purchased and issued in lieu of any component part of the ration." This was, at best, a grudging admission that such produce served a useful purpose in maintaining soldier health; it was far from an endorsement for a regular issue. Ironically, hundreds of army surgeons had long before then reported how readily scorbutic tendencies disappeared from regiments that increased the issue of fresh vegetables and fruits. Moreover, a large proportion of Union volunteers found the limited supply of vegetables, fruits, and legumes detrimental to their health. Many of them reported in their letters, diaries, and memoirs how seriously their energy levels, digestive systems, and resistance to stress and disease were impaired by a diet overly heavy in meat products.[9]

The army tried to emulate the French Crimean experience by issuing large amounts of desiccated vegetables produced by firms in the United States. These consisted of a wide and healthy variety of vegetables chopped into a mix, dried, and then compressed into cakes. Most Civil War soldiers had had no exposure to or even knowledge of this product and usually were puzzled or appalled when told to eat it. In fact, it has become one of the iconic aspects of Civil War history that all soldiers hated the thought of desiccated vegetables and made fun of this new product of industrial America. Civil War sanitarians strongly supported the concept and noted that soldier antipathy largely stemmed from the fact that they were not taught how to properly cook it. "When thoroughly soaked, sufficiently boiled, and properly seasoned, they are generally relished," reported Franklin B. Hough of these desiccated vegetables.[10]

Coffee was the most thoroughly enjoyed item on the army ration list, even more so than fresh beef. It was the beverage of choice for the majority of soldiers, and many of them appreciated the fact that their government provided beans of the finest quality. They did complain about condensed milk, which was universally condemned. Some men cautioned against overindulgence, arguing that a pint of coffee in the morning and another in the evening was "as much as it is healthy to drink each day." That is one reason why Congress inserted tea as an approved substitute for coffee on a voluntary basis. Although more expensive and less widely consumed in the American civilian public of the day, tea did not contain the same natural oils as coffee. Most Americans and the soldiers they sent to the army were committed coffee drinkers. "I verily believed that but for coffee, the rebellion would never have been crushed out," wrote William B. Lapham of the Seventh Maine Battery.[11]

Civil War soldiers were well aware that the quantity and quality of their food depended on whether they were on the move or held in stationary camps for an extended period of time. Army logistics varied widely in the two instances. When in semipermanent camps, it was possible to obtain the full array of food items unless the sites happened to be located too far from convenient railroad lines or river channels. But on the move or before proper lines of communications could be established, this proved impossible. As a result the army had developed the marching ration to be issued during active campaigns. This involved a severely reduced allotment that was largely carried by the soldier himself and by the limited wagon transportation allowed field armies. According to John Billings, the marching ration consisted only of a pound of hardtack, three-quarters of a pound of salt pork or the usual issue of fresh beef, and some of the so-called short rations (sugar, coffee, and salt). Under difficult conditions, the fresh beef tended to be the first to be eliminated since slow-moving cattle herds could not keep up with the army. The marching ration contained nothing in the way of vegetables or legumes. Living for an extended period of time on it was injurious to health, and there were many campaigns in the Civil War that forced men to rely on it for months at a time.[12]

FIFTEENTH CORPS MEDICAL INSPECTION REPORTS

The Fifteenth Corps medical inspection reports reveal how well the troops fared when they were temporarily in one place during an active campaign. In April 1863, while camping in the Louisiana bottomlands with direct access to river steamers, the men lived largely on bread and fresh beef, both of which they received in good supply. First Division regiments were widely supplied with portable camp ovens and baked their own bread. It was not of particularly good quality but was hot and fresh. Those regiments often supplemented the bread with hardtack, which they both ate in camp and took along when sent away to some field assignment. Vegetables, however, were in very short supply. The commissary sometimes issued them, and the Sanitary Commission contributed a limited quantity. Some soldiers managed to find and purchase vegetables locally with private funds as well.[13]

The food situation remained the same in some ways but changed in others when the Fifteenth Corps camped at the Big Black River in September 1863. Here, it did not have direct access to river or rail transport, relying on wagons from Vicksburg, ten miles to the west. Once again the emphasis was on soft bread and fresh beef, with vegetables in extremely short supply. Many regiments had no vegetables at all, while in others the men purchased a few with their own funds. Whereas the commissary had issued some vegetables here and there the previous April, in far too many regiments he issued none at all during September. In other regiments "a few vegetables are provided at long intervals." The Eighth Wisconsin fairly represented most other units of the corps in this way. "Soft bread daily and fresh beef 2 to 3 days in the week. No vegetables excepting a few purchased."[14]

Both in April and September 1863, the Fifteenth Corps was camped in the field at a distance from major supply depots. Although in direct touch with river steamers on the bottomlands, those boats were strained to supply everything Grant's army needed. At the Big Black River, the men did not even have direct access to any modern means of transportation. But in June 1865 they were stationed at Louisville, one of the huge supply nodes of the western theater of operations. Here, the problem was an inundation of local women and boys bringing pies and cakes to sell to the soldiers. The quality of these desserts was not high, but after Fifteenth Corps men were paid, they spent lavishly on them. Sutlers also offered sour beer for sale to the men. John M. Woodworth, the medical inspector of the Army of the Tennessee, was convinced that there was less illness among Seventeenth Corps troops than in the Fifteenth Corps only because the former had not yet been paid off and could not spend so much money on these pies and cakes.[15]

The Fifteenth Corps record in food quality was nothing to brag about. The overemphasis on fresh beef and the severe lack of fresh vegetables would have appalled Civil War sanitarians. It did not seem to negatively impress the corps medical inspectors, however, who simply reported it as a matter of fact without much effort to rectify the situation. Inspectors failed to investigate why commissaries were issuing so few vegetables. Neither the private purchase of vegetables by the men or the efforts by the Sanitary Commission could make up for this drastic differential between the two basic food groups available to Civil War units. No matter whether the regiments were stuck in the bottomland mud, enjoying the camps along the Big Black River, or swallowing poorly made desserts offered by civilian vendors at Louisville, they mostly ate bread and fresh beef while suffering for vegetables.

SANITARY COMMISSION CAMP INSPECTION RETURNS

As with every other subject area, the Sanitary Commission camp inspection returns offer a wider survey across the Union army than do the Fifteenth Corps medical inspection reports when it comes to food quality. The best standard form contained fourteen questions relating to the topic. These questions covered many aspects, including whether company officers supervised the quality of rations and whether they were required to taste the food the men ate, or if they simply left those responsibilities to noncommissioned officers. The quantity and quality of rations; how often fresh meat and fresh vegetables were issued; how often desiccated vegetables, dried meat, soups, and dried fruit were issued; and whether tea was sometimes drawn rather than coffee were all included. The commission wanted to know if soft bread was served and whether it was of good quality. It also wished to know if company funds were being set up and utilized to supplement army issues of various food items.

Overwhelmingly, the majority of units inspected by commission agents reported the quantity of army rations as adequate to plentiful. There was no effort by officers to teach the men moderation in their eating habits. Capt. John D. Frank of Battery G, First New York Light Artillery thought "they need all their rations & encourages them to eat them all," as reported by Henry Oliver. All indications show that most men had no difficulty wolfing down everything issued to them. In only a dozen of the 280 returns used in this study did the inspector indicate any soldier dissatisfaction with the quantity or quality of military food.[16]

When it came to fresh meat, the returns indicate that this was the prime food item on the ration list. It was not issued, or only rarely issued, in 13.5 percent of the 280 units, while in the rest it was provided in varied frequencies. The most common was an issue twice a week, as it was for 35.4 percent of the 242 units that received fresh beef. The second-most-common frequency was three times a week, the standard for 26.1 percent of the units. Other frequencies included once, four times, and five times a week. For 8.9 percent of the 242 units, fresh beef arrived every day, a truly beneficent situation as far as most Civil War soldiers were concerned. In many regiments the commissaries issued fresh beef "as often as men want it," fulfilling congressional instructions to the letter.[17]

Issues of fresh vegetables fell far below that for fresh beef. Of the 241 returns that mentioned this topic, 117 (48.5 percent) indicated that no fresh vegetables were issued or that they were issued rarely. That means that only slightly more than half—51.5 percent—of the units received fresh vegetables regularly or occasionally while in their semipermanent camps, most of which were located within reasonable distance of major supply lines.

The camp inspection returns reinforce what many personal accounts of Civil War soldiers indicate, that a large proportion of Union soldiers wanted more vegetables than they received. Instead, they were compelled to find other ways to obtain them. A common practice was to purchase them from local civilians with their own funds or to trade parts of their army ration for them. M. P. Buel found when visiting the First Nebraska that the men bartered their coffee for cabbage, Irish potatoes, and sweet potatoes. Supply arrangements were particularly difficult for those regiments stationed in the Department of the Gulf. Members of the Twelfth Connecticut traded their beef ration for fresh vegetables because the poor civilians who lived near Camp Parapet north of New Orleans had "no meat." In a few cases friends on the home front or even the governor of the home state provided some vegetables for the troops. Members of the First Louisiana Native Guards (US) near Thibodaux had no fresh vegetables and instead munched on sugar cane, which no doubt tasted sweet but was no substitute nutritionally for a full array of vegetables. To some degree, a plant-based diet was a matter of culture. William M. Chamberlain noted that the Thirty-Ninth New York, filled with men of European birth, placed far more emphasis on fresh vegetables than American regiments.[18]

The short rations of fresh vegetables led to widespread disgruntlement among a large proportion of Union soldiers. "*Complain generally of want of vegetables,*" Bernard J. Bettelheim emphasized in his return covering the Ninth Kentucky near Murfreesboro in March 1863. There was a seasonal aspect to this problem in that fresh vegetables tended to be most scarce during the winter and early spring months. That was why Edward A. Crane saw signs of scorbutic tendencies for the first time in January 1862 while visiting the Seventh Maine in the Washington, DC, area. In fact, "fresh vegetables have nearly disappeared from among the articles of food" in its entire division. But many inspectors blamed the commissaries rather than the seasons for the lack of fresh vegetables. Frederick Law Olmsted thought that not only vegetables but also dried fruit should be on the required part of the army ration rather than left to the choice of commissaries.[19]

Providing desiccated vegetables went a long way toward ameliorating this deficiency, and in that way the army did surprisingly well. Of 170 returns that specifically mention this item, 51.2 percent confirmed that it was issued regularly, while 48.8 percent indicated no issue of it at all. Three other dried foods were available to the Union army, but authorities did not do well at all in giving them to the troops. Of 131 returns mentioning dried meat, only 4.5 percent received it and 95.5 percent did not. Of 100 mentioning dried soup, only 5.0 percent tried it and the rest had no experience with the product. Of 145 mentioning dried fruit, only 17.2 percent consumed it and the rest had none at all. There is no explanation for why dried vegetables assumed such a relatively high profile in army issues in contrast to other dried food items. All of them held tremendous advantages in terms of long-term storage and ease of transportation that fresh vegetables lacked. Dried vegetables and fruits were especially good to combat the onset of scorbutic symptoms. Of course, soldier resistance to desiccated food of all kinds was a significant factor. Commissaries tended to be closely attuned to providing the men what they wanted and avoided issuing the foods that they disliked—and more likely to go to waste—as much as possible.

Soldier dislike of desiccated vegetables has always had a high profile in our awareness of Civil War army food. Those men who found it disgusting were quite vocal and wrote about it in such humorous ways that historians could not resist emphasizing their viewpoint. But the Sanitary Commission camp inspection returns do not support the idea that dried vegetables were universally rejected. Of 280 returns, only 28 indicated active dislike by the men. Camp inspectors did what they could to educate officers and troops about how to properly prepare dried mixed vegetables, for that was the true problem. Soldiers tended to not soak them before cooking and then to boil them in too little water and for too short a time. Proper preparation produced a tasty meal that was rich in important nutrients. And dried vegetables solved many of the procurement and transportation problems inherent in providing fresh produce.[20]

Tea was introduced into the army ration as a substitute in August 1861 and was issued quite often. Of the 183 returns that specifically mention the subject, 56.8 percent indicated that the men received at least some quantities at regular or irregular intervals. In 43.2 percent of the returns, no tea was issued at all. Personal preferences played the largest role here. Men who had grown used to drinking tea before the war tended to want it in the army as well. Ethnic preferences also came into play. George L. Andrews thought that the Germans in Lt. Col. Andrew Brickel's First New York Artillery Battalion strongly preferred coffee over tea, and Franklin B. Hough reported that even among the American-born members of the Nineteenth Indiana, a cup of coffee two to three times daily was the norm. Yet tea made some inroads into soldier food ways, "gaining ground in most regiments, by the efforts of surgeons," as Aigner reported of the many infantry, cavalry, and artillery units he inspected near Cairo during the fall of 1861.[21]

Soft and fresh bread was readily provided the men while in their semi-permanent camps. Of the 280 returns, a total of 161, or 57.5 percent, indicated some degree of issue. For the most part, soldiers preferred fresh bread over hardtack, but some would rather receive flour in lieu of baked bread. That way they could carry it for some time and make it into flapjacks over a campfire as an alternative to hard bread.[22]

Eating habits also became a factor in army food. The young men who flocked to the colors seemed to have unusually healthy appetites in the view of many observers. "The surgeon says all the men eat too much," Robert Collyer wrote about Alfred L. Castleman, then the surgeon of the Fifth Wisconsin. One consequence of overeating was waste of food. More than one camp inspector found uneaten bits of rations littering the inside of tents, the areas outside them, company streets, and the drains as well. Men of the Fourth New York Battery complained that they did not get enough to eat, and yet Henry Oliver found wasted food all over the unit's camp.[23]

Sutlers fed this inordinate appetite in order to make a profit off the volunteer army. Civilians given permission to accompany regiments, usually bringing a supply of food items to supplement the army ration, they easily became a problem as far as sanitarians were concerned. "Many times the men throw away their rations and feed at the sutlers," Hough commented of the Nineteenth Indiana. The food offered by these men tended to be sweets and delicacies that were not only expensive but also unhealthy. Even worse were the many local peddlers who flocked to army camps. They usually brought homemade cakes and pies for sale that varied widely in quality.[24]

A better way for soldiers to supplement their rations was through the system of company funds, which the army had established long before the war and now applied to the volunteer force as well. This organized system required the leadership of company commanders and the cooperation of the rank and file; officers had to administer it and the men had to eat in moderation to save rations and receive credit from the commissary with which to obtain items of choice. The problem was, however, that very many company officers did not know about the company fund, were uninterested in it, or found it too time consuming to take on. According to the camp inspection returns, there was a noticeable trend in that regiments serving in the East very often had a thriving company-fund program, while regiments serving in the West did not. Aigner cynically ascribed this to "the stupidity or laziness of captains & the wasteful habits of the men" in the units he inspected near Cairo. The officers thought of ration economy "with even greater contempt than of camp police & military hygiene." There seems to have been little improvement in this deficiency over time.[25]

Officers did not provide as much oversight of their unit's food system as they were required to do. Of 209 returns that specifically mention this topic,

23.5 percent indicated no oversight by officers of any kind. In these cases the officers allowed commissary sergeants to handle everything. Among the rest, 139 returns indicated that an officer-oversight program was mandatory in the unit, and an additional 21 returns indicated that such oversight was voluntary. This supervision mainly consisted of witnessing the receipt and distribution of ration items by noncommissioned officers and tasting the men's cooked food on a regular basis. Overall, 76.5 percent of the returns reported some degree of supervision by officers, but how effective it was is questionable. Commission inspectors usually did not have the time or opportunity to dig deeply into this issue, relying for the most part on what officers told them or on a cursory examination of stored rations. There were only a couple of exceptions among the 280 returns. In the Twenty-Eighth Illinois "almost all captains eat with their men," while in the Tenth Iowa a standing commission of one captain and two lieutenants assumed full responsibility for such oversight. The Tenth's surgeon was required to taste the food and reported that the quantity was "more than necessary."[26]

Despite the limited oversight by officers, the camp inspection returns support the idea that the quality and quantity of food issued to the Union army was widely satisfying to officers and men alike. Some complained of the monotonous character of army rations; the congressionally approved table of August 1861 was not strong on variety. For example, when E. J. Dunning visited the Twentieth New York, he found that the regiment received soft bread, hardtack, and flour every other day; fresh meat, pork, salt beef, and bacon in alternating cycles over every ten days; and rice, beans, and desiccated potatoes or mixed vegetables every ten days. There was no dried fruit and very few fresh vegetables, but tea and coffee were issued in equal amounts. This was varied enough to satisfy most men for the short term, but followed for months at a time, it could become wearing.[27]

The worst problems arose when units were positioned in areas poorly served by railroad and steamboat communications, such as the mountains of western Virginia. Edward Mead found serious concerns among the Union regiments wintering in that region during 1861–62. "Old Pork-bad Crackers Coffee bad," he noted of the Seventy-Fifth Ohio, which was camped near Huttonsville, Virginia. "Dysentery & Diarrhea caused by bad food some cases unmanageable." Even when food arrived, it sometimes was in bad shape. "Potatoes 4 Days during month some barrels of Pots frozen." The regiment only had four days' issue of desiccated vegetables during the past month as well. Commission agents strongly tended to assume that unusual levels of illness in a unit were a natural consequence of poor-quality rations.[28]

If one considers the evidence in the camp inspection returns from the standpoint of Civil War sanitarians, the results are not complimentary to the army system of feeding soldiers. Only 25 percent of the 280 returns could be counted as reflecting good results, while 32.2 percent are fair and 42.8 percent are bad. But this largely was because of the general failure of providing a balanced diet for the troops. Sanitarians were not vegetarians but they firmly believed in a balanced and varied diet, and commissaries simply could not, or chose not to, issue enough vegetables or legumes to achieve that goal. Their negligence in providing fruit of any kind was even worse. Scurvy appeared far too often in the ranks as a result. Scorbutic tendencies were best alleviated with foods rich in vitamin C such as fruits, but during the Civil War, vegetables became the main antiscorbutic food. The military food system was deficient in both these categories.

Soldiers were a captive population, dependent on a national system of provision that was authorized and executed by governmental and military layers of authority. The setup was a good case study of institutional diet. Congress and the army failed to incorporate advanced dietary reforms current in civilian society, but they largely succeeded in providing a minimally healthy diet for soldiers within an arguable definition of what that meant. Their success was severely limited, however, and provided no cause for celebration as far as Civil War sanitarians were concerned. The diet was only partially balanced, too heavy on meat, too light on vegetables, and almost devoid of fruit. Quality tended to range from fair to good, but in some cases it was quite bad. Yet considering all the challenges of feeding an army that, by 1865, mustered more than a million men spread out over half the nation, commissaries could congratulate themselves for at least managing to keep the armies moving on their stomachs.

COOKING

Providing raw food items was one step in army sustenance; the next was preparing them for consumption. In this the army did little to help the soldier other than provide minimal cooking utensils and urge officers to organize messes or to arrange for dedicated cooks to prepare meals for entire companies. After that the men were largely on their own as far as cooking was concerned. Of course, in large installations such as hospitals, rendezvous camps, and convalescent camps, the cooking usually was organized from the top down, with plenty of cooks and communal dining halls. But most soldiers spent little time in these installations in contrast to their regimental homes. In these semipermanent regimental camps that the Sanitary Commission inspectors visited, the men either did their own cooking or clubbed with a handful of comrades in a mess. A third option was to either enjoy or simply put up with whatever dedicated company-level cooks managed to offer them.

THE ARMY, THE SANITARIANS, AND THE SOLDIERS ON COOKING

Civil War sanitarians widely recognized the army's limited interest in soldier preparation of their rations. Even though cooking was "one of the most important of considerations," John Ordronaux decried the indifference of the military system to the issue. He urged the army to train a corps of cooks and distribute them across the force "in order to prevent disease, waste of food, and to extract the best possible good from it." One such trained cook assigned to every company with a helpful assistant was his preferred solution.[29]

Other concerned observers realized, however, that a corps of trained cooks was never a possibility. They instead tried to reach out to the rank and file. "Every soldier should make the art of cooking his study," wrote August V. Kautz, a cavalry division commander. "More disease and deaths are occasioned in an army by bad cooking than by any other cause." Other authors provided soldier recipes for the making of healthy meals and described how to improvise cooking arrangements in the field. A typical army method was to dig a trench two feet deep, three feet wide, and ten feet long; build fires along the bottom; and arrange camp kettles along the top for company-level cooking. Everyone tried to wean the soldier away from frying or roasting and toward stewing or boiling meat. Sanitarians might have taken some comfort in the fact that cooking in the British Army was no better than in the American force. Continental armies tended to have better cooking regimes, and the only way the British could improve was to educate the common soldier much in the way concerned Americans were trying to do for their own army.[30]

It is not that the Federal military system was completely immune to the importance of cooking, but it simply did not do very much to address the issue. Army regulations required "the greatest care" in washing cooking utensils and rotating men in and out of kitchen duties on the company level. They also instructed company officers to closely supervise cooking, messing arrangements, and the cleanliness of kitchens and eating areas. As far as cooking instructions, regulations mentioned that bread must be

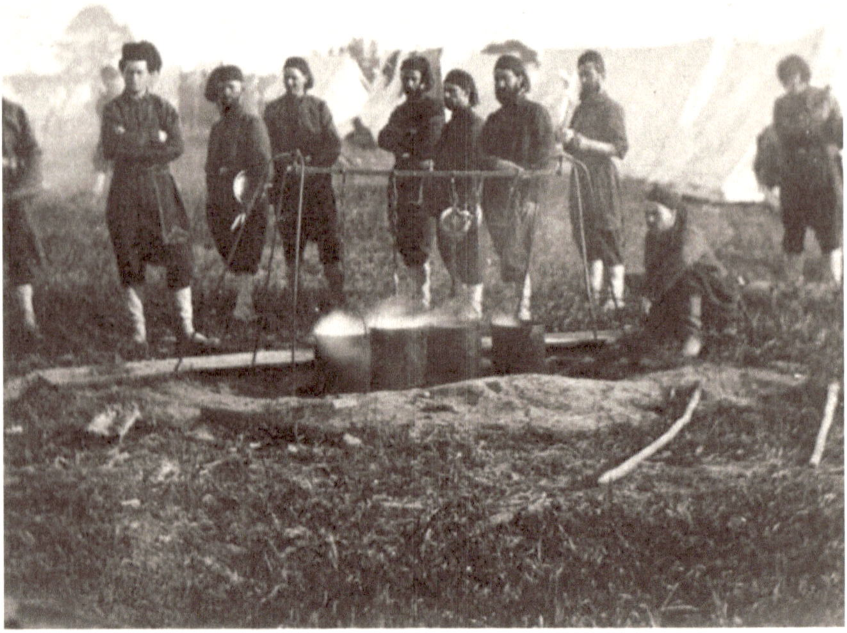

Cooking over a Trench. Members of the Fifth New York show the way to cook, as the army and sanitarians recommended, by digging a trench, laying coals along its bottom, and suspending pots above it. The Fifth was Gouverneur K. Warren and Gordon H. Winslow's regiment, here posted at Fortress Monroe, Virginia, in a photograph taken by George Stacy. (Library of Congress, Prints & Photographs Division, LCDIG-stereo-1s01798)

"thoroughly baked," soup boiled at least five hours, and vegetables well cooked "to be perfectly soft and digestible."[31]

While encouraging in their general tone, these few and simple directions about cooking were inadequate in addressing such a significant and complex feature of army life. One can see faint reflections of these regulations in practice, but the limited implementation of those injunctions is more glaring. Samuel Gridley Howe castigated nearly everything in army cooking when he inspected Massachusetts regiments early in the war. The detailed cooks had no training at all, and their culinary arrangements were minimal at best. He found that their cleaning of cooking utensils was quite poor and also thought the army's camp kettle was inadequate.[32]

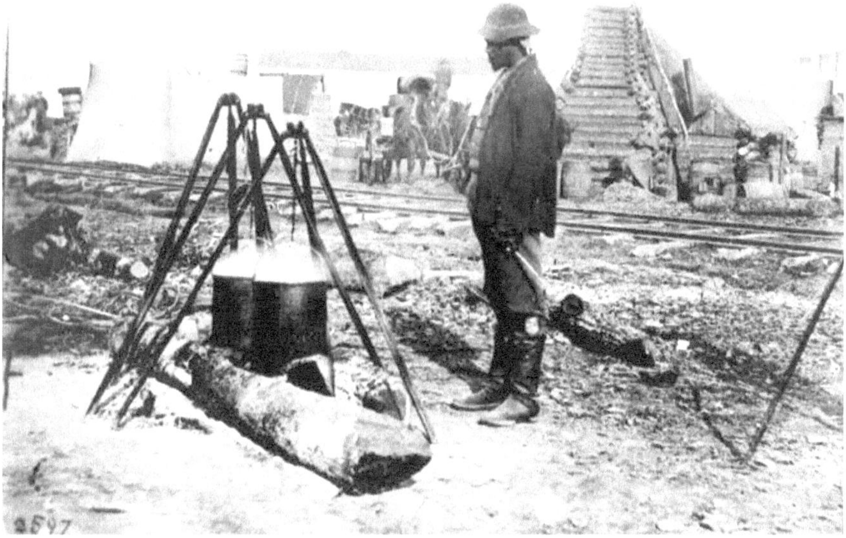

Cooking on the Surface. With two big pots slowly boiling while placed directly on a slow-burning wood fire on the surface of the ground, this man, who probably was a servant for an officers' mess, demonstrates a common form of cooking in the Union army. The image was exposed at City Point, Virginia, sometime between June 1864 and March 1865. (Library of Congress, Prints & Photographs Division, Civil War Photographs, LCDIG-ppmsca-33096)

As with nearly everything else in army life, the initial period of service was a time of adjustment until most soldiers found a niche in which they were comfortable. When it came to cooking arrangements, they tended to be found in forming small groups of men into a mess. Rice C. Bull of the 123rd New York explained this well. Three men who could get along with each other, usually sharing sleeping arrangements as well, pooled their individual rations and did their own cooking with a few simple utensils they could easily carry on the march. The advantages were that they could eat when they wanted and fix the food in any way they chose, neither of which was possible with company-level cooking. "Under this system of feeding the men were more independent, well satisfied, and much better fed."[33]

This view was not shared by sanitarians or the inspectors sent to the field by the Sanitary Commission. They overwhelmingly favored an organized system of cooking from the top down, with company-level cooks

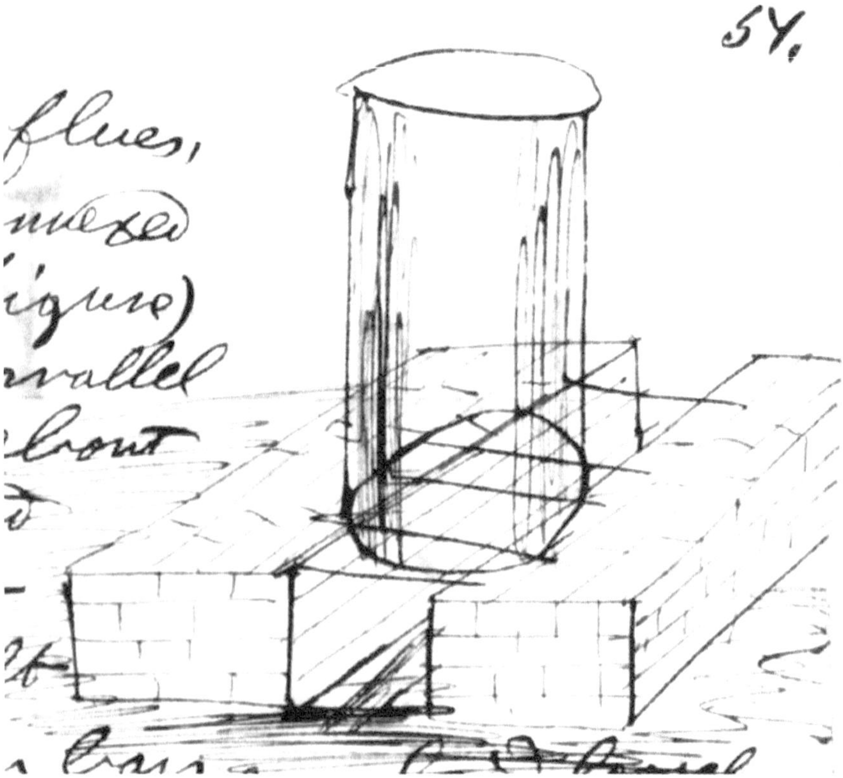

Cooking with a Brick Flue. Franklin Benjamin Hough kept a journal while he was a Sanitary Commission camp inspector in which he not only wrote entries but also drew many sketches illustrating camp life for "the Little Folks at Home." Here, he depicts a brick cooking flue. The basic concept is the same as cooking over a trench, except that everything is above ground, with a narrow valley to hold the fire, metal rods extending across it, and a large pot resting on the rods. ("Sketches of the Field and Camp in a Series of Letters from a Sanitary Inspector to the Little Folks at Home, Vol. 1, Washington, Feb. 1862," 51, Franklin Benjamin Hough Papers, from the collections of the New York State Library, Manuscripts and Special Collections, Albany, New York)

closely supervised by officers. This disjunction between the theory of cooking arrangements and what the men in the field preferred is striking. Much of it can be explained by quality of execution; in both methods of cooking, good preparation would have gone a long way toward acceptance.

Failure of executing the cooking process with common sense and attention to detail also dogged the care of utensils. These instruments were few and simple, but the willingness of men to take the trouble of scouring them clean after every use was limited at best. One of the most persistent facts to emerge from this story is the lack of good care regarding cooking vessels. These were neglected, reported Lewis H. Steiner when looking through the camps of Banks's division. "Instead of really scoured vessels, filthy, fat bedaubed kettles and pans meet the eye."[34]

Many soldiers testified that the true problem was not the quality of rations issued by the army, but the want of knowledge about how to prepare them for meals. Most men simply did not know how to cook anything when they volunteered. And at the beginning most companies had detailed cooks with no more knowledge of the art than the men they served. Potatoes still had a raw core in the middle no matter how long they were boiled, coffee was barely palatable one day and absolutely unbearable the next, and rice and beans were not properly soaked before being cooked. When it

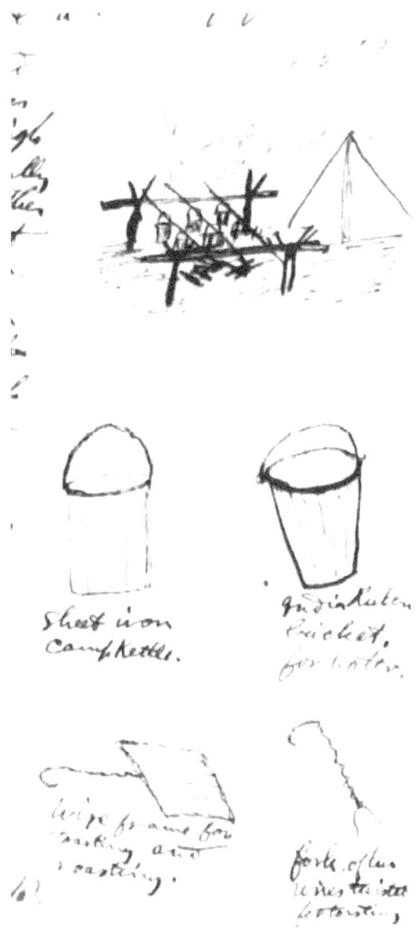

Cooking Utensils. A variety of handy tools and vessels for cooking in camp can be seen in these illustrations by Franklin Benjamin Hough. At top, he drew a view of several pots cooking over a fire built on the surface of the ground. Below that he drew two items. Under the left one he wrote, "sheet iron camp kettle," and under the right, "India Rubber bucket, for water." On the lowest row Hough drew two utensils. Under the left he wrote, "wire frame for toasting and roasting," and under the right, "fork of two wires twisted for toasting." ("Sketches of the Field and Camp in a Series of Letters from a Sanitary Inspector to the Little Folks at Home, Vol. 1, Washington, Feb. 1862," 47, Franklin Benjamin Hough Papers, from the collections of the New York State Library, Manuscripts and Special Collections, Albany, New York)

came to meat, company cooks in semipermanent camps typically boiled it in water, while individual cooks typically fried it in grease. On campaign, soldiers tended to broil it over a campfire while stuck on a stick. Individuals often fried hardtack in a skillet soaked with grease.[35]

The army failed to issue regulations about cooking and failed to publish an official cookbook for soldiers. All it did was to saddle supervisory requirements on company-level officers and the regimental surgeon. A general order issued by headquarters, Department of the South midway through the war stated that cooking was "a matter of great importance" that had "not yet received from a majority of the officers in our volunteer service that attention which is paid to it in the Regular Army of the United States and by the armies of Europe." The order went on to repeat the responsibility of officers to supervise cooking but only stipulated that meat should not be fried. There is evidence that at least some officers in the Department of the South took this directive to heart, but it was only one of a couple of dozen military departments in the Union army. As far as cooking details were concerned, Surgeon General Hammond included some good directions about preparing a variety of foods in his treatise on hygiene, published in 1863. Surg. Jonathan Letterman put together "Directions for Cooking in Camp," which was issued in August 1862 for the Army of the Potomac, of which he was medical director.[36]

Army officials agreed with sanitarians that the best way to organize cooking in semipermanent camps was on the company level. There, dedicated cooks could gain experience about how to prepare meals, and officers had more opportunities to supervise and control the process. Individual cooking was the worst method from the standpoint of both the army and sanitarians, while messes, an intermediate level of organizing food preparation, was allowable if necessary. The army had to give in on this issue because cooking by company was utterly impossible on campaign. Even in semipermanent camps it sometimes was impractical, and the men generally did not like it. Thus, messing and individual cooking became the more common methods of organizing food preparation in the Civil War.[37]

FIFTEENTH CORPS MEDICAL INSPECTION REPORTS

There often was a disjunction between what the army wished its soldiers to do and what they actually did, and cooking was no different. Soldiers had enough leeway in their daily habits to settle into a routine comfortable for themselves regardless of general orders or sanitary principles. Fifteenth

Corps medical inspectors paid a good deal of attention to food preparation in the semipermanent camps they investigated in April 1863 and found that the harsh environmental conditions of the Louisiana bottomlands produced poor cooking reports. For almost every regiment in the corps, the inspectors found a high level of ignorance about good cooking and eating regimens. In regiment after regiment, the comments were similar. While a couple of them cooked by companies, most did so by messes of five to twelve men each. There was little and often literally no officer supervision. The messes were allowed to cook in whatever method they wished and eat when they desired. In many regiments the men cooked and ate in filth. "Cooking very bad in this regiment," wrote the medical inspector about the Fifty-Seventh Ohio, a statement that also applied to several other regiments. Cooking utensils tended to be in poor shape in the Fifth Minnesota as well.[38]

The living environment was far better in Fifteenth Corps camps along the Big Black River in September, but the men's habits were no different. The medical inspector found that all regiments except the Fifth Minnesota cooked by messes. Even batteries, which were the same size as infantry companies, cooked by messes rather than by companies. All men drew their individual rations and stored them, along with unwashed cooking utensils, in their sleeping quarters, creating a very unclean and, in the eyes of the inspector, unhealthy living space. It was "'every man for himself,'" reported Surg. Edward O. F. Roler. That included eating times, which were highly irregular. Roler considered regular mealtimes "one of the essential conditions in hygienic nutrition."[39]

The situation was noticeably better in February and March 1864, when the corps spent the winter in northern Alabama. About half the regiments enforced cooking by companies rather than messes. While some received high marks for keeping their sleeping quarters clean, many of the units cooking by messes continued to allow the men to store their provisions where they slept. Those regiments received low marks for cleanliness. Several others were poorly supplied with cooking utensils, which their men failed to keep clean. Only in a small number of units did the medical inspector declare the cooking to be well and systematically conducted. For the majority, even among those where company-level food preparation prevailed, it was deemed either mediocre or poor. A handful of units had constructed a cookhouse, but in most the men cooked outdoors or in their cabins and tents. Only two companies of the Tenth Missouri kept their quarters clean and conducted cooking with regularity, while the other eight companies were a mess. "Quarters quite dirty," the inspector, Surg. John M.

Woodworth, wrote of the Fifty-Sixth Illinois. "Cook and eat in quarters." Woodworth found in March that his suggestions for improving the cooking arrangements in the Second Division of the corps had been ignored, in contrast to the units in the Third Division, which took his advice to heart. In the latter he found "great improvement . . . in the manner of cooking" except for the Sixty-Third Illinois and the division pioneer corps. That improvement mainly was in the form of constructing "good cook houses" and enforcing food preparation by companies. When this was brought to the attention of the Sixty-Third Illinois commander, he promised to build a house and "break up squad cooking in his regt. at once."[40]

Fifteenth Corps medical inspectors tabulated the results of their visits to the camps with numerical ratings. In April 1863, with twenty regiments included, eight (40 percent) rated good, two (10 percent) rated fair, and the remaining ten (50 percent) rated bad in the category of cooking. This improved a good deal by September 1863, when once again twenty regiments were rated. This time twelve (60 percent) achieved a good score, five (20 percent) were fair, and only three (15 percent) rated bad.[41]

It is interesting that after three years of field service, most of these Fifteenth Corps regiments still were not practicing the basics of good food preparation, camp cleanliness, and regularity in mealtimes. Much of this can be ascribed to a general laxity of rules enforcement that plagued the volunteer army of the Union throughout the war. But it was more acute in the area of food preparation because that depended so much on individual taste and convenience. The officers felt they could easily afford to let the men have their way in these areas. It was a good safety valve for releasing pent-up frustration with the restraints of military life to let the men mess in squads and to store their food where they could keep an eye on it, given soldier tendencies to pilfer things from their comrades. The men also generally preferred to fry their food.

SANITARY COMMISSION CAMP INSPECTION RETURNS

Sanitary Commission inspectors had their own take on the quality of cooking in Union army camps. Their standard form included ten questions relating to the subject. The commission wanted to know about the cooking facilities; whether the men used portable stoves, brick or earthen flues constructed on site, trenches, or simply a campfire on unbroken ground; how carefully they maintained their cooking utensils; and whether food preparation was conducted by dedicated cooks or the men frequently rotated in and out of such duties. The inspector was supposed to judge how well the cooks performed their task, which was the most difficult question to answer unless he happened to visit at mealtime and was willing to smell and taste the food.

But camp inspectors recorded enough information to fruitfully answer many of these questions. They noted the cooking personnel in 188 regiments and concluded that in 147 (78.2 percent) of them, it was done by dedicated cooks who often were assisted by men who rotated in and out of their positions. In another 35 regiments (18.6 percent), the primary cooking was performed by men who rotated frequently, and in only 6 (3.2 percent) was there no systematic effort by regimental or company officers to manage the cooking personnel. In other words, it was every man for himself in those last regiments as far as food preparation was concerned.

As for cooking facilities, 226 returns mentioned exactly what the cooks prepared their food on. For most, 102 (45.2 percent), it was on the unbroken surface of the ground. For 94 (41.5 percent), this was done with trenches dug for the purpose. And 30 (13.3 percent) inspected units used some sort of brick or earthen flue. Another 43 returns indicated the use of portable stoves, but they were not the exclusive cooking platform. These stoves often were used by some men in a given regiment and not others because they usually were individually purchased. When it came to utensil care, inspectors were rather generous. Out of 191 returns that mention this aspect, 148 (77.5 percent) rated good, 28 (14.7 percent) rated fair, and 15 (7.8 percent) rated bad.

Inspectors contributed quite a few comments on the returns that reflected their personal reaction to cooking in the camps. They paid much attention to the method of organizing the food preparation, reporting all three ways of doing so: company-level cooks, small messes, and individuals. The inspectors often commented that the lower the level, the worse the results. In a tiny number of regiments, a professional cook had been hired by the officers, receiving in one case 12.5 cents per soldier per week as a wage. In these favored units the cooking was excellent, "better than they had at home in most cases," Hough stated of men in the First Connecticut Artillery. In terms of cooking facilities, inspector comments reflect the small number of regiments that had been provided with good cooking stoves, often through the help of state rather than Federal authorities. Some others used "brick flues, open tops with iron bars across." Virtually all units baked bread or had it shipped in daily from a nearby depot. When inspectors tasted the men's food, their reactions were split between admitting it was quite bad to praising it when they could. They at times offered summary comments about the overall success rate of regimental cooking. When Bettelheim had to do so for the artillery attached to Horatio Van Cleve's division, Army of the Cumberland, he answered with a bit of sarcasm. "The boys are fat at any rate."[42]

Bettelheim found an interesting attitude in the Twenty-Second Indiana when he visited its camp in April 1863. "Company cooks spoke against by many officers," he wrote in his return. "On march the men must take along cooked rations. They eat even raw bacon. Each sits down cooking his own. It is a kind of amusement to the men." No one better expressed a very common conceit among Union soldiers; they much preferred to be in charge of their own food preparation. It gave them many opportunities to make their own decisions. They loved the freedom from supervision by their officers that messing by squads or by individuals offered them.[43]

Sanitary inspectors found a wide range of cooking conditions and results among the camps they visited. Some surgeons and company-level officers supervised rigorously, and cooks in some regiments seriously learned how to perform their tasks to produce good meals. But these units cannot be taken as typical. Overall, the camp inspection returns reveal a picture of, at best, middling results in food preparation as far as good sanitary principles were concerned. The chief problems were the strong tendency to arrange for food preparation to be done by messes and by individuals, with the consequent low level of officer supervision. Even when arranged on the company level, officer oversight was mediocre at best. Lesser problems included the minimal cooking facilities provided units in camp and the army's negligence in providing the men with detailed instructions about how to prepare their meals.[44]

Despite all this, the overall ratings in the camp inspection returns gave the volunteer army pretty good marks for cooking. Slightly more than half the units—51.7 percent—scored a good rating, while 33.6 percent received a fair rating, and only 14.7 percent earned a bad rating. Inspectors tended not to hold the units to strict accountability according to sanitarian principles regarding group versus individual food preparation, cleaning cooking utensils, and officer supervision. They were rather lenient; as long as the men seemed content, they gave cooking a passing grade.

Based on their comments, however, the returns strongly view food quality and cooking as uneven and officer supervision as lacking. The army appointed company-level officers and regimental surgeons as the primary agents in regulating both important areas of soldier life. It can be said that most of them either failed or at best only partially fulfilled that duty. The

Union army marched on its stomach, but that stomach was too often filled with fried meat rather than a variety of wholesome foods properly prepared. It managed to win the war but could have suffered less if its volunteer officers had taken better care of the army's collective stomach.

7

Water, Alcohol, and Morale

What the soldier drank was just as important to his health as what he ate. The body actually needs liquid reinforcement more frequently than nourishment from food, but arranging for the former in Civil War camps and especially during an active campaign was in some ways more difficult than arranging for provisions. Coffee and tea were part of the army ration and therefore arrived through the logistical system that supported troops in the field, but water was not part of that system. Soldiers, with the aid of officers, were expected to find it on their own. They relied mostly on natural sources and found water in varied degrees of purity, usefulness, and wholesomeness. Even when the soldiers used civilian sources of water, they had to deal with varying quality. The US Sanitary Commission reported on all these aspects of drinking water.

Continental Army rations included wine and brandy during the American Revolutionary War, but the Union army's did not.[1] Soldiers had to find their own sources of alcoholic refreshment if they were inclined to do so. The army did provide whiskey on a very limited basis for therapeutic and medicinal purposes, and then only on the recommendations of surgeons and officers. Nevertheless, those men who craved liquor managed in many ways to acquire it through informal means. Alcohol played a role in soldier life during the Civil War, but how widely it was consumed is the question, and the Sanitary Commission camp inspection returns offer one of the best insights into the topic.

Finally, morale in the ranks became a matter of concern on the part of Civil War sanitarians. In this they were well ahead of their time, at least as far as the American military experience was concerned. While the more advanced military systems of major Continental powers in Europe paid significant attention to what sanitarians often called "amusements" in the ranks, the US Army paid limited attention to the matter. Even sanitarians went only so far in arguing that soldiers needed to be kept entertained in order to divert them from harmful influences such as liquor and to avoid what the era termed "nostalgia," or severe homesickness. They were, however, aiming in the right direction. Within fifty years after Appomattox, the US Army would devote a great deal of attention to shaping morale among its soldiers during World War I.

The Sanitary Commission was highly concerned about all three of these subjects, devoting many questions on its standard camp inspection form to them. Sanitarians in and out of the army agreed on the importance of clean water for soldier health. Fortunately, most inspected regiments chalked up a good record for accessing clean water. Commission members, however, deplored the consumption of liquor except for purely medical uses. They preferred that it be doled out rather like a prescription from surgeons than freely available to all who wished to imbibe. The camp inspection returns offered commission members encouraging news in that regard. They contain convincing evidence that the thirst for alcohol was less widespread among the troops than they feared and much less than historians have previously assumed. When it came to morale, though, Civil War sanitarians had rather limited ideas. Musical entertainment in the form of regimental bands and hours spent in reading a variety of literature, not just material of a religious nature, was about all they could suggest. The results of the camp inspection program indicated that the Union army did very poorly when it came to institutional methods to shape soldier morale, which must have been a disappointment to the commission.

WATER

No matter how many types of potable fluids might be available to Civil War soldiers, water was the most widely obtainable and the most important. The human body cannot survive without regular infusions of it. Water came from a variety of sources that included springs, surface runoff into streams, and manmade wells. As a result, its quality varied widely, with important effects on health. Sanitarians made a study of water from this perspective, and they had definite ideas about what sources were better than others and how to treat impure water to minimize health risks.

SANITARIANS AND THE ARMY ON WATER

John Ordronaux noted that changes in drinking water had a direct effect on a person's digestive system. He advised that adding a bit of vinegar to water taken from a stream, or even adding coffee or tea to a canteen filled with water, would help counteract any ill effects of impurity. He also told readers that they should not drink immediately after a heavy exertion, especially in hot weather, but cool off gradually first. William P. Craighill, a military engineer, wrote of filtering muddy water and boiling or mixing it with charcoal to counteract impurities. He also urged soldiers to drink early in the morning but not during strenuous marches. They could keep the mouth moist during these times by chewing on a straw or a leaf. Tying a wet handkerchief around their necks helped allay thirst until they had cooled off after a march.[2]

Surgeon General Hammond devoted a good deal of attention to water because it was "never found in nature in a state of absolute purity." Rainwater came closest to that ideal, but it still contained "traces of organic matter, nitric acid, and ammonia" from the atmosphere. Well and spring water had "soluble materials present in the strata through which they pass," and stagnant water was the most impure. Hammond cautioned soldiers to look for running water, citing springs, streams, and rivers as the best choices. He recognized that large rivers were problematic, as they often contained "decaying vegetation and animal remains, the sewerage of cities, [and] the refuse of manufactories." Every element of civilian society tended to be drawn to rivers for multiple uses, and armies were no different. They relied on rivers as transportation routes, sources of drinking and cleaning water, for bathing, and for the disposal of human and animal waste.[3]

Surg. Benjamin Woodward of the Twenty-Second Illinois made a particular study of water and army life that he shared with the Sanitary Commission soon after the war. River water posed special problems because it was saturated with impurities from tributaries and all manner of other materials swept into the current by erosion. The Twenty-Second Illinois was stationed at Cairo, Illinois, and Bird's Point, Missouri, during the fall and winter of 1861–62, and thus the men drank much water from the Mississippi River. Many of them complained of loose bowels, and Woodward, who performed several autopsies on deceased soldiers, often found a "dense deposit which on a microscopic examination proved to be the mud of the river water" that coated their stomachs and intestines. Filtering the river water through gravel and charcoal in barrels helped a lot. Even when the regiment ascended the Tennessee River in April 1862, the water of that stream led to diarrhea. Because the Twenty-Second was on the move, it could not easily filter the water, so Woodward had the men boil it, which also helped a good deal. Despite all this, he concluded that the water of the Mississippi River, at least, was actually quite good if one could properly filter out the impurities. Woodward kept a sample in a bottle for several months and found that all unpleasant elements settled to the bottom, leaving the water clear and healthy.[4]

During subsequent moves of the Twenty-Second Illinois, Woodward continued to examine water sources through a microscope. He found that some infantry officers scoffed at this instrument, while others took his research seriously. When the regiment was camped at Cowan, Tennessee, during July 1863, the local water caused much diarrhea. Woodward found that it was impregnated with nitrates, alum, and soda salts from caves at the base of the nearby Cumberland Plateau. When he informed division commander Philip Sheridan of this, Sheridan ordered the camps moved to the top of the plateau, where the men enjoyed good air and springs of soft water.[5]

Woodward tried to regulate the water-drinking habits of his men. They tended to be so thirsty on hot marches that they rushed to the nearest pool or well and drank heavily no matter how impure the water might be. "It has always been my endeavor to break up the habit, convinced that it is injurious even if the water is good, which it seldom is on the track of large armies." He was a firm believer that adding some cornmeal purified the liquid. The resulting mixture could "quench thirst far better than even the purest water."[6]

SOLDIER PERSONAL ACCOUNTS ON WATER

Civil War soldiers laced their personal accounts with descriptions of water, both good and bad. It was a subject of abiding and universal importance. They tended to agree that water from a spring was the best. But all sources contained some degree of contaminants, and when heavy with them, it was noticeable to the taste and in the effect on their digestive systems. Sulfur and iron were noted in soldier accounts of their water intake, with consequent illness that, according to some, even led to eventual death. They knew that the worst type was swampy water and any stream connected with swamp land. "We are drinking water a little better than poison," reported Chauncey H. Cooke of the Twenty-Fifth Wisconsin about his camp experience at Snyder's Bluff, Mississippi, on the edge of the Mississippi Delta. Regiments transferred from the uplands of southern Missouri to participate in the

Vicksburg siege were stunned at the difference in water quality between the two regions. Civilians in the Vicksburg area used cisterns—underground storage pits to collect rainwater—but the Union army quickly used up all the water in them after moving in to lay siege to the city.[7]

The large Federal force operating against Vicksburg mostly drew its drinking water from the Mississippi River, which flowed muddy and rapid but was generally considered better than the adjacent Yazoo River. The latter channel drained the lower part of the Mississippi Delta and flowed into the Mississippi just above Vicksburg. It was notoriously unhealthy because of its slow current and the amount of swampy water that fed it. The water in the Yazoo "smells and tastes of all manner of filth and decayed vegetation," William T. Shepherd of Battery B, First Illinois Light Artillery told his mother. "Dead alligators and fish and the greenish slime from swamps, with the occasional ancient remains of Army mules and horses do not add to its flavor in the least." Steamers carrying troops up the Yazoo often stopped in the Mississippi midchannel to let the men fill their canteens with water there before ascending the tributary.[8]

In short, the Federals relied heavily on the Mississippi River for drinking water during the Vicksburg operations. They were well aware that it contained many sediments and even saw dead animals floating downriver with the current. "It was the sewer for all the filth of the northern states," as Cooke wrote, but they drank from it anyway, and most found it palatable. While some knew that filtering or letting the water settle removed most of the impurities, the majority did not have an opportunity to do so. The residents of St. Louis reportedly did not filter or purify the Mississippi River water in any way before using it. Although the river's water tended to produce diarrhea in some soldiers, it had a general reputation for healthiness.[9]

Union soldiers typically took their water as they found it, impurities and all. That was not only true of the Mississippi River but also of all natural water sources. One soldier blamed the iron content of water used near Ironton, Missouri, for the outbreak of boils over his body. The surgeon of the Twentieth Indiana noted the presence of the "usual Lime Salts" in water found near Cockeysville, Maryland, while sulfur content seemed to make men of the First Rhode Island Cavalry ill.[10]

There were various methods of dealing with less than pristine water if one had the time to do so. Clarifying involved letting it settle for some time so that unwanted elements fell to the bottom of the vessel. Surg. John G. Perry of the Twentieth Massachusetts patiently allowed water to settle for half an hour before using it. Adding a little vinegar was useful as a way to purify it further. Various ways to filter out impurities also were available. John D. Billings recalled two different filtration devices that were sold to soldiers, but neither of them lasted very long under field conditions. Hammond had much faith in carbon-based filtering systems. He also endorsed filtering water through sand, gravel, and charcoal. Adding alum and permanganate of potassa was an option, as was distillation. The latter involved boiling the water in a copper still and collecting the resulting condensation; it was the method used on board sailing vessels.[11]

Given the trouble involved in any water treatment, it is not surprising that relatively little of it took place in Civil War camps. Typically, soldiers looked for running water on the assumption that it contained fewer problem elements than stagnant pools. In fact, in the Army of the Potomac, taking water from running streams and "living springs" was mandated by general orders, which also warned the men to avoid water from surface drainage. The latter was widely viewed by commentators as containing all sorts of impurities in a concentrated form because they were not mixed yet into a large stream, where they became more diluted and manageable.[12]

The quality of well water varied a good deal. Some of it was quite good, but this depended much on the topography. Civilian wells were usually dug in good places and could be used by the men, but when the soldiers sank their own wells, they usually had little choice in the location. On the Atlantic coast one did not have to dig more than a few feet to find water, but it tended to be brackish. The men shored up the sides of their wells with empty barrels and cracker boxes. If they were willing to dig deeper, hitting and pushing through a stratum of gravel or blue clay, water of "generally a good quality" could be found. Springs also proved to be a good source of water, probably the most favored of all natural sources for Union soldiers. Of course, if the spring was located on low ground with surface drainage feeding it, the purity declined a great deal.[13]

FIFTEENTH CORPS MEDICAL INSPECTION REPORTS

Despite the many complications of finding palatable water, Union soldiers managed to do so well enough to keep them going. It was far easier to locate natural sources when selecting a semipermanent camp than when moving through the countryside. Therefore, camp inspectors typically reported that good water was used. In the Fifteenth Corps, for example, out of eighteen regiments of the Second Division camped along the Big Black River in September 1863, seventeen were rated as having good water and only one as fair.[14]

SANITARY COMMISSION CAMP INSPECTION RETURNS

The Sanitary Commission included water quality in its standard camp inspection form. Nine questions covered exactly what type of source was used, whether the water was clear and apparently wholesome, and whether it had a local reputation among civilians as being of healthy quality. The results were highly encouraging for any sanitarian. Because some regiments used water from two different sources, the total listed on the 280 returns used in this study amounted to 305 sources. Springs accounted for 154 (50.4 percent) of the total. Wells were the next most popular, with 76 (24.9 percent). Small streams represented 12.1 percent, while rivers accounted for 9.5 percent of the total. Only three regiments were able to use city water, two relied on a pond, and another two simply collected rainwater. Another two regiments relied on Bayou La Fourche in Louisiana.

Those regiments that used more than one source typically divided them into categories. Drinking and cooking water came from wells and springs, while water for washing came from streams. The Third Wisconsin was one of the regiments using city water; the men simply turned a tap on a hydrant at Frederick, Maryland, to access the town reservoir.[15]

It is not surprising that water quality rated very highly in the view of camp inspectors. Among the 280 returns, 72.5 percent managed a good rating, while 20.0 percent rated fair and only 7.5 percent bad. But again, one must keep in mind that it was easier to find good sources of water when selecting a semipermanent camp than when bivouacking in an active campaign. The commission made no attempt to gauge or monitor field experiences on the operational level.

ALCOHOL

Liquor obviously was a fluid of choice in Civil War America that supplemented water for many men who enlisted in the army. But the conflict took place at the end of a long period in which societal reforms raised awareness of the harmful effects of overindulgence in alcohol, leading many thousands of Americans to swear off or limit their use of intoxicating beverages. The temperance movement neared the end of its first great phase by 1861, after accomplishing much over the previous thirty years. The big question was whether the young men who made up the Union army would be tempted to indulge now that they were away from home for the first time. To what extent did the volunteers reflect societal attitudes toward liquor? Was the Union army awash in alcohol?

Sanitarians were keenly interested in these questions because the Civil War was by far the biggest conflict to occur since the onset of the temperance movement of the early 1830s. It provided a marvelous case study of alcohol use in the military. Consumption of liquor in American society generally had fallen a great deal by 1861. It had been on a steady rise from 1790 to 1830 because of a general belief that alcohol was "healthful, nutritious, stimulating and relaxing," and whiskey in particular was in plentiful and cheap supply. In addition to several economic factors, the temperance movement, which began as an effort to moderate rather than eliminate alcoholic consumption, led to a steady decline of drinking from 1830 to 1860. From that point consumption remained relatively stable for a long period of time. Thus, the Union army was created when the temperance movement, which by now had largely morphed into a movement to prohibit alcoholic consumption rather than just reduce it, still had potency.[16]

LIQUOR AND THE ARMY

Historian Megan Bever points out that the culture of restraint in alcoholic consumption penetrated noticeably among the enlisted men of the Union army but was not dominant. She believes that officers indulged far more freely and openly than their subordinates, which was why evidence in personal accounts tend to depict the Civil War military as a drinking army. The regular army had moved to align with the basic goals of the temperance movement long before the war. Congress dropped the regular issue of liquor in 1832, reserving whiskey rations only for certain circumstances, such as hard labor or exposure to cold weather, or as a nutrient.[17]

The idea that alcohol was a healthy drink pervaded the prewar United States, but it was on the wane. In Britain physicians engaged in a raging debate over that point during the 1860s; those who argued against alcohol's therapeutic value partially won that debate by the 1870s, although they conceded that liquor could lower the temperature of a patient suffering from fever. In the United States the question also was discussed but with less heat. "Ardent spirits are not necessary to health in the healthy," wrote John Ordronaux. "All authorities agree that . . . the soldier is everywhere found to be better without them." He believed alcohol should be strictly regulated as a prescribed medicine under the surgeon's control. Ordronaux saw no benefits of any kind other than in limited hospital use. In sharp contrast

Hammond argued that alcohol was food. He even experimented on himself with a series of three exercises that involved consuming alcohol with his meals. When he ate the prescribed amount of food, liquor only mildly disturbed his system. When he ate less, alcohol helped compensate for the reduced amount of food. When he ate more, liquor made him feel worse. These limited and highly subjective experiments led the surgeon general to extoll "the real hygienic and physiological advantages" of alcohol.[18]

Fortunately, everyone ignored Hammond's ill-considered view on the use of liquor and generally adhered to official army policy. Now and then a barrel of whiskey was requisitioned for distribution to men who had endured hard physical conditions of military labor or who were compelled to serve in unhealthy locations. Surg. Thomas S. Hawley was convinced that issuing whiskey reduced the sick list in his Eleventh Missouri from seventy to forty-eight men in a week. In contrast, Surg. Abner Hard refused to authorize whiskey for the Eighth Illinois Cavalry in cold and wet conditions. He pointed out that the Fifty-Third Pennsylvania, camped nearby and in similar circumstances, did issue whiskey, after which its sick list dramatically increased, with a death rate three times higher than the Illinois unit.[19]

Assertions that the Union army was awash in alcohol are misleading. Whiskey rations were comparatively rare, even for prescription use. John Billings could not recall more than three or four times during the entire war when his battery received an official issue, although he admitted that veterans in other units could remember more times. Even so few issues were too many in the view of some men. Whatever power liquor possessed as a stimulant quickly wore off, thought Capt. John W. De Forest of the Twelfth Connecticut, with the result that one felt even worse than before. Another negative result of its use as a stimulant was that some men drank several rations, taking them from those who refused to imbibe, and their drunken antics were visible for all to see. While there is plenty of evidence that a large proportion of men in a given unit accepted and enjoyed the infrequent issue of army whiskey, there is just as much evidence that an equal or higher percentage refused to touch it. Fifteen to twenty men, or about half of Company F, Twenty-Second Iowa, for example, turned down the issue when offered. On the other end of the spectrum, Billings knew of two or three men in his battery who "were always on the scent for something to drink." There is equally strong evidence that widespread but temporary tipsiness in a regiment led to enormous problems of discipline for a few hours.[20]

The official army take on this issue was to document the treated cases of alcoholism in the Union force. Defining alcoholism as including inebriation, delirium tremens, and chronic drunkenness, it concluded that on average there were nearly 5 cases per 1,000 white soldiers annually. The rate was higher at the start and the end of the war, and it increased when units were stationed near large cities. The rate among Black troops, at 1 case per 4,500 men, was much lower. "As a matter of fact," concluded the compilers of the *Medical and Surgical History of the War of the Rebellion,* "the campaigns of the civil war were made on hot coffee, with a rare issue of whiskey under special conditions of fatigue or discomfort."[21]

The Sanitary Commission took a public stand in favor of the army's policy. It sought to eliminate individual drinking of liquor by soldiers but allowed that alcohol could be prescribed for medicinal purposes by surgeons. But commission authorities also urged that any consumption take place after, not before, heavy physical exertion. Many regimental surgeons in the volunteer force agreed with this position and pushed it even further. The commission circulated a questionnaire right after the war to these medical personnel that contained many questions about their experience with military medicine. One related to alcohol use. While all regimental surgeons who answered that question agreed that liquor should only be issued on the order of a competent medical officer, many went on to voice their opinion that physicians should refrain from authorizing it at any time. "I do not believe the whisky ration is of any advantage to a soldier," stated Surg. Henry Manfred of the Twenty-Second Kentucky. They opposed alcohol use by officers as well, always preferring good coffee as the most important fluid to be consumed by army personnel.[22]

SANITARY COMMISSION CAMP INSPECTION RETURNS

Seven questions related to alcohol appeared on the commission's standard camp inspection return. The organization wanted to know if sutlers sold intoxicating beverages and if peddlers were allowed to cater to the drinking inclinations of the men. Did the troops gain access to alcohol through other means? Was there much intoxication in the regiment? This last question was answered by the regimental officers and surgeons. But the camp inspector was also required to ask for details, such as how many men on average were in the guardhouse and whether those cases were primarily caused by problems associated with drinking. The standard form included the right kind of questions for both the commission and later the interested historian to gain special insight into alcohol use and abuse on the regimental level in the Civil War.

The answers to those questions are a bit surprising. A historian who has read numerous personal accounts by soldiers that emphasize drinking and its riotous consequences would find it odd that so many regimental officers claimed that intoxication was not a problem for their units. Based on his visit to the Seventy-Fourth Illinois, Bernard J. Bettelheim praised it as a model regiment because only one officer had imbibed, and he had resigned sometime before the inspection. In the Third Maine Battery, "insolence to noncommissioned officers" rather than intoxication was the main reason for men to be put in the guardhouse. At times, the inspectors questioned the glowing reports of sobriety offered by regimental officers. Godfrey Aigner was surprised at the low number of men sent to the guardhouse, although the officers readily admitted that most were there because of drunkenness. Edward A. Crane did not believe regimental officers who told him alcohol abuse did not exist when he interviewed them at Baton Rouge in December 1862. "So I have been told in every camp which I have visited, and yet I have seen numbers of drunken soldiers about town, drunk [with liquor] purchased some where in the place."[23]

Camp inspection returns certainly do provide evidence of alcohol use and abuse, as do other documents collected by the Sanitary Commission during and after the war. Surg. Orpheus Everts informed the commission that "several instances of insubordination, followed by severe punishments," resulted from an issue of whiskey to the Twentieth Indiana while it occupied Hatteras Island, North Carolina, in the fall of 1861. It became clear from the returns that many inspectors connected ethnicity with elevated levels of alcohol consumption. The multiethnic Thirty-Ninth New York had a system, according to William M. Chamberlain, whereby each man paid the sutler thirteen cents a day in exchange for an ounce of brandy morning and evening and three half-pints of beer at noon. Louis Blenker's entire division gained a widespread reputation for imbibing in the fall of 1861. Even army commander George B. McClellan noted the convivial atmosphere in that unit whenever he visited, and he was feted by champagne. "All of them are Germans, and hard drinkers," Franklin B. Hough noted of Blenker's men in a missive home.[24]

Persistent discipline problems linked to alcohol abuse existed in virtually all regiments inspected. But, it is important to add, those problems were limited. In most regiments only a handful of men were placed in the guardhouse for intoxication. This ranged from only one per day on average, as in the Fifth Vermont, to fifteen per day as in the First Connecticut Artillery. In the latter unit Hough found the lieutenant colonel livid with anger at

Blenker's division for providing a poor example as well as a source of liquor for his artillerymen. Some regimental commanders admitted that alcohol abuse was the cause for all, or most, of their disciplinary headaches. But in the hard-drinking Thirty-Ninth New York, Col. Frederick G. D'Utassy believed that it accounted for only 5 percent of disciplinary infractions.[25]

The majority of camp inspection returns do not support the view that alcoholic consumption was endemic or a universal problem. Some regimental officers noted that it rose and fell according to circumstances. "No opportunities lost by some men" to acquire it, reported parties in Col. Hiram Berdan's two US sharpshooter regiments to W. S. Hough. "No, haven't learned the ropes yet," commented officers of the First Wisconsin Artillery to Robert Ware when telling him that the Second and Fourth Battalions had just arrived a week before from Racine to Fortress Monroe and had not yet found a source of liquor. Payday tended to lead to higher levels of intoxication in some regiments, while in others, "every chance they get they are drunk." In addition, those habitual drinkers tended to be public spectacles. When Dr. Elisha Harris inspected Camp Sprague near New York City, he was appalled at the sanitary condition of the entire compound. But on looking into the guardhouse, he found "more drunken men and more neglect of personal cleanliness than need to exist in an Army of 100,000 men."[26]

But the most striking lesson from the camp inspection returns is not the occasional sarcastic comment about soldiers longing for drink, but the many assertions that, even though some troops were habitual drinkers, the majority were sober most of the time. And for a few regiments at least, complete abstinence was the rule. George L. Andrews noted his impression that the men of Lt. Col. Andreas Brickel's First New York Light Artillery Battalion drank "more frequently than is usual in the vol. service generally" and that problems associated with intoxication were "more than common in the army." Yet he also mentioned that only two or three men of that unit were in the guardhouse on a daily basis due to intoxication. For a battalion-sized formation, that was a very low level of men locked up for infractions of the drinking rules. John H. Douglas noted an important point in his inspection of the Second Missouri, that "men drink but not to intoxication." The regimental sutler sold hard liquor, wine, and beer, and the Missourians also obtained alcohol from other sources, but the regiment rarely suffered any problems from it. In some units, such as the Seventh New York, officers worked hard to limit their men's access to the varied sources of liquor and succeeded. For a handful of units, the inspectors reported nearly complete sobriety. "A very temperate regiment," Alex McDonald wrote of the First

Maine Cavalry. In the Third Maine a group of soldiers staged a demonstration to tell their colonel that they did not appreciate the fact that the sutler was selling alcohol. They brought "several bottles of champaigne" and spilled them on the ground in front of their commander's tent, which led to the stopping of that sale.[27]

This is a part of the story of alcohol in the Union army that receives little attention from historians. A sizeable proportion of the force strongly adhered to principles of sobriety, reflecting the continued strength of the temperance and prohibition objectives of the antiliquor movement before the war. Soldiers like Lucius W. Barber of the Fifteenth Illinois and Jenkin Lloyd Jones of the Sixth Wisconsin Battery filled their personal accounts with evidence that they were disgusted by alcoholic consumption and its effects on the health and behavior of their comrades. A wide swath of other soldiers hovered in the middle ranges of the spectrum; sober most of the time, they drank to excess on the rare occasion when circumstances offered them the opportunity to imbibe more than was advisable. The true problem drinker, the man who habitually sought alcoholic stimulation, made up only a small proportion of each regiment. If John Billings was right on that score, then the proportion was close to 2 or 3 percent. In an unusual case, a Union medical inspector noted that 160 members of the Sixteenth Illinois were bona fide members of a temperance society.[28]

If historians look for evidence of riotous drunken behavior, they will have no trouble finding it in Civil War sources.[29] But there is an equally large body of primary evidence that paints a picture of sobriety. That is one of the more important values of the Sanitary Commission camp inspection returns. They take a more comprehensive view of the subject, cover a wide range of army units over time, and include thoughtful comments by outsiders looking into the regiment's life. These returns do not support the idea that Civil War armies were awash in liquor or were heavily taxed with the burden of dealing with drunken soldiers. Of 242 returns that specifically mention what regimental officers said about liquor in their commands, 51 (21.1 percent) indicated that there was no problem associated with intoxication or that the men did not obtain liquor to any appreciable degree. The rest, 191 (78.9 percent), indicated a willingness on the part of regimental officers to admit that intoxication did exist in their units at a level that was manageable. But the camp inspector did not just rely on the testimony of the unit's officers; he asked for statistics on the number of men held in the guardhouse on a daily basis and why they were incarcerated. Overwhelmingly, those guardhouse cases were caused by intoxication; but they involved only a handful of men. For a regiment with eight hundred or nine hundred men to have so few of them held for infractions of discipline associated with alcohol does not amount to a significant liquor problem. There are no readily available statistics such as these for civilian society in the Civil War era, but it is difficult to believe that this army ratio of drunkenness could be higher than that to be found among citizens.

The camp inspection returns reflect the conclusion that drunkenness was not endemic in the Union army. The inspectors gave an overall rating based not only on what the regimental commander told them about the topic but also on what they tried to objectively observe on their own. The good rating is 41.4 percent, the fair rating 38.5 percent, and the bad rating 20.1 percent. Rather than hopelessly mired in overindulgence, the Union army's experience with alcohol was decidedly mixed and much better than one would expect.

MORALE

Of all the fifteen subject areas encompassed by the Sanitary Commission camp inspection program, attention paid to soldier amusements is the most surprising. Civil War–era sanitarians concentrated on a man's physical health and paid limited attention to his morale. For that matter, no Civil War historian has yet identified this as an important topic of discussion. But the commission really pioneered in efforts to create soldier morale as a major subject of interest. It saw this as one part of a multilayered effort to shape an effective and healthy military organization. The commission's perception of soldier morale was crude by twentieth-century standards, but that merely heightens its significance as a pioneer of social engineering in the army.

The American army lagged behind the Continental European forces in efforts to shape morale. The French army served as a model of more advanced ideas. It had developed a system of gymnastic exercises that the Americans ignored when copying many other aspects of the French military system. In fact, a school of gymnastics was created near Vincennes to which every regiment sent a noncommissioned officer for six months of "scaling walls, swimming, fencing with the bayonet, singing, dancing, reading, [and] writing," as McClellan reported. Upon returning to his regiment, that noncommissioned officer was supposed to train his comrades along those lines. The British Army also ignored the gymnastics program but instituted instead a system of barrack libraries and reading rooms for troops stationed at permanent installations. British military bands were only partially funded by the government, which paid the salaries of musicians, but the other expenses were underwritten by stoppages from the salaries of officers and by annual subscriptions on the part of other army personnel.[30]

SANITARIANS AND THE ARMY ON SOLDIER AMUSEMENTS

"Much may be done to induce cheerfulness in an army," wrote Surgeon General Hammond. "Games of various kinds, especially such as require exercise in the open air, should be encouraged." The Sanitary Commission agreed. "When practicable," wrote W. H. Van Buren, such things as "running, leaping, wrestling, fencing, bayonet exercise, cricket, baseball, football, [and] quoits" could play a large role in relieving the boredom of camp life and diverting the men from harmful habits such as drinking. Hammond also urged that books "of a light character," amateur theatrics, and especially military music become part of a general program of amusing the men. He placed most emphasis on regimental bands. "We have never seen an intelligent soldier who did not take pleasure in the music the bands afforded."[31]

The Union army never instituted a program of morale boosting among the volunteers. One of the few nods in this direction appeared in July 1864, when Brig. Gen. Christopher C. Andrews issued a general order on the subject for his Second Division, Seventh Corps, which was stationed at Devall's Bluff, Arkansas. "The health of the soldier depends much upon the mental and moral influences around him as well as the physical," he informed his subordinates. Officers were saddled with the responsibility of "keeping up a cheerful and hopeful state of mind among the men; [they] should encourage amusements and diversions" in addition to maintaining a high level of camp sanitation so as to cover both the emotional and physical aspects of soldier maintenance.[32]

We have no idea how seriously Andrews's subordinates assumed their responsibility for amusing the troops, but judging from a broad survey of personal accounts by officers across the volunteer army, very few of them bothered to do so. Surg. John G. Perry of the Twentieth Massachusetts was very unusual in his effort to build a gymnasium at the regiment's winter quarters. "The officers are interested in the plan," he wrote, "and already we fence, box, and exercise every day, and feel much better for it."[33]

But for virtually all other regiments in the Union army, the men had to amuse themselves. For the most part, they did a decent job of it. When the Eighth Illinois Cavalry went into winter quarters at Alexandria, Virginia, early in 1862, the men "proceeded to enjoy themselves as well as they could, with such amusements as came to hand." That primarily meant reading and writing letters home. Another readily available source of diversion was an influx of newspapers and magazines into the semipermanent camps. Frederick W. Wild of Alexander's Baltimore Battery usually read them aloud to the four comrades with whom he shared a hut. "Checkers, dominoes and cards also helped to pass away the time," he recalled, "and a congenial happy group we were."[34]

Providing a band for each regiment was the only institutional support for a program of morale boosting offered by the government. But even there the officers and men were given the chance to contribute to its maintenance with their own funds. How important it was for the officers, especially, to publicly support the band was illustrated by the case of the First Rhode Island Cavalry. Early in the war no officers took an interest in it, at least according to bugler George Sargent, and as a consequence "the band took no interest in the regiment." Sargent noticed that at dress parade he often saw only half the band members playing while the rest were out "skylarking." Then Col. Alfred Duffié took command of the regiment and changed everything. He so enjoyed the band's performances that he established a fund for its benefit and required each company commander to contribute every month. The money was then divided among the band members as extra pay. Now they had every reason to take an interest in the regiment. The band also entertained at military hospitals, where surgeons praised its effect on the morale of the sick.[35]

Despite evidence that regimental bands played a significant role in soldier morale, the government decided to eliminate them in July 1862. This move had been building for several months. As early as December 1861, Benjamin F. Larned, the paymaster general of the US Army, complained to Sen. Henry Wilson of the Military Affairs Committee that regimental bands were "far more ornamental than useful, and should be abolished." He estimated it would save the government $5 million. Secretary of War Simon Cameron thought the bands should at least be reduced in size because "their usefulness [was] not at all commensurate with their heavy expense." On August 9, 1862, the army instructed its commanders to muster out of service all regimental band members. They were allowed to create brigade-level bands of no more than sixteen members by transferring the regimental musicians to the brigade band or by recruiting new musicians. This shortsighted move largely took military music out of the Union army, severely reducing its only real institutional support for soldier morale.[36]

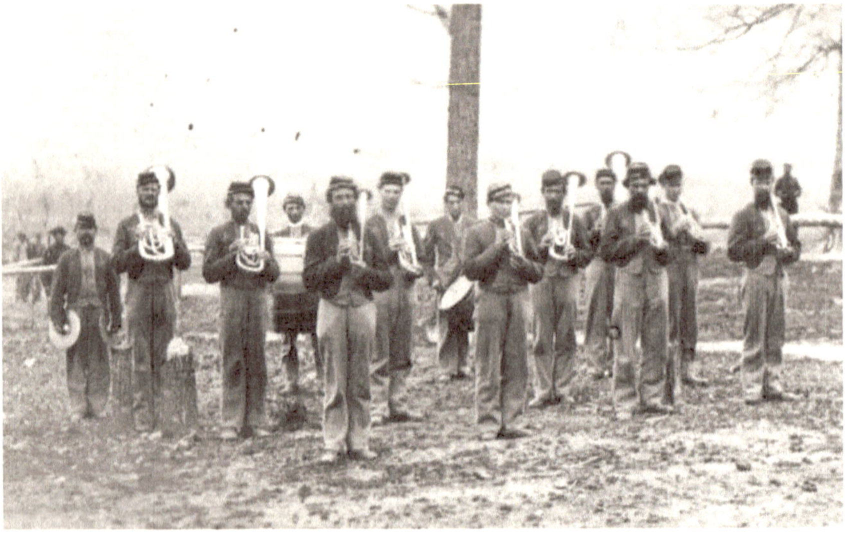

Twelfth Indiana Band. This photograph gives a good impression of what a scruffy field band on the regimental level looked like during the Civil War. The men are ready but look like they have seen hard service. They have deployed two drums, ten horns, and one cymbal. Col. Reuben Williams indicated that this band contained sixteen pieces by mid July 1863 and was one of only two regimental bands in the Fifteenth Corps at that time. (Williams, *General Reub Williams's Memories,* 108; Library of Congress, Prints & Photographs Division, LCDIG-ppmsca-71740)

The only other institutional element in the Union army that could be considered a diversion for the men was target practice. This normally would be regarded as an essential element of training, but the truth was that very little target shooting took place during the training phase of a regiment's war service. Officers of the army as well as the Sanitary Commission also viewed weapons firing to be an aspect of morale boosting because it naturally drew the interest of the men away from boredom. But the extent to which target shooting was pursued depended almost entirely on the regimental commander and thus varied widely across the Union army. A handful of officers took it seriously. For example, in the Twenty-Second Maine a firing range was created, with targets six feet tall and five feet wide placed "in front of some obstruction of timber, earth or other material." Guards used it when relieved so they could discharge their muskets while supervised by a noncommissioned officer between nine o'clock in the morning and one o'clock in the afternoon. But such an arrangement was unusual across the army's regiments, most of which set up no systematic approach to target shooting.[37]

SANITARY COMMISSION CAMP INSPECTION RETURNS

To gauge what if anything the army was doing to amuse the men, the Sanitary Commission standard camp-inspection form included ten questions under the heading "Recreations." The list began with, "Are the men generally in good spirits?" It then continued to question whether the regimental officers had instituted any systematic effort to arrest their boredom; if there was a band and whether the officers and men contributed funds for its maintenance; if a regimental library existed and whether it consisted mostly of religious reading matter; if there was no library, whether newspapers and other material circulated through the ranks; and whether target shooting constituted any part of a morale-boosting effort.

Of 280 returns, information specifically about anything that could be termed a regimental system of soldier amusements appeared in only 179. Of that number, only 29 units (16.3 percent of the total) could lay claim to such a system. These included regiments in which the chaplain did something special, usually collecting books for a regimental library. In contrast, for 150 of the 179 regiments (83.7 percent), inspectors reported there was no system that attempted to instill soldier morale.

Despite that very poor showing, the returns offer overwhelming evidence that the men were in generally good spirits. Of course, this may have involved a good deal of exaggeration, for how can a regimental officer accurately characterize the mood of several hundred men? Plus, there could have been some degree of wanting to create a good image of the regiment for the commission inspector. But we cannot go too far in questioning the results of these returns. We can assume that the men were typically happy to rely on their own resources for amusement and felt no real need for the army to divert their attention. Specific information about the troops' mood was mentioned on 246 returns—of that number 228 (92.6 percent) indicated they were cheerful, while 9 (3.7 percent) were listed as in fairly good spirits and another 9 (3.7 percent) in poor spirits.

As the only institutional support for morale, the regimental band figured prominently on the standard inspection form. It was specifically mentioned on 171 returns dated from the start of the war to August 1862. Of that number, 94 (54.9 percent) indicated that the unit had a regimental band, while 77 (45.1 percent) did not. That is a bit astonishing, but one must remember that it was difficult to find competent musicians willing to volunteer for army service. Moreover, 8 of the 171 returns dealt with artillery batteries, which were not allowed a band by army regulations. Still, it is telling that even during the first fifteen months of the war, when regimental bands were allowed, nearly half the volunteer units did not have one. After August 1862, when regimental bands were no longer allowed, 23 of 25 returns that specifically mention bands indicated that the regiment had none. Ironically, two regiments in that time period still maintained a band, somehow managing to retain their musicians without anyone in the army administration objecting.

There is evidence in the returns that many men appreciated the music of regimental bands and regretted their absence even during the first fifteen months of the war. Robert Jones visited the Fortieth New York, which had no military music. "If we only had a band I should like camp life better," one of the regimental sergeants told him, "but now I get wearied." The value of military music was appreciated so much by the Twenty-First Illinois that even after August 1862 it maintained a band on its own resources. The colonel detailed men from the ranks who were willing to try their hand at playing and hired a civilian to lead them, paying him seventy-five dollars per month. The officers and men raised more than one thousand dollars to purchase instruments. While the brigade enjoyed the playing of this regimental band, it did not contribute to its upkeep. In the First Kentucky, which did not have a band, officers encouraged the drum-and-fife men assigned the unit to give concerts. The star was Louis H. Hoeke, a gifted musician who played a silver fife given him by Brig. Gen. William Sooy Smith on the occasion of his promotion to second lieutenant in December 1862. Bettelheim was enchanted by Hoeke's playing when he visited the regiment.[38]

Hoeke's example highlights the fact that many Civil War soldiers not only valued music in the army but also were willing to find ways to gain access to it. In the Second and Fourth Battalions of the First Wisconsin Artillery, a company of Germans created their own private band by bringing instruments from home. A privately obtained melodeon supported the efforts of a glee club that was created among First Connecticut artillerymen, and the First Minnesota must have had music because John H. Douglas found the men "dancing every evening" when he visited the regiment. Officers and men of the Forty-Fifth Massachusetts footed the bill to maintain a regimental band in early 1863 in defiance of the government's refusal to support such things. Of course, these were the rare exceptions. The majority of regiments accepted the absence of a band without a murmur.[39]

The only other major topic addressing soldier amusements in the returns related to the creation and maintenance of libraries. Few units bothered to create one. Only 83 returns refer to regimental or company libraries or to the informal circulation of reading matter such as newspapers, magazines, and books from one man to another. In other words, reading was highlighted as a significant feature of camp life in only 29.6 percent of the units represented by the 280 camp inspection returns. Target practice held an even lower profile, with only 20 of the 280 returns—7.1 percent—mentioning it.

"The spirits of the men are excellent, as a general thing, but as to the means of keeping them in that state, they are left entirely to their own resources." Thus concluded Godfrey Aigner of the many regiments he inspected around Cairo in the fall of 1861, and his comment applied to the majority of all units visited by commission agents. In a handful of regiments, the troops engaged in sports and other athletic competitions. Although the chaplain of the Fifteenth New York Engineers told William Chamberlain that the men were "too *old* to play" games, inspectors found them playing football in the Thirty-Sixth New York, baseball in the Second Rhode Island, and quoits in Battery A, New Jersey Light Artillery. Other men were engaged in "considerable card playing" in the Seventh New Jersey; performing gymnastics in the First Minnesota; and rolling "ten pins" in the First Michigan Engineers and Mechanics.[40]

Regimental chaplains were in a position to play an important role in soldier morale, but they did not take full advantage of it. The majority of units that had no reading material was largely a fault of the chaplains. They had more time and opportunity than regimental officers to gather in books and manage their distribution. Of course, most of their time was spent in religious matters, which also were components of soldier morale. For example, the Second New Jersey had "a large prayer tent, Prayer meetings regularly," reported Franklin B. Hough. But the Sanitary Commission was not interested in the men's religious life; it included no questions on that topic on any of the standard inspection forms. Nevertheless, Hough recorded in detail the many activities of Chaplain Edward A. Walker for the First Connecticut Artillery, which ranged from holding prayer meetings to supplying the men with blankets from their home state. But Walker did nothing of a secular nature to amuse the troops. Bettelheim frequently advised regimental chaplains to be active in finding reading matter for the men, but as an overzealous missionary himself, he tended to urge them to secure religious tracts. The Sanitary Commission preferred a body of reading material of a more varied and secular kind.[41]

In a small number of regiments, inspectors found libraries similar to the type that the commission wished to see. The Forty-Eighth Pennsylvania had company-level libraries with twenty-four books in each, although the volumes were mostly of a religious character, while Battery A, New Jersey Light Artillery had a library contributed by the "Ladies of Jersey City," which was not mainly religious. "There is considerable reading," reported Edward A. Crane about the Second Vermont, which had a library of one hundred volumes. That collection paled in comparison with the First Connecticut Artillery, the chaplain of which collected five hundred books and boasted that fewer than 10 men out of the 891 in the regiment were illiterate. Of the Thirty-Sixth Illinois, Douglas reported that only 9 of 1,158 men were unable to sign their payroll. The chaplain in charge of the regimental library of the Tenth Iowa noted, "Men very fond of reading, but also of retaining books & magazines." Troops who desired a library in the Thirty-Sixth Illinois managed to raise three hundred dollars from their comrades to create one. Most regiments without formal libraries still had reading matter; four hundred New York newspapers were sold daily to the First and Second US Sharpshooters in February 1862. But in some units the desire for books overrode newspapers as a source of reading interest.[42]

As with music, examples of efforts to establish unit libraries were comparatively rare. Most regiments had no library of any kind. Both Bettelheim and Alfred L. Castleman remarked on the scarcity of regimental libraries. Bettelheim, in fact, noted that the Fifth Indiana Battery received a small library from a Mr. Clark in Indianapolis, but the men "traded off the books for one thing or another, because of their [the books] being too religious." When Castleman asked the Thirty-Sixth Illinois chaplain what kind of books the men wished to add to their privately financed regimental library, he found they included "*Dick's Works* McCauley, Bancroft, Addison, Fielding and a list of others which would have graced the library of a literary Savan." But most units relied on private means and peddler sales for any influx of books, magazines, and newspapers. Marvin M. Marsh believed that all New England units received a good deal of periodical literature from their friends at home, which enlivened their days in camp. But he also suggested regulating the men's exposure to certain kinds of politically controversial reading. Marsh recommended excluding the *New York Express* and the *New York World* from the camp of the 174th Pennsylvania at Beaufort, South Carolina, because their antiwar tone was eroding morale among the troops. Over and above considerations of how newspapers influenced morale, another factor came into play. The desire to read any kind of material was to a great degree limited among the young men who formed the volunteer army of the Union. "Not reading men generally," noted Aigner of the Thirty-First Illinois; the same undoubtedly applied to many other regiments as well.[43]

As mentioned earlier, commission inspectors overwhelmingly reported that the men were in fine spirits, and we must give a good deal of credence to that conclusion. On rare occasions did the inspectors report poor spirits. These instances usually stemmed from long delays in receiving pay (six months in the case of the Second Pennsylvania Heavy Artillery), recent defeat in battle (as with the Third Maine after First Bull Run), or poor clothing (as with the Second Iowa Battery). Morale in the First Regiment, Corps d'Afrique was low because the government shamefully paid Black troops less money than white soldiers. In some instances there was just a general feeling of depression, as with the Ninth New Hampshire, which occupied a horrible camp in January 1863. In others the men could more clearly identify what made them discontent. Henry W. Warriner recorded the list he found among members of a battalion of the First Nebraska Cavalry at Benton Barracks, St. Louis. "They grumble about Barracks clothing, cooking (at times) and the absence of arms. Amusements meager irregular & drills." The battalion had no band, no library, and only a few odd newspapers circulating through the ranks.[44]

The majority of camp inspection returns reveal that the men relied on their own resources to pass time in the army. Inspectors noted that they "amuse themselves" and at times delineated the many ways the more enterprising among the troops could do so. In the Twentieth New York, E. J. Dunning reported "evening entertainments, illuminations, music, [and] games," noting, "there is in their movements and the expression of their faces a certain vivacity that I have not observed in other regiments."[45]

If most of the returns had reported hopeful signs as those Dunning found in the Twentieth New York, the Sanitary Commission would have been delighted. But the camp inspection program failed to delight on the score of soldier morale. It was encouraging that most regiments seemed to be in good spirits but not helpful that the army did so little to shape those spirits. The important point as far as the Sanitary Commission was concerned was to urge the army to take an active role in creating troop morale, and in that sense the army largely failed. Of the 280 returns used in this study, in only 26.7 percent did the unit rate good in the area of encouraging soldier morale. For the rest, 38.6 percent rated fair and 34.7 percent rated bad. The men may have been generally happy, but the army had done very little to make them so.

After the war, when army surgeons compiled the multivolume *Medical and Surgical History of the War of the Rebellion,* they admitted that depression was a significant factor in soldier health. Everyone was subject to dejection at the "discomfort, hardships, and exposures" of army life, but when temporary depression became morbid, it was designated as nostalgia. "This must therefore be regarded as a camp disease of the war period," the authors concluded. But they asserted that nostalgia was infrequent, with 2.34 cases per 1,000 white troops annually. The authors encouraged the army in future to identify those men who were "leading spirits" in every command, men who could carry along their comrades into sports or amateur entertainments. They envisioned the appointment of an officer in every command to serve as "Superintendent of Public Amusements," who would manage all efforts along this line. This was particularly important during the long months spent in semipermanent camps. Support for institutional measures to encourage soldier morale also came from regimental surgeons. O. W. Long of the Eleventh Illinois wrote to the Sanitary Commission soon after the war to share his views. "Music and cheerful games generally beget a cheerful frame of mind, improve and invigorate all the functions of the Body and are valuable as a Prophylactic. Nearly all the Maladies of Camp may be much alleviated by these means." In short, for at least some members of the military system, there was much that could be done to avert nostalgia and encourage a positive attitude among soldiers.[46]

The war experience had heightened the army's institutional awareness of soldier morale and how important it could be for officers to take an interest in shaping it. But that heightened awareness came too late to have an effect during the war. Moreover, it had no effect on current or future practice in the post–Civil War army. The culture of mid-nineteenth-century America was not conducive to the idea of social shaping by large institutions, even though only a few decades later that idea would firmly take root with the developing corporate culture of the industrial era. The concept found fertile ground in the US Army only during World War I. Until then, American soldiers largely had to shape their own emotional well-being.

From water to alcohol to morale, the army devoted greater or lesser degrees of care in soldier health. Officers strove to find enough potable water to sustain the troops and limit the supply of liquor to reduce disciplinary problems, but they paid little attention to diverting the men when lying idle. The environment of the semipermanent camp was especially conducive to success in water supply because there was an opportunity to select campsites that were within easy reach of good natural sources of water. But the camps, with their opportunities for idleness, also became environments conducive to the infiltration of liquor into army life. Officers had to be extra vigilant to cut off that supply. In addition, this idleness increased the importance of tending to the mood of the men. As with so many other challenges concerning soldier life, the army largely succeeded in supplying decent water and limited the supply of alcohol well enough to get by. Its comparative lack of support for soldier morale was offset only by the native tendency of the young volunteers to find their own happiness.

8

Recruit Examination and Vaccination

Two subject areas on the Sanitary Commission standard form dealt with important issues relating to the induction of volunteers into their regimental service. The notion that surgeons had a responsibility to thoroughly examine the physical and mental condition of the enlistee before he was mustered in, rejecting the unfit to save the government the expense of caring for a soldier unable to perform his duties, was well established both in Europe and the United States before 1861. The other responsibility, also requiring a conscientious approach by surgeons, was to make sure that all enlistees were protected from smallpox by vaccinating those not already immunized. This idea also was very well established in Europe and in the United States and, in fact, had deep roots in the civilian societies of the Western world. Blessed with time and opportunity, the prewar US Army did a good job of handling both requirements. But with the onset of the Civil War and the need to quickly raise a huge volunteer force, both of these necessary medical tasks were only partially performed.

RECRUIT EXAMINATION

Civil War surgeons had plenty of information readily available to guide them in examining enlistees before muster in. The European experience in this regard was a potent example. No matter whether they used a comprehensive system of conscription or relied on volunteers, all major European armies emphasized medical examination as a key filter to weed out the unfit before their government invested funds in training recruits. All of them publicized in detail the standards used in their examinations, which were quite similar to those adopted by the US Army long before the outbreak of the Civil War. Britain's policies came closest to those of the United States because both countries relied fully on volunteering to fill the ranks before the war, and the Federal government largely continued to do so during the conflict itself. In Britain surgeons distinguished between recruits from towns and those from the countryside. They preferred the latter because rural men's physical development at the chest and the extremities was more advanced. City recruits tended to have less endurance and a generally lower standard of health.[1]

Statistics on the ratio of rejection at enlistment reflect a thorough job of applying military standards for physical and mental development. For example, of 13,949 recruits examined at Dublin for British service, 3,032 were rejected for poor health, "weakness of intellect," and other causes. In France 5,818,944 men were examined from 1816 to 1835, with 1,076,130 rejected. In the United States the mandate was for a thorough inspection that resulted in some very high rates of rejection. In 1852 army surgeons examined 16,064 enlistees and turned away 13,338 of them—nearly 2,500 because they could not speak English—accepting only 2,726 (16.9 percent) of the men who volunteered. This was an especially low rate of acceptance; on average, a bit more than 5,000 men had been accepted yearly from 1849 to 1855. American statistics, on average, were well within the average rate of rejections in Britain and France from the 1830s to the 1860s.[2]

RECRUIT EXAMINATION IN THE VOLUNTEER FORCE

Authorities tried to enforce the same high standards for enlistees into the volunteer Union force as it had maintained for the regular army. Recruits were to be "minutely examined by the surgeon and assistant surgeon of the regiment." If someone slipped past this filter and was discharged within three months of muster in "for a disability which existed" at enlistment, he would receive no pay or allowances except for food and transportation home. "Any free white male person" who was eighteen to thirty-five years old; at least five feet, three inches tall (no maximum height was specified); and "effective, able-bodied, sober, free from disease, of good character and habits, and with a competent knowledge of the English language, may be enlisted." The age and height standards did not apply to those who had previously served in the army or to musicians. Most of these basic requirements were included in army regulations and promulgated through a general order issued on August 3, 1861. The minimum-height regulation was promulgated through a separate general order dated August 17, 1861, and represented a reduction from the prewar standard of five feet, four and a half inches. By November 28, 1864, Secretary of War Stanton reduced the standard height further to just five feet.[3]

The problem was that relatively few volunteer surgeons fully performed their duty in examining recruits. It was a mistake to rely on doctors without military experience, who joined the service at the same time as the regimental officers and men, to perform this important task. It was best done by a medical officer who had experience and no connection with the regiment, but the regular army simply did not have enough surgeons to go around. The system relied on a self-regulated process by men who had many incentives not to be too critical about examining enlistees. Officers wanted to keep regimental numbers high so that the unit did not fall below the minimal strength required for muster in. They outranked the surgeons and could apply pressure on them to quickly and uncritically look over the men before the mustering officer swore them in.

Godfrey Aigner noted this problem after visiting many units around Cairo in the fall of 1861. All of them, except those raised in Missouri, had something like a medical inspection at enlistment, but none of those checks were thorough. The regiments that underwent a retro-examination after enlistment also were not thoroughly scrutinized. Aigner estimated that at least one out of ten men should have been rejected and probably would be discharged for medical reasons before long. It was more difficult, however, to get a discharge for medical reasons approved than it was to reject a recruit before muster in, and Aigner feared that this problem would raise the mortality rate among these regiments in the following few months.[4]

Surgeon General Hammond was well aware of this problem. He had heard of many instances wherein the regimental surgeon simply walked along the line of men, looking at them along the way, before muster in. One surgeon told Hammond that his colonel absolutely refused to let him have the men strip to be properly examined. Surg. De Witt C. Peters, in an article titled "Remarks on the Evils of Youthful Enlistments," castigated regimental officers for their shortsightedness. "Instead of being anxious to obtain numbers, all officers should be governed by a desire to select none but serviceable men."[5]

Surg. Abner Hard knew that the examination he conducted for the Eighth Illinois Cavalry was not according to regulations, but he had no choice in the matter. The men marched past him, and if he saw any with obvious physical defects, he pulled them out of the column and rejected them. "This was the only examination," and Hard was convinced he could have saved the government much money if he had been allowed to conduct it as the regulations stipulated. Roberts Bartholow also experienced the difficulties faced by conscientious surgeons when it came to examining recruits. A regular army surgeon, he was allowed only a "hasty and most superficial examination" that consisted of walking along the ranks with the colonel and looking at the men. Some were obviously unfit, but if he rejected too many of them, the colonel complained about it. Even when a surgeon examined recruits according to the rules, it was possible for the recruit to circumvent him. George Sargent tried to enlist in the Twenty-Fifth Massachusetts, but the surgeon advised him to reconsider. "You had ought to be put out to pasture in order to fatten up a little," the medical officer told him. "Your bones are too prominent. I will give you until tomorrow to think of it." Sargent did think of it but decided to enlist instead in the First New England Cavalry, which was later designated the First Rhode Island Cavalry, and its surgeon readily accepted him.[6]

This problem was not confined to the initial phase of the war but persisted throughout the conflict whenever new regiments were raised. It inflicted a noticeable burden on the military system because thousands of men unfit for field service had to be taken into the hospitals and eventually discharged after performing little if any duty for the government. In some cases, admittedly, those physical defects were not apparent at muster in but became evident after a few months of service. But in others it should have been obvious from the start. Bartholow saw the result of all this. While serving as surgeon in charge of a military hospital at Fort Schuyler, New York, he encountered many patients who were underage or overage and should never have been allowed into the army.[7]

In contrast to the "loose system" of recruit examination in volunteer units, Bartholow discussed the proper way to filter enlistees before muster in while writing a book sanctioned by Surgeon General Hammond and published in 1864. Bartholow advised examining surgeons to make the enlistee walk briskly three or four times around the room and then hop for a while, after which the physician ought to pay close attention to the man's hearing, speech, sight, ears, mouth, and intellect. He wrote that a thorough examination included the recruit stripping and that his chest, abdomen, and legs should also be examined. The ideal recruit in Bartholow's view was of medium height and compactly built. He warned against men of unusual height or weight and favored those between five feet, six inches and five feet, ten inches tall. Bartholow thought that anyone over six feet, three inches was less able to endure field service. He noted that Americans tended to be taller and thinner than Europeans, blaming it on tobacco use. The army did not correlate weight with height in its induction standards, but Bartholow thought this was important. Anyone who was five feet, three inches tall should weigh at least 120 pounds at muster in. On the other end of the spectrum, anyone more than 220 pounds without some "corresponding height and muscular sufficiency" should be rejected.[8]

Hammond also criticized the recruit-examination process in his own book. He was sure European armies did a better job of weeding out the unfit than did the volunteer system of the United States. One difference was the minimum age, typically higher in Europe than eighteen years. "Boys do not make good soldiers," Hammond wrote. He admitted seeing many of them younger than eighteen years in the army. Many physicians argued that a man did not achieve full physical maturity until age twenty-five, but Hammond allowed that, at least in the United States, the threshold could be set at age twenty. By the time one reached their thirties, their personal habits were set, making them poorer candidates for army service, and between thirty-five and fifty-five, their ability to perform arduous service in the field steadily declined. One could not expect anyone over forty-five to endure campaign and battle. Lung power, measured in part by chest capacity, was a vital element in soldiering, although physicians were divided on how best to judge this. As a rule, men over six feet, three inches did not make good soldiers unless they had commensurate development in their muscles and lung capacity. Hammond suggested that the army set twenty as the minimum enlistment age and 125 pounds as the minimum weight, increasing the ratio five pounds per inch so that at six feet, seven inches, the corresponding ideal weight should be 195 pounds.[9]

Unlike other commentators on recruitment examination, Hammond paid attention to the temperament of the enlistee as a filtering element. He divided this topic into four categories. Men of a sanguine temperament, he believed, were good at making charges but less able on the defensive. They were hopeful and influenced others to be as well. Men of phlegmatic temperament were slow and indecisive but would do well serving in heavy artillery units. Those of choleric temperament were firm and determined, making them "admirably qualified for military service." But those of nervous temperament did not make good soldiers. "The nervous temperament itself is almost a pathological condition," Hammond declared.[10]

When the Federal government instituted a national draft in March 1863, it relied on the Provost Marshal General's Bureau in the War Department to handle it. This bureau not only managed conscription but also was charged with managing new men who volunteered to serve in preexisting volunteer regiments. It instituted a thorough system of physical examination of both drafted and volunteer men very much in line with prescribed standards. The men undressed, and the surgeon paid attention to a long list of items concerning their fitness for soldiering. Each physician could process forty men a day, taking more time with drafted men because they tended to feign illness. The Medical Branch of the bureau was created in January 1864 to maintain records of the 1,014,776 men who were examined during the last half of the war.[11]

SANITARY COMMISSION CAMP INSPECTION RETURNS

But the system of thorough examination created by 1863 was not applied to the majority of volunteer regiments that fought the Civil War. Our best insight into the process whereby they entered Federal service is the result of the Sanitary Commission's camp inspection program, which is weighted toward the early part of the war before the Provost Marshal General's examination program was created. The standard form contained seven questions regarding this topic. They helped inspectors establish whether an examination was conducted before muster in and whether it was thorough. They also directed his attention to whether a follow-through examination was conducted after muster in and how thorough it might have been.

The returns indicate that a thorough examination was conducted in only 18.5 percent of the 280 units inspected. For 57.2 percent of the units inspected, some partial degree of examination occurred, and no examination was indicated for 24.3 percent. By army regulations, all regiments were supposed to do a full and thorough examination, and the fact that less than one-fifth of them fulfilled that requirement says a great deal about the laxness with which the Union's volunteer army was created. A heavy majority of regiments instituted what can be counted as little more than the form of an examination, which also reflects negatively on the volunteer force. As far as the army and the sanitarians were concerned, a partial examination was only slightly better than no examination—it fell very far short of orders and expectations. The returns reflect negatively on the volunteer regiments when it came to remedial examinations after muster in as well. Only 25 regiments conducted a meaningful physical examination of the men after the unit was sworn in to Federal service. That represented only 11.1 percent of the 225 returns that mention the important topic of remedial examination.

Some regimental surgeons were frank with commission inspectors about this issue. They tried to ameliorate the negative consequences of failing to properly examine recruits by noting that they readily discharged men who reported health conditions that obviously predated their enlistment. This occurred during a remedial examination or when the men reported at sick call. The number discharged after enlistment for health conditions that either obviously or probably had been contracted before enlistment ranged from 8 to 117 men in any given regiment. In two units surgeons provided enough data for the inspector to report on the percentage of men thus discharged compared to the strength of the regiment. In the Third New York Cavalry that was 3.4 percent, and in the Second Pennsylvania Heavy Artillery it was 14 percent. In a rare instance, the surgeon of the Second Louisiana (US) had conducted a thorough examination just before muster in and rejected 10 percent of the enlistees, a percentage that fell well within the rejection rate for the remedial examinations conducted in the Third New York Cavalry and the Second Pennsylvania Heavy Artillery.[12]

A number of regimental surgeons stressed to the inspectors that they conducted a "weeding out" process after muster in. No one conducted this remedial program better than Surg. R. W. Hazlett of the Second Virginia (US), which later was designated the Second West Virginia and still later the Fifth West Virginia Cavalry. He rejected 122 men out of 1,040 men, or 11.7 percent. Hazlett found among the dismissed men many hernias, ulcers, and rheumatism as well as some who suffered from defective sight and hearing. A dozen of these rejected men were later returned to the regiment by his superiors in the medical chain of command, but Hazlett also sent a number of regimental members to the general hospital for conditions that probably had been contracted before enlistment.[13]

The statistics on the percentage of enlistees found unfit for military service confirm the necessity of a good examination, and those regimental officials who fulfilled army directives were happy to tell commission inspectors about it. The surgeon of the First Wisconsin Artillery informed Robert Ware that the "men stripped" for the examination. Officers of the Eleventh New York Battery and Twelfth New York Battery told Franklin B. Hough that their units adhered to army regulations in the filtering process. The Twentieth New York had not one but three examinations. The first took place just before muster in, when thirty-seven men were rejected. Then the state ordered another examination, which led to eleven men being rejected. A US officer conducted the third examination, rejecting three additional men.[14]

For those regiments that failed to examine the men properly, a number of reasons were offered. With the Nineteenth Indiana, it was considered "too expensive." Officers of the Second New York Light Artillery blamed the surgeon, who "was a poor physician. Passed some improper men." But the most common complaint was that the surgeon was not given the opportunity to properly inspect the recruits. "He merely looked at & asked them whether they had any diseases. This was all," wrote Bernard J. Bettelheim about how Dr. A. W. Hiese examined the men of the 100th Illinois.[15]

The problems resulting from lax enforcement of the physical examination became apparent pretty quickly. To a greater or lesser extent, every regiment had to deal with a percentage of its personnel who could not meet the physical challenges of camp life. In the Nineteenth Indiana Surg. C. J. Woods estimated that 150 men were "not fit for service." He discharged 100 of them by the time Franklin B. Hough visited the regiment and was working on the remaining 50 cases. "Men were enlisted who had crooked feet, hernias, scropula & c & c." Col. Solomon Meredith of the Nineteenth Indiana "thought Medical Inspection superfluous. Those who should be discharged are hollow hearted feeble, and frail men, some with constitutional diseases." James Gall found about thirty personnel in the First US Colored Troops to be boys under age fifteen who "have never been able to do soldier's duty, have done nothing in fact but enlarge the expense of the government & swell the sick list of their regiment."[16]

Overall, the volunteer regiments did quite poorly in the important task of weeding out physically unfit enlistees. The primary reasons for this stem from the hasty way in which the regiments were organized, the fact that their officers were as green as the men in understanding what the regular army had long known, and the officers' unwillingness to quickly learn from the army establishment how important it was for the government not to be burdened with soldiers unable to perform their duties. There were a number of subsidiary reasons for this failure, but the most important stemmed from the very nature of the mobilization policy the nation had followed since its founding nearly a century before.

The real problem here was that the bulk of the Union army was raised in an atmosphere of spirited volunteerism in several gushes over the course of the war. Few officials wanted to curb that enthusiasm by telling men they were not welcome in the army, and regimental officers wanted to have the largest numbers on their enlistment rolls as possible. But this was not the only way in which the Union army was raised; much of it was done in a less hurried, less frenzied manner that allowed the medical staff to properly examine prospective soldiers. Even in distant California, enlistees underwent a proper medical examination. After the Provost Marshal General's Bureau in the War Department exerted control of mobilization, thorough examinations became the norm. They were largely performed by civilian surgeons adhering to army standards who rejected volunteers and drafted men at the proportion of 319 per 1,000 by November 1863; the average in Britain and France at the time was 451 men per 1,000. Col. James B. Fry, the provost marshal general, noted that by October 1863, the army had medically discharged 200,000 men since the start of the war. He estimated that half of them probably had been unfit for service from the start and, based on that, assumed the Federal government had spent $40 million on those soldiers who gave little and in some cases no real service to the cause.[17]

Fry's estimate that 100,000 men had been discharged for causes that should have been weeded out at muster in is probably too high. Rather than half, it could have been up to one-third of the 200,000 discharged by October 1863. But even that more limited proportion might have saved the government $26 million and a lot of trouble. Recruit examination was an important gatekeeping mechanism fully understood by the army establishment and the sanitarians but not by the volunteer officers or the rank and file throughout the Civil War.

VACCINATION

The need to protect the men from the dangers of smallpox also proved to be important in the molding of an effective volunteer army for the Union. But in this case that importance was far more widely understood and taken seriously than recruit examination. The Civil War occurred at the end of a long period of American history in which smallpox had greatly declined due to widespread vaccination, but the disease was by no means eliminated. Volunteer officers and surgeons were relatively careful to vaccinate the men early in their unit's service and reacted swiftly at the first indication of any outbreak in the rank and file.

SMALLPOX IN AMERICA

Smallpox was truly a scourge of humanity, leading to death in some cases and terrible suffering and scarring among those it spared. Armies were especially susceptible to this disease. British soldiers had suffered horribly from it during the Seven Years' War (1756–63), when about a quarter of those affected died. This experience led to mandatory inoculation in the British force during the American Revolutionary War. Inoculation, or the transfer of matter from a sore to a well person to prime his body's defenses, had been practiced in the British colonies since the 1720s. Its efficacy was demonstrated in an outbreak of the disease in Boston in 1721, when 2 percent of those inoculated died in comparison to 14 percent who had not been inoculated. George Washington mandated inoculation for the Continental Army in 1777. He had survived a bout with smallpox at age nineteen and pushed inoculation against some resistance from the rank and file.[18]

The symptoms of smallpox were very serious. Twelve days after exposure, one broke out with "headache, chills, backache, high fever, vomiting, and anxiety." Then four days after the start of symptoms, a rash appeared on the "face, chest, arms, back and legs." Then sores developed in the mouth, throat, and nasal passages, followed by more sores on the skin, including the palms of the hands and soles of the feet. In the worst cases these sores "ran together into an oozing mass." It took ten days for scabs to form over these sores, and permanent scarring often resulted. Spread by physical contact, the victim was contagious from the first appearance of symptoms to the end of the outbreak four weeks later.[19]

English physician Edward Jenner played an important role in the war against smallpox. Mostly, his contribution lay in scientifically analyzing the process of inoculation and popularizing it in the Western world. He also used cowpox as the agent rather than material from a smallpox-infected person. Jenner was not by any means the originator of either concept, but his persistent advocacy of inoculation (a term that was interchangeably used with vaccination) from 1798 on proved to be a watershed in the struggle against this disease. In the United States vaccination became so widespread that by the 1840s, many felt smallpox had largely been eliminated. Mandatory vaccination programs in many European nations bore fruit; no epidemic outbreak of the disease had occurred in Austria or Prussia, for example, during the half century before the Civil War. But some degree of opposition against vaccination arose by the 1850s. That opposition included an argument that it did not work, that poor procedure could lead to unintended health problems, that it could introduce new diseases, and that compulsory vaccination was repugnant to an individual's control over his or her own body.[20]

The US Army practiced vaccination during the 1850s. All recruits were required to be vaccinated unless they showed signs of prior immunization, which was a scar on the arm. The vaccine used originated from cows, but by the 1850s, it had been propagated from person to person like the older system of inoculation. Called "vaccine," this matter tended to be generated by individuals who recruited people, especially poor children, to serve as the producer. When pustules formed on the skin, the liquid could be used for a quick inoculation or the scab could be taken and dried for later use. Scabs became the primary method of vaccinating soldiers because of their long period of potency. They were moistened, mashed up, and then placed into newly made small wounds in the person to be vaccinated. If many soldiers had to be treated, it was common to vaccinate them in waves so that scabs from members of the first wave could be used for treating men in subsequent waves, thus limiting the need for more scabs to be shipped to the army.[21]

It was not a foolproof system. Spurious vaccinations were those that did not take properly. Instead of the normal small pustule, a sign of success, more serious ulceration developed and in some cases syphilis as well. Even without these serious complications, it was found that the first man to be vaccinated typically received the expected immunity, but the effectiveness of the material declined when it was taken from him to his comrades. The more often vaccine was replicated wave to wave, the lower the level of effectiveness. In addition, some of the original matter received from the vaccine farms was inert and proved to be useless.[22]

Statistics provided powerful evidence that a proper system of vaccination was a lifesaver. A team of physicians writing in the *Transactions of the American Medical Association* in 1866 argued for the "immensely protective" nature of inoculation, which provided "almost perfect" protection against death by smallpox. Among adults who had "good marks of vaccination," 40.5 percent could be considered "perfectly protected" because they did not develop pustules on additional inoculations. The rest could be brought up to that stage with more vaccine. The team recommended that everyone be revaccinated at least every five years and whenever they were exposed to the disease. Evidence indicated that vaccination was effective even if administered as many as four days after exposure.[23]

THE ARMY AND SMALLPOX

Despite the problems and limitations, vaccination had reached a stage wherein it severely reduced the scourge of smallpox in mid-nineteenth America. With the raising of the huge volunteer army, deep concerns about a renewed threat from the disease emerged early in the war. Sanitarians strongly advised the vaccination of all enlistees who lacked signs of prior immunization as soon as possible. The Sanitary Commission assigned F. G. Smith and Alfred Stillé to write a paper on the value of vaccination for military service. Quickly put together and published in 1861, this report noted the lingering doubts entertained by many Americans about the efficacy and safety of immunization and sought to allay that resistance by marshaling statistics to prove its worth in battling the disease. Those statistics spanned the continent of Europe, extending decades into the past. At the least, this data indicated that vaccination lowered the mortality rate of those exposed to smallpox even if it did not grant complete immunity. Smith and Stillé argued that repeated vaccinations greatly increased the body's defense against the disease, although admitting that over a long period of time, even repeated doses wore off. All armies in Europe practiced initial vaccination of recruits previously unvaccinated, and most of them also practiced revaccination to increase immunity. Smith and Stillé recommended that the Union army revaccinate all soldiers who could not prove they had been vaccinated within the previous five years.[24]

The Federal government required that all volunteers be vaccinated at least once at muster in, but it left revaccination up to the discretion of the regimental surgeon. In a small number of cases, those physicians examined all men of their unit for signs of previous inoculation and maintained thorough records. In the Twenty-First New York, for example, Surg. Charles H. Wilcox and Asst. Surg. Joseph A. Peters found that 644 of 706 men (91.2 percent) showed signs of previous vaccination. They noted that 167 men had been vaccinated within the past seven years, and 477 before that time. This data strongly indicates how widespread vaccination was practiced in civilian society before the Civil War, a point that New York Surg. General S. O. Vanderpoel reinforced when he reported that 7,765 of 9,548 men examined (81.3 percent) showed signs of previous inoculation.[25]

Revaccinating those previously inoculated provided an opportunity to see how resistance to smallpox could be reinforced by repeated applications of the vaccine. If it produced pustules, the man was considered to have been susceptible to both the vaccine and the virus, and the new application was considered to have strengthened his immunity. Wilcox and Peters found, however, that a relatively small proportion of men in the Twenty-First New York showed no signs of prior vaccination even though they insisted they had been inoculated. But for most, this process of gauging resistance seemed to be valid. Vanderpoel reported that of 2,292 men found susceptible on revaccination, 1,338 of them (58.3 percent) had marks of previous vaccination.[26]

The authors of the *Medical and Surgical History of the War of the Rebellion* also weighed in with conclusions about vaccination and smallpox. They charted the level of susceptibility among selected regiments, noting that in the Sixty-Sixth New York, 325 out of 738 men (44 percent) erupted with pustules when revaccinated. In the Fifty-Third Pennsylvania the rate was 593 out of 818 men (72.5 percent). Differentials such as these seemed to indicate to the authors that the home territory of each regiment had a role to play in the percentage of men who had already built up immunity to smallpox, either through prior exposure or more thorough inoculation. Regiments raised in cities, such as the Second New York, had much lower rates of susceptibility than those raised in rural areas, such as the First Minnesota. The authors also noted that Black regiments seemed to suffer much more from smallpox outbreaks than white units.[27]

So much of the evidence about smallpox and how to prevent it depended on the pustules serving as a sign. But physicians had developed through experience a method of reading those signs to detect spurious, or failed, vaccination attempts. Surg. Claiborne J. Walton of the Twenty-Second Kentucky described this method. In a genuine, or successful, inoculation the inflammation began two or three days later and was "well defined." In contrast, the spurious vaccination produced inflammation immediately, and it was diffused across wide areas of the skin. The genuine inoculation produced a scab that "presents a *rich glossy (waxy)* appearance, of a light *mahogany* color, *depressed* in the *center,*" that detached by the twentieth day. In a spurious inoculation the scab had "a *dingy ashy* appearance and is *fibrous* in its structure. It is very rough and continues to grow larger and higher from the accumulation of matter beneath." The scab in this case remained until accidently knocked off the skin. In the final stages the genuine sore was "circular and *neatly* pitted," and it healed by itself. In the spurious version it was "*irregular* & Rough around the edges" and required treatment.[28]

In other words, army surgeons had a rich storehouse of prior knowledge about smallpox, vaccination practices, and effectiveness of treatment to draw from when dealing with this problem in its military context. Statistics spoke powerfully about how to gain a handle on controlling it. But people differ in their bodily reaction to stimuli, and that included smallpox inoculation. Robert Beecham of the Second Wisconsin had been inoculated several years before the war and had a good reaction, indicating sound protection. But the order in his regiment was for everyone to be revaccinated on enlistment. Beecham later regretted it, for he did not react well to the second inoculation. He remembered that it produced "woe and wretchedness that surpassed any case of genuine smallpox, taken naturally, on record." His tentmates also suffered for ten days, and nothing the surgeon gave them or that they could purchase from the local town alleviated their symptoms. Even after the immediate effects wore off, Beecham continued to have scars from that second inoculation for several years. "No more vaccination for me," he concluded.[29]

Beecham's reaction was unfortunate but not typical of all Union soldiers. Most of them took to revaccination well. A few hated the idea of deliberately injecting poisonous matter into their system and resisted all vaccination, but this was the army, after all, and they were forced to submit. One man in the Eighth Illinois Cavalry "declared he 'would die first'" but yielded when threatened with punishment.[30]

Officers and surgeons alike understood that at the first indication of smallpox in any unit, immediate action was necessary. Even if only one man showed signs of infection, vaccination for all was the rule. Surgeons concentrated on revaccinating everyone within reach of the infected man as soon as possible. In such cases any holdouts in the rank and file felt threatened enough to agree to inoculation. These outbreaks often resulted from a man returning to the regiment from furlough and having been exposed to the disease in transit. If only a handful of men were infected, they could be shunted to a specially created smallpox hospital. If that was not possible, the unfortunate men had to camp outside the picket lines.[31]

When Capt. Henry Romeyn's Company B, Fourteenth US Colored Troops experienced an outbreak after exposure to the disease in Nashville, his men were unceremoniously told to leave camp. Col. Thomas J. Morgan stood at a distance and shouted his order to Romeyn. "'Captain, strike your company tents at once and get out of camp. Go anywhere you please, not less than half a mile away; make requisition for anything you want and it will be filled, but get out.'" It was a strict quarantine; all supplies and mail were left on and near a stump halfway between the regimental camp and the company camp. Forty of Romeyn's men came down with smallpox, and two of them died. When the quarantine finally ended, all the surviving company members burned their clothes and rejoined the regiment.[32]

The evidence from personal accounts strongly indicates that, despite the high level of inoculation, smallpox affected very many units in the Federal army in at least limited ways. It could have been much worse except for the alertness of surgeons and unit commanders who took effective measures to contain small outbreaks before they got out of hand. Detection, isolation of infectious individuals, and emergency inoculation were the key elements in that containment strategy.

SANITARY COMMISSION CAMP INSPECTION RETURNS

The Sanitary Commission wanted to know basic information about the program of vaccination in all regiments, including six questions about the subject area on its standard camp inspection return. It asked if all men had been inoculated since enlistment, how many had not yet been vaccinated, how many showed signs of previous inoculation, and how many times had they been previously vaccinated. The commission also wanted to know how many new vaccinations were successful, dividing this number into those who had been previously inoculated and those receiving the vaccine for the first time.

What information the commission received as a result of these questions was limited. Inspectors could document whether regimental vaccination programs took place at enlistment or later, and they could generally note if all or part of the unit had been covered. But they failed to provide any amount of data on the details. The reason was that the army did not require surgeons to compile statistics on how many men had been previously vaccinated or whether new treatments seemed to be successful. A handful of regimental surgeons did this on their own but were far too few to constitute a meaningful data set. In some cases the physicians had accumulated such records but could not readily put their hands on them when the inspector visited. The commission also limited its opportunity to learn about this subject area by dropping all questions about vaccination from one of its several versions of the camp inspection return; fortunately, it was a form that was not used for long.

Among the 280 returns used in this study, only 49 specifically mentioned whether the men were fully inoculated at enlistment, and only 7 of those (14.3 percent) indicated it had been done. Another 33 (67.3 percent) indicated it was not done at all on induction, while 9 (18.4 percent) indicated partial vaccination at enlistment. But the returns show that much more had been done after enlistment in an effort to make up for that very poor showing. A total of 164 returns contained information about retro-vaccination, of which 62 (37.8 percent) indicated that all men had been inoculated by the time of the inspector's visit. Whether that was because of full vaccination at enlistment or after was usually not specified. But another 40 returns (24.4

percent) indicated that no retro-vaccination had taken place. Finally, 62 returns (37.8 percent) indicated that the surgeons had administered partial retro-vaccinations.

The returns shored up the idea that a large percentage of Americans accepted inoculation by the middle of the nineteenth century. In the Fifth New York, of 950 men vaccinated, 758 (79.9 percent) showed clear signs of prior inoculation, of whom 200 had been vaccinated more than once before enlisting. In the Ninety-First New York, 83.3 percent of the 300 men vaccinated since enlistment had shown signs of previous inoculation, and 48.0 percent of those previously inoculated had been vaccinated more than once before enlisting. Many men had been inoculated when young, and many members of ethnic regiments had been vaccinated in their home countries. The willingness to take the vaccine thus was widespread and deep in American society.[33]

In a few cases considerable numbers of men in certain units actually requested additional vaccinations. "All who had not been vaccinated & perhaps ½ rest revaccinated at their request," reported Surg. Thaddeus Hildreth of the Third Maine. Confidence in the process of inoculation led to virtually every member of some regiments, such as the Fiftieth New York Engineers, being vaccinated "2 or 3 times."[34]

But there were a handful of individuals who absolutely refused to be vaccinated. Two men in the Eighth Illinois Cavalry "had to be tied" before the surgeon could apply the vaccine. Although not reported on the camp inspection returns, two regimental surgeons told the commission just after the war of further cases of resistance. Four men had "evaded vaccination through prejudice" in the Twenty-Second Kentucky, wrote the unit's surgeon, and all of them contracted smallpox, with two of them dying from it. One man in the Nineteenth Illinois was allowed to refuse inoculation when his company was vaccinated; he also contracted the disease after two and a half years of service.[35]

The returns also indicated signs of complications associated with the inoculation process. In a few cases the logistical system to supply vaccine failed. Surgeon Hazlett tried for five months to requisition matter for the Second West Virginia, while it was serving in a mountainous region, but with no success. Even though the Seventy-Ninth Indiana was at Murfreesboro, easily within reach of a railroad, Surg. Lewis Manker filed three requisitions for vaccine that went unfilled. When material was available, as it was with the large majority of units, a small percentage of men in every regiment suffered from sore arms after the vaccination. In some cases "obstinate ulcers with diffused inflammation," apparently caused by bad vaccine matter, were observed by regimental surgeons. Much more seriously, syphilitic symptoms appeared after inoculation in a few men. Complications such as these led at least one doctor, Surg. Charles N. Ellinwood of the Seventy-Fourth Illinois, to disapprove of revaccination as taking an unnecessary risk with the man's overall health.[36]

Complications and doubts about the safety of inoculation remained a marginal element in the story of smallpox during the Civil War. Widespread acceptance of vaccination was the mainstream opinion, both in civilian society and in the Union army. And still, the volunteer force did not do a very impressive job of administering vaccine in the way that sanitarians or even the army establishment desired. Considering all 280 camp inspection returns, only 29.3 percent indicated full compliance—that is, full inoculation at enlistment. What could be considered essentially complete failure to do so applied to 36.4 percent of the regiments, while 34.3 percent applied the program to a limited degree, mostly through retro-vaccinating after enlistment. This could well be a sufficient cause for the widespread occurrence of smallpox outbreaks across the Union volunteer force, although none of those events reached epidemic proportions thanks to vigorous responses by regimental and medical personnel.

THE ARMY'S SPIN ON SMALLPOX DURING THE CIVIL WAR

The authors of the *Medical and Surgical History of the War of the Rebellion* had a vested interest in slanting this story. As career army medical officers, they sought to blame the outbreaks of smallpox on civilian society. No civil authority had mandated a compulsory vaccination program for citizens, and few state authorities spent much time or energy on assuring that volunteer regiments were inoculated before offering their services to the Federal government. The authors estimated that, as a result, perhaps every fourth or fifth man in the volunteer force was susceptible to smallpox. Yet the army vaccinated many men during the course of the war and obtained vaccine matter from civilians, who developed it mostly from children; they were supposed to send a certificate to note the name of the child and the date of removal. Much material was provided by Dr. Ephraim Cutter of Woburn, Massachusetts, "who raised crusts from the calf by vaccination with humanized virus" as opposed to deriving it directly from cowpox. Problems in supply included attempts to produce vaccine matter on the arm of an adult through revaccination, which tended to produce "impure virus" that led to spurious vaccination. Problems in application included sores and ulcers. When the First Middle Tennessee (US) was inoculated, one-third of the men developed ulcers, and many of those were still not healed a month later.[37]

The *Medical and Surgical History* documented the extent of smallpox outbreaks, noting that it could "be said to have been present in every department during every year of the war." At least 12,236 cases were treated during the conflict, averaging 5.5 cases per 1,000 men annually. Of those, 4,717 died, or 1.95 per 1,000 men annually. That these statistics were not higher was due to effective measures of containment, according to the authors of the compilation. They were able, in the end, to praise their colleagues for preventing a medical catastrophe.[38]

Prudent systems of preventive healthcare stress measures to avert problems that could be expected in the course of events. Examining the enlistee for existing health conditions not conducive to the performance of military duties certainly fell squarely into that category. Employing a proven method of averting smallpox certainly fell into that category as well. Both systems of preventive healthcare were well established before 1861, and yet neither was fully implemented by the volunteer officers and regimental surgeons who tended the bulk of Union soldiers. In both areas most of those responsible tried to partly fulfill their duties, but many factors impeded their efforts, while some did not even try, and still others fully complied with directives. At most, one can only say that the majority of those held responsible for the health of the men did enough to contain but not prevent problems associated with prior health conditions or with smallpox from significantly affecting the Union army.

9

Regimental Hospitals and Officer Supervision

The last two subject areas covered by the US Sanitary Commission camp inspection returns related decisively to the efforts of regimental officers and medical staff. Both areas went to the heart of unit effectiveness. Regimental hospitals offered the first level of institutional medical care in the Union army. They were typically the first stop for a man whose condition seemed to his unit's surgeon to warrant institutionalized care. The condition of this hospital therefore became of great interest to the commission. The second subject area, officer supervision of many aspects of preventive healthcare in the regiment, measured how well the unit's authorities paid attention to their duties. Both subject areas pointed directly to the twin themes of this study—preventive healthcare and military effectiveness in the Union army. Despite the fundamental importance of both subject areas, volunteer regiments did not fare well in either of them.

REGIMENTAL HOSPITALS

The Union army had a multilayered hospital system during the Civil War. The most fundamental tier was created and administered by the surgeon and assistant surgeon of each regiment, with the aid of the unit commander. Members of the regimental medical staff were the first contact for a soldier who felt ill or who had been injured. The surgeon could give him some medicine or other topical application and send him back to duty, or he could admit the man to the regimental hospital. An intermediate stage was to excuse him from duty without admitting him to the unit hospital, which meant he was "sick in quarters" for a while.

Beyond the regimental hospital, which was supposed to be permanent as long as the regiment was in service, the Federal army established brigade, division, and corps hospitals on a temporary basis. Above that intermediate level, the general hospitals constituted the highest tier of the military healthcare system. They were located all across the Northern states and in occupied Southern territory. As the name implies, these facilities accepted men from all units in the Federal army. The regimental and the general hospital were the permanent facilities that bracketed the temporary hospitals on the brigade, division, and corps levels, which could be established and disassembled whenever medical personnel felt it necessary to do so. Typically, these middle-level facilities were created during and after a major battle to handle the large influx of wounded and then consolidated and eventually dissolved as the number of cases declined. Those patients remaining almost always were transferred to the higher level, the general hospitals, rather than down to their respective regimental hospitals.

For obvious reasons, the army required that all regiments maintain hospital facilities. The majority of cases in them were medical rather than surgical—in other words, they resulted from illness rather than battle injuries, thus making these establishments important in the daily health of the men. Regimental surgeons and their facilities were the first response to waves of illness that affected new volunteer regiments early in their service. The Army of the Potomac had 130,000 men on its rolls during October and November 1861, and 7,932 of them were ill with various fevers. That was a sick rate of 6.1 percent, which was a bit higher than average. In the division commanded by Nathaniel P. Banks in early 1862, 388 of the 17,000 men (2.2 percent) were ill in regimental, brigade, and general hospitals. But another 454 soldiers in the division were sick in quarters, making the overall illness rate 4.9 percent. In fact, there was a strong tendency for more men to be ill in quarters than to be placed in the hospital system, a decision made entirely by regimental surgeons. For example, in the Eleventh Massachusetts, while 17 men were admitted to the regimental hospital, 145 were sick in quarters during December 1861.[1]

The equipment and supplies needed by a regimental hospital were many and varied. It began with a tent specially designed for hospital use. The concept of housing and treating ill soldiers in a tent dated back at least as far as the Napoleonic Wars. In the Civil War the Union army used wall tents to accommodate six to twenty cases on cots, although at the higher end of occupancy they would be very crowded. The walls were four feet, six inches tall, which, with the A-frame on top, allowed for eleven feet of clearance at the middle. Two or more tents could be joined at the ends to form a long corridor. The Army of the Cumberland carried with it 250 such hospital tents during the Tullahoma Campaign.[2]

Some method of conveying sick or wounded men was considered necessary. By 1859, the army had authorized both a two-wheeled and a four-wheeled ambulance, but providing usable ones to the huge volunteer force of the Civil War was not easy. Unlike the standard army wagon, the ambulance had springs and was a more delicate vehicle that often broke down. Surg. Alonzo J. Phelps, as medical director of Brig. Gen. Thomas Wood's division, inspected 101 ambulances belonging to the division in late 1862 and found that only 39 were serviceable. These were all he could use during the upcoming Stones River Campaign. The army also authorized the use of a cacolet, which was a litter mounted on a horse or mule. This was capable of carrying one or two men, but the patients were "strapped tightly to the body of the animal" and thus "felt his every motion." As John D. Billings correctly noted, the horse litter was "used but very little" in the Union army.[3]

THE SANITARY COMMISSION AND FIFTEENTH CORPS MEDICAL INSPECTORS ON REGIMENTAL HOSPITALS

Sanitary Commission workers discussed many problems associated with regimental hospitals. Godfrey Aigner studied the facilities created by the regiments gathered in the District of Cairo during the fall of 1861. He noted "slow but steady improvement" in the management of these hospitals by regimental medical personnel. They dealt with a wide variety of ailments, especially those associated with the illnesses suffered by fresh recruits adjusting to camp life. Aigner concluded that housing the sick in wooden buildings was preferable to tents because the "boarded roofs with ridge ventilation" increased air circulation. He also criticized the tendency of regimental physicians to allow large numbers of ill men to remain in their quarters. Citing the Crimean War experience, Aigner contended that the French initially favored the sick remaining in their quarters but soon found it was counterproductive and shifted them to hospitals. "In quarters," he argued, "the sick soldier is under no control in regard to his diet & hygiene; in 9 cases out of ten he continues to be exposed to the very causes which have produced his disease; if removed in time to the hospital, the latter cease to operate on him while the effects, already provided by them, are counteracted by a better atmosphere, appropriate diet, comfortable rest, & always ready assistance."[4]

Aigner worked against the flow on these important issues. Most sanitarians favored tents over buildings as accommodations for sick soldiers, and unit physicians overwhelmingly tended to favor allowing the mild cases to remain in living quarters. But reports filed by the medical inspectors in the Fifteenth Corps reveal that hospital tents were an item of great interest on the part of everyone in a regiment. They often were used for many purposes other than housing the sick and by many personnel other than the medical staff. These corps-level reports reveal that regimental quartermasters, commissaries, and other staff regularly used hospital tents for their own purposes. In many cases those hospital tents were in terrible condition but had not yet been replaced. In more than one regiment, the medical staff had to borrow tents from regimental sutlers to house their cases. When the inspector found a regiment using regulation hospital tents for the purpose they were intended, he made a point of noting that in his report because it was comparatively uncommon. This was one reason why so many mild cases were allowed to remain in their quarters; there simply was no separate housing facility for them.[5]

SANITARY COMMISSION CAMP INSPECTION RETURNS

The camp inspection returns of the Sanitary Commission offer another perspective on how Union regiments handled the important task of maintaining a hospital. Out of 280 returns used for this study, 223 specifically deal with regimental medical facilities, and out of that number, 207 (92.8 percent) indicated that a regimental hospital existed, leaving only 16 (7.2 percent) without one.

This situation was different when addressing artillery batteries, for they were typically not allowed a surgeon or a hospital. About the size of an infantry company, the battery was too small a unit for the government to provide staff and hospital equipment. They were typically assigned to infantry units and expected to make do with sharing the infantry's medical resources. But the camp inspection returns reveal an interesting twist on that topic. Of sixty-one batteries covered by the topic of hospital resources, eleven (18.1 percent) actually had a surgeon, and most of these, plus a few more, had a hospital; so, a total of fifteen (24.5 percent) had their own medical facilities. The regular artillery units all had these facilities, but few volunteer batteries possessed them. Still, thirty-five batteries, or 57.4 percent of the total, had no hospital or medical staff. They relied on physicians from other units to drop by and see to their sick personnel, sending them to infantry regimental hospitals when needed.[6]

While almost all infantry regiments had a hospital, how well stocked it happened to be was another story. Of 212 returns that specifically mention this topic, only 135 (63.6 percent) could be said to have been well stocked with equipment and medical supplies. That meant that 77 (36.4 percent) had little or even no equipment or supplies. The chief reason was logistical in nature. Medical personnel had been lax in filing requisitions in a timely manner or they had repeatedly filed them only to have them unfilled for months at a time.

Shelter for the sick also proved to be complicated, which reinforces the discussion of this problem already mentioned in the Fifteenth Corps medical inspection reports. Of 180 Sanitary Commission inspection returns that specifically mention this topic, 95 (52.7 percent) of regimental hospitals used tents. Another 58 (32.2 percent) used nearby civilian houses or specially erected wooden huts, and another 27 (15.1 percent) used a combination of tents, houses, and huts. The commission also considered it important that the cases in the regimental hospital use a separate sink from the rest of the men to prevent the spread of illness. For the most part, regimental medical staff honored this requirement. Of 98 returns that specifically mention it, 78 (79.5 percent) had separate toilet facilities for patients in regimental hospitals, while 20 (20.5 percent) did not.

Camp inspectors did not spare criticism when they found particularly bad regimental hospitals and usually blamed the unit's medical staff. When George A. Blake visited the Twelfth Connecticut at Camp Parapet north of New Orleans, he found the hospital "a disgrace to all connected with it." Surg. William R. Brownell had been detached to other duties, and the hospital was managed by two assistant surgeons. One of them was "too old—too slow—a sloven passing no good qualifications," and the other was "incompetent." Inspectors also praised good hospitals when they saw them, such as the arrangements made by Surg. Luther G. Thomas for the Twenty-Sixth New Jersey, whose hospital tents were "the neatest and kept in the best order of any I have yet visited," as F. U. Johnston declared.[7]

The camp inspection returns provide data on the number of men treated in the three places a regimental surgeon could send a sick man. In virtually every instance those sick in quarters were far more numerous than in the regimental hospitals or in general hospitals. In a small number of cases, the surgeon did not approve of letting sick men stay in their quarters. In a few other cases, staff did not approve of sending them to general hospitals because "none are again heard from," as Surg. Elisha Griswold of the Second Pennsylvania Heavy Artillery told T. B. Smith. John H. Douglas reported that in the Twelfth Missouri only half the cases sent to general hospital returned to duty within a reasonable amount of time. In other regiments the men themselves did not like to go to the general hospitals, preferring to remain with their comrades while recovering. Edward A. Crane found that in the Fifty-Second Massachusetts, Surg. Frederick A. Sawyer was prescribing medicine for a dozen men who reported at sick call but were "not excused from duty," creating yet another category of treatment that did not require rest in quarters or in any hospital.[8]

The returns also reveal that, while many regimental hospitals were not fully equipped with ambulances or stretchers, they tended to be better supplied with medicines and surgical instruments. Very few of them, however, possessed a horse litter. Ironically, even cavalry regiments usually did not have a cacolet. It was not by any means a popular piece of equipment.[9]

While a minority of regimental hospitals had no separate sink for the patients, in some cases the surgeon mandated a degree of care in disposing of human excrement. In the Fifth Vermont, for example, hospital attendants emptied bedpans into the slop barrels that syphoned off kitchen waste. In the Tenth Iowa, camped near the Mississippi at Bird's Point, Missouri, the contents of bedpans were "thrown into river."[10]

Relatively few sick men in regimental hospitals suffered from dangerous ailments because the more serious cases typically were sent on to general hospitals. But when soldiers died in the regimental hospital, they were either buried nearby or their remains were sent home. In the First Connecticut Artillery, according to Franklin B. Hough, the surgeon made a point of stating that all were "sent home 'tenderly,' at expense of companies, and friends. None buried in Virginia." But in the Twenty-Seventh Illinois, five deceased comrades were interred in the nearby Cairo city cemetery, while three others were "sent home."[11]

Relatively few regiments had a formally organized ambulance corps that was trained and drilled to perform its duties. Perhaps one reason for this was revealed in the inspection of the Eighth New York. William M. Chamberlain reported that its band members "refuse[d] to act" as the ambulance corps. But one can only assume that unit commanders and surgeons in the others did not think there was any need to organize such a corps.[12]

Camp inspectors provided much detail about the medical officers in charge of regimental hospitals. Most of the unit doctors mentioned had studied at good universities and had chalked up respectable amounts of practical experience before joining the army. Several held degrees from European universities, while others had earned degrees in the United States at the University of Michigan, Rush College in Chicago, the University of Pennsylvania, and St. Louis Medical College. Most regimental surgeons had enough prewar experience in their profession to inspire confidence. For example, Abner Hard, surgeon of the Eighth Illinois Cavalry, received his medical degree from Iowa University in 1854 and had practiced in small towns for eight years, even though he had only limited hospital and surgical experience. James McNair of the Fifteenth New York Engineers, a graduate of a London university in 1839, had racked up twenty years of town practice. Edward O. F. Roler received his degree in 1859 and had but two and a half years of practice and little hospital experience before becoming surgeon of the Fifty-Fifth Illinois.[13]

In a handful of cases, regiments and batteries made do without surgeons by finding men in the ranks who had some experience related to medicine. Chamberlain met "a very nice little man" who was trying to fill the medical needs of Battery A, First New York Light Artillery. He had been detached from the ranks of the Twenty-Ninth New York and, although pleasant, was "so doubtful of his own position that he does not go near Headquarters." Capt. Nelson T. Spoor faced a similar problem in his Second Iowa Battery and solved it by placing a private as acting surgeon, detailing another private to help him. Surg. Jotham Donnell had no assistant surgeon, so he appointed "a Medically Educated private" to help him in the Fifteenth Maine. Emergency measures such as these seemed inevitable, considering both the lack of medical staff assigned to batteries and the difficulty of replacing staff in those units where they were allowed.[14]

Occasionally, camp inspectors found doctors who were uncooperative or simply ignorant. Chamberlain was surprised at the attitude of Surg. Francis L. Wheaton in the Second Rhode Island, who refused to share statistics about illness rates in the regiment. Instead, Wheaton "spent the time of our interview in abusing the Commission." On the other end of the spectrum was Dr. Henry M. Crouse of the Fifty-Seventh Indiana, who "did not know of Sant. Com.," reported Bernard J. Bettelheim. A small number of physicians seemed ill suited for field service. Crane was disgusted with Surg. Louis Darling of the 161st New York. An 1829 graduate of Dartmouth, Darling appeared to be "a fossil" to the critical inspector.[15]

Only 18.2 percent of the returns gave regimental hospitals a rating of good, while 36.1 percent were rated as fair and an astonishing 45.7 percent as bad. The primary reason for this poor showing was that regimental hospitals required a variety of equipment and supplies as well as good management by medical personnel. Both were in short supply in the volunteer force. Regimental commanders were important in this, too, because they and their staff had to make sure the surgeons received all that they required. Unfortunately, these men more often failed than succeeded.

OFFICER SUPERVISION

As in so many aspects of military life during the Civil War, effectiveness boiled down to the quality of personnel. Preventive healthcare measures could not work if regimental officers and medical staff failed to follow procedures known to be effective in limiting sickness in the ranks. This was a fundamental problem of the volunteer force: the ability of its officers to take seriously the military regimen and to see that measures were adopted to protect their men's health. It was a demanding call to duty. Officers had a long list of things to do on a regular basis while in camp; tending to soldier health was far too often placed low on the list. This was a major cause for the reduction of military effectiveness in the Union's volunteer army.

Both the sanitarians and the army took officer supervision seriously. John Ordronaux advised surgeons and assistant surgeons to conduct a sanitary inspection of living quarters, rations, kitchens, and sinks at least twice a week. Some conscientious army officers advised daily inspections of the rations and food preparation routine, but in contrast, George B. McClellan felt that the Russian army policy of monthly inspections by the regimental commander was sufficient. In some cases volunteer officers did their job well. Dr. Ira Russell was impressed with Col. William Blaisdell, who was "ever watchful of the health of his men" in the Eleventh Massachusetts. He cooperated with the surgical staff "to improve the sanitary condition of the men."[16]

But Blaisdell was exceptionally good at sanitary work. Aigner was convinced that few volunteer officers truly understood how important it was to pay attention to sanitary matters after visiting several units around Cairo in the fall of 1861. He concluded that most regimental surgeons were general physicians with little training or experience, yet they had not been instructed to deal with the special health risks of army service. Worse, "the ignorance & recklessness of many volunteer surgeons" appalled Aigner. After interviewing several regimental surgeons, he found that too many were ignorant of basic knowledge, such as how to stop bleeding or how to treat typhoid fever. He found levels of ignorance "unequalled by anything except the coolness & indifference with which the most heroic remedies are administered by these very men."[17]

The army tried to counter this problem by creating the post of medical inspector on the corps level. This officer was charged with "all that relates to the sanitary condition of the Army," as the War Department put it. He also was to cooperate with infantry officers and unit surgeons to correct problems. Dr. Charles Tripler, medical director of the Army of the Potomac, wanted to go a step further and increase the number of surgeons assigned to units. He felt that there should be at least one surgeon for every 250 men instead of one for every 500 men, plus the assignment of one assistant surgeon for every artillery battery. Tripler noted two problems associated with sanitary care. Most fundamental was the "want of military habits and training" among the regimental medical personnel. "The general impression among the people seems to be that a good citizen physician is fully competent to discharge the duties of a regimental surgeon." The other problem Tripler recognized was the reluctance of many regimental commanders to work with their medical staff. They protected their turf by not allowing surgeons "to meddle in any way with the police customs of the camp, or to insist on any measures for the preservation of the health of the men." McClellan saw both problems emerge from the very beginning of the Army of the Potomac in the late summer of 1861.[18]

Tension between regimental and medical staff existed throughout the Army of the Potomac. Sometimes it originated from the unit commander and at other times from the surgeon. In both cases it readily assumed a fight for greater control over their spheres of responsibility. The colonel believed he should be in charge literally of everything to do with the regiment, while the surgeon believed he was exclusively responsible for anything to do with healthcare matters. As with the case of Surg. Alfred L. Castleman and Col. Amasa Cobb in the Fifth Wisconsin, personality clashes made the situation worse.[19]

FIFTEENTH CORPS MEDICAL INSPECTION REPORTS

In the Fifteenth Corps, medical inspectors found that a certain degree of tension between medical staff and regimental officers existed in the Army of the Tennessee as well. In some units there was full cooperation and regular inspections of the cooking arrangements. But in others this system completely broke down. "Police of camp is bad," reported Surg. Edward O. F. Roler about the Third Missouri during the week ending September 12, 1863. "In this regt. there exists an unfortunate lack of harmony between the medical and Field and other officers." A wider problem had everything to do with the shortage of medical personnel rather than with lack of cooperation. Corps medical inspectors documented how many regiments did not have a full staff on duty because of illness and detachment of surgeons away from their units to perform other needed tasks. As mentioned, artillery batteries and pioneer companies were not authorized to have a surgeon and usually had to make do with visits from regimental physicians stationed nearby. Roler found that a pioneer corps of 116 detached white troops, supplemented by 230 Black laborers, was tended by the assistant surgeon of the Thirtieth Iowa, who came by now and then to see how they fared. It was not uncommon for many regiments in the corps to have only one rather than two surgeons on duty at any given time.[20]

The strain placed on the health of a regiment by the absence of a full medical staff was very evident to the Fifteenth Corps medical inspectors. Surg. Charles L. Chambers of the Thirty-Fifth Iowa had resigned a couple of months before Roler inspected the regiment; Asst. Surg. Stephen M. Cobb, assisted by a contract surgeon, tried to fill in, but he was not up to the task. "A good Physician is badly needed," warned Roler, "one who can discriminate in the variety of diseases occurring in camp, and prescribe treatment adapted to the pathology of the case." Dr. John M. Woodworth took over as corps medical inspector by early 1864 and particularly noted the frequency with which he encountered resistance to medical-staff advice among regimental commanders. In the Eighteenth Wisconsin Surg. Erastus J. Buck received "little encouragement to look after the sanitary condition of his regt., as I am led to believe that his suggestions are lightly regarded, if not considered wholy out of place, by the comd'g officer." Referring generally to the Second Division of the corps, Woodworth bemoaned the fact that commanders "too often denied or indifferently" followed through with suggestions made by their medical staff. Even when an acceptable level of cooperation existed, Woodworth found that many surgeons were poorly provided with blanks and books for the keeping of proper medical records.[21]

PERSONAL ACCOUNTS

These Fifteenth Corps medical inspection reports reflect conditions on the ground, so to speak, at the regimental level and reinforce the notion

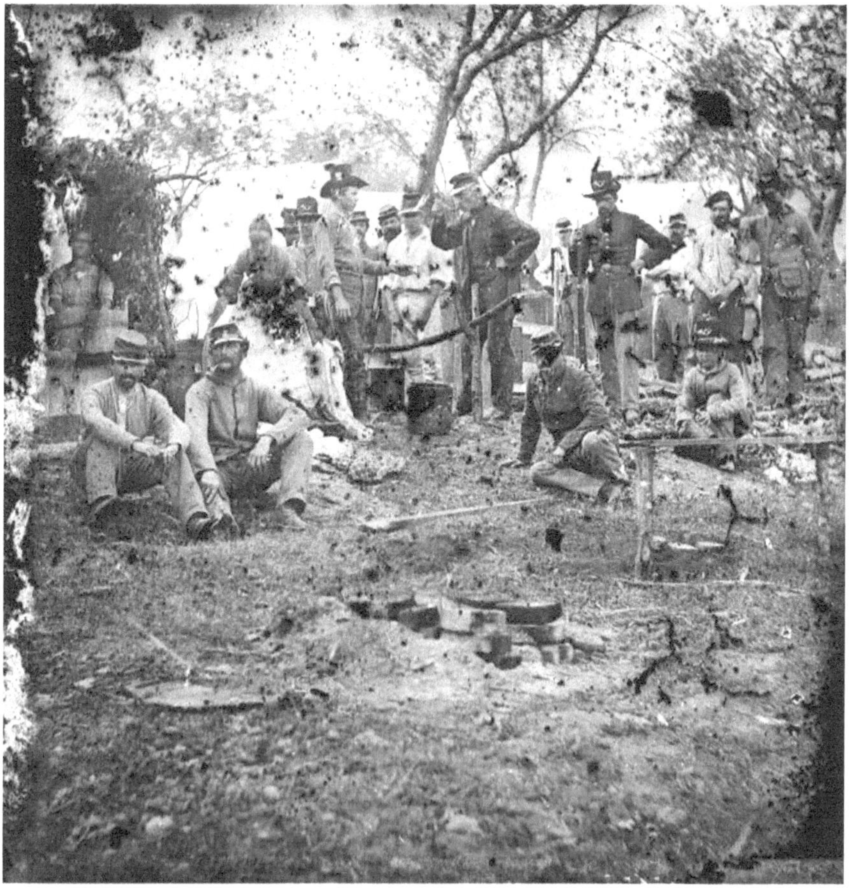

Officer Tasting the Men's Food. This image mentions "Capt. Ballerman's Kitchen, Tasting the Soup," but the good captain cannot be further identified; his name does not appear in any readily available primary sources. That is too bad, for he was demonstrating what all conscientious officers were supposed to do—take an interest in the quality of their men's cooking. (Library of Congress, Prints & Photographs Division, Civil War Photographs, LCDIG-cwpb-01680)

that proper sanitation rested heavily on the quality of officers. Personal accounts also support this notion. Col. Emerson Opdycke was tickled at the high praise accorded his 125th Ohio, part of the Army of the Cumberland, for camp cleanliness. He noted that other regiments nearby received low ratings, "and some of the regiments were scolded severely" by the medical inspector. A volunteer officer, Opdycke was impressed by the regular officers he encountered, believing them to be more attentive to the sanitary condition of their commands than the typical volunteer officer. In the Army of the Potomac, Alpheus S. Williams made a point of visiting most of the regiments in his brigade on a daily basis "to examine the condition of the camps, hospitals, kitchens, etc." Regimental commanders such as Alfred N. Duffié of the First Rhode Island Cavalry and Abel Smith of the 165th New York inspected quarters and kitchens regularly. Smith also began company funds for the purchase of vegetables and "encouraged amusements, together with strict sanitary regulations."[22]

Other conscientious officers can be found here and there if one looks for them. Lt. Goodwin Atkins Stone of the Second Massachusetts Cavalry took great pride in his company kitchen, "as neat and clean as possible; plenty to eat, nicely cooked. There is a good deal of pleasure in taking care of your men, so much can be done for their health and comfort that is commonly neglected." Capt. Sidney Willard temporarily commanded the Thirty-Fifth Massachusetts after the Battle of Antietam (September 17, 1862). "I have intense satisfaction in my position for two reasons,—it enables me to enforce cleanliness, and prohibit swearing; which last I have checked to a considerable extent, to a degree which I never thought I should be able to."[23]

SANITARY COMMISSION CAMP INSPECTION RETURNS

The standard camp inspection return included nine questions under the heading "Preventive Duty of Surgeon." They started with a direct question about whether the surgeon understood that duty and went on to find out whether he conducted daily inspections of the camp "with reference to its cleanliness." Did he inspect the food and the cooking? Did he report to regimental officers and advise them on measures to be taken? Did he administer anything to serve as prophylactics to prevent malaria? Did he allow the men to drill before eating breakfast? The standard form did not include other regimental officers, but it could easily have done so because the surgeon was not fully in charge of these matters. He had to cooperate with the regimental commander, and to a lesser degree with company commanders, if he hoped to fully implement a program of preventive healthcare in camp. The regimental commander was officially in charge of everything, and he was, in turn, expected to cooperate with the surgical staff on medical matters.

The overall results of the camp inspection program reinforced the view that conscientious officers were relatively rare. When referring to medical staff, the inspectors provided enough commentary on 226 returns to offer an evaluation, and only 62 (27.4 percent) of the officers could be rated as good in supervising the health of their men. Another 123 (54.4 percent) could be rated as fair, while 41 (18.2 percent) were bad. When it came to regimental officers, inspectors provided proper evidence for 253 returns, rating 37 (14.7 percent) as good, 129 (50.9 percent) as fair, and 87 (34.4 percent) as bad when it came to camp supervision. While medical staff came off better than regimental commanders in the eyes of commission inspectors, it could not have been a source of pride to know that only a bit more than one out of four surgeons could be considered good at fulfilling their responsibilities for preventive healthcare.

Commission inspectors severely criticized doctors in their returns. "The surgical staff of the regiment is in a complete state of demoralization," wrote George L. Andrews about the Fifth Wisconsin—at the time when Castleman was having his troubles with Cobb—and "the opinion of the inspector is, that it is almost entirely inefficient." That was on October 21, 1861. Two days later Andrews again visited the regiment and reported hopeful signs of resolving the troubles between medical staff and commander. But William Chamberlain could offer little hope for improvement in the Eighth New York, which had an "inefficient Surgeon" in Dr. Mertz Froelich, a graduate of the University of Tübingen with a practice in New York City. "He is not a prepossessing person," wrote Chamberlain, who noted that Froelich inspected the camp "from a considerable distance." Company officers "leave the room when he enters."[24]

George A. Blake could not restrain his frustration with some medical personnel while completing his returns. Surg. A. H. Van Orstrand of the Fourth Wisconsin was "a careless, listless sloven—unpopular with the regiment and unfit for his position. It was impossible to obtain *accurate* information—he *guesses* at everything, and the spirit of accommodation is not in him." Asst. Surg. S. W. Wilson "hardly knows whether he understands his responsibilities or not!" When Blake visited the First Louisiana Colored Heavy Artillery, which later was redesignated the Seventh and then the Tenth US Colored Heavy Artillery, he found no regimental hospital, ambulances, or stretchers and learned that no requisitions had been filed for missing supplies. The regiment had no surgeon either but was tended by Asst. Surg. John Fish. "Advised the Surgeon to learn his duty and do it! And told him how!" wrote Blake.[25]

James Gall found a worse situation in the First US Colored Troops, which had been raised mostly in the area around Washington, DC. The men were in pretty good shape physically, and he judged that "anything like proper care" was all that was needed to avoid serious health problems. But the regiment had never had a good medical staff before Gall visited in September 1863. After organizing two months before, it was under the care of a contract surgeon who refused to accompany the regiment when it was ordered to North Carolina. An assistant surgeon was temporarily assigned who, "disliking the duty, of course, neglected it." When the First US Colored Troops reached North Carolina, Pvt. John King of the Twenty-First Connecticut, "who pretended to some medical skill," was detached to serve it. But King habitually left the regiment on the pretense of seeking medical supplies while really looking for whiskey and often came back drunk. He was soon returned to duty in the Twenty-First Connecticut. Then the First US Colored Troops received another contract surgeon, Dr. Yellotty, who relied heavily on W. H. Andrews, a Black man with three years of drugstore experience, to act as hospital steward. Andrews kept the regimental hospital in "pretty good order," but Yellotty was irresponsible. He "gets drunk occasionally & at the time of my inspection had a bruised nose & black eye" from a fall while tipsy on whiskey. "The Col. intends the next time Yellotty gets drunk to put him in an ambulance & cart him over to the Medical Society for examination," Gall reported with amusement. The regiment finally managed to find a competent and stable medical staff after September.[26]

Commission inspectors praised good regimental commanders when they saw them, but not necessarily for their upholding of sanitary principles. Col. Solomon Meredith seemed to have a hold on the attention and respect of his men in the Nineteenth Indiana, even though the sanitary condition of that regiment was pretty dismal. Likewise, Col. McLeod Murphy was able to handle the rowdy men of the Fifteenth New York Engineers, and Col. Gouverneur K. Warren turned his Fifth New York into a model regiment as far as discipline and instruction were concerned. But the inspectors who praised these officers did not even mention their attention to sanitary measures. T. B. Smith wrote of company officers in the Second Pennsylvania Heavy Artillery who maintained neat quarters among the men, even though "some minor Sanitary nuisances are overlooked." Col. Oliver O. Howard came in for unusual praise when Robert Jones visited the Third Maine. Howard "was remarkably frank" while answering Jones's questions. The colonel was "conscious of the defects of his camp" and accepted full responsibility for them. In fact, Howard was giving a lesson in tactics to his officers when Jones interrupted him to ask those questions. "The answers on this report which are the least complimentary are given in his own words," Jones wrote.[27]

In rare cases inspectors found regiments with a regular system of supervision in place. For example, the officers of the Thirty-Ninth Ohio had created "a board of inspectors," consisting of the surgeon and two captains. "They inspect Camp every day & report on Sunday," wrote William W. Estabrook. "If the quarters of any squad are found dirty, the Segt. In charge of the squad is reduced to the ranks."[28]

But the inspectors inevitably found many regimental officers who did not take sanitary precautions seriously. Those officers felt it was not their responsibility to make sure their soldiers bathed regularly. Blake found that this indifference extended into higher levels of command when he spoke to Brig. Gen. Israel Richardson while visiting the Thirty-Seventh New York. Blake "mildly suggested means for improving the Sanitary condition of his brigade." But Richardson frankly replied that the "sanitary condition of his camps [was] of minor importance compared to building forts and perfection in drill."[29]

Henry W. Warriner unloaded much of his frustration with Lt. Col. Matthewson T. Patrick in his return. Patrick's battalion of the First Nebraska Cavalry was in sorry shape when Warriner visited the men at Benton Barracks and found that the commander "obviously fails to appreciate the full range of his duties & responsibilities. He could not tell me where the sinks were; knew nothing of the cooking, not even the system by which it was done; could give but very slight information as to the personal habits of the men, and so on. He is exemplary in his own habits, good natured but knows nothing 'about war.'"[30]

Making all this indifference on the part of unit officers far worse was a widespread spirit of antagonism between them and the medical staff. It is true that in some units there was effective cooperation, but the commission inspectors found too many instances where fighting rather than cooperating was the rule. Alfred Castleman vented his frustration to Robert Collyer in August 1861, telling the inspector that he wanted to resign as surgeon of the Fifth Wisconsin because of Cobb's opposition to his control of the regiment's health matters. Castleman admitted that Cobb was in most ways a good colonel, but he "does not care about sanitary matters," as Collyer wrote. Cobb once told Castleman "that there was too much bother about the sick any how." Andrews called the root of the trouble "a habitual conflict of jurisdiction" when he also visited the Fifth Wisconsin in November 1861. After Castleman resigned from the regiment and became a Sanitary Commission inspector, he noticed the same problem on his visit to the Seventy-Ninth Pennsylvania in March 1863. "A difference exists, as is often the case, between the military and surgical Departments, & it is to be regretted that something can not be done to define the rights of these departments."[31]

Indifference and conflict characterized many other units as well. Andrews noticed "an entire absence of harmony & cooperation between the

Regt., Co., & Medl. Officers" in the Ninth Maine. Surg. William A. Webster told F. U. Johnston that he had "used all efforts to get the tents properly spaced" in the camp of the Ninth New Hampshire, "but the officers will not give their attention to the proper care of the men." A widespread complaint was that the officers in many regiments simply ignored the sound sanitary advice of the surgeons in choosing campsites. Inspectors often phrased this problem as the surgeon having no influence with the officers.[32]

Only 15.3 percent of the 280 returns could be considered as rating good in the subject area of officer supervision, while 52.5 percent rated fair and 32.2 percent bad. A bad rating in this area essentially meant that there was no officer supervision worth mentioning, and the fact that almost one out of three regiments fell into this category was an indictment of the low level of professionalism among volunteer officers, at least in the area of preventive healthcare.

Maintaining well-organized and well-stocked hospitals on the regimental level and taking seriously their responsibility to supervise all aspects of preventive healthcare were fundamental tasks of regimental and company commanders and the medical staff that was supposed to cooperate with them. But it is surprising how many men in both categories took their responsibilities so lightly in these areas. As in many other subject areas covered by the Sanitary Commission camp inspection returns, some officers and surgeons did enough across the board to enable their regiments to muddle through, but it did not need to happen that way. Far too many officers considered sanitary duties a choice rather than an imperative. Their men suffered for it.

10

Confederate Sanitation

In contrast to the Union side of the Civil War, the Confederates never mounted anything that could be termed a sanitarian movement. Sanitary principles were known among some Confederate army officers, some members of the Richmond government, and a handful of civilian physicians in the South. But the number of individuals who discussed these principles was quite small, and they never attempted to form an alliance with each other. There was nothing like a nongovernmental organization similar to the US Sanitary Commission in the Confederacy. As a result, preventive healthcare and military effectiveness in terms of preserving Rebel soldiers had poor showings in the Confederate army.

One of the few Southern voices raised in a public way to promote sanitary ideas was that of John Stainback Wilson. Born in Augusta, Georgia, in 1821, he obtained a degree from the Medical College of Georgia twenty-five years later. Wilson practiced in Marengo County, Alabama, and in Columbus, Georgia. He began writing about various aspects of healthcare, strongly advocating medical education for women beginning in 1854. Wilson believed them to be better physicians for female patients than male doctors. He authored a comprehensive treatise in his first book, *Woman's Home Book of Health,* which appeared in 1860. The next year his short booklet titled *Southern Soldier's Health Guide* was published in Columbus. It contained advice mostly about diet and health for Confederate soldiers. For example, Wilson praised rice as one of the "most wholesome and nutritious of all foods, and it should form a large part of the dietary of Southern soldiers." Rice was especially good for stopping diarrhea. Wilson also praised the traditional Southern ash cake, bread prepared over hot stones and covered with ashes while cooking, as "the most wholesome form of bread, and is well suited to camp life." He believed, along with many in the North, that coffee had important medicinal benefits and should be taken as a restorative rather than as a regular drink. Although it jolted the body's system, coffee had "little or no nutriment." Wilson warned against all liquor, the effects of which were "evil—evil only, and that continually. The apparent strength and animation imparted by them is fictitious and delusive, the transient and temporary excitement arising from their use being invariably and necessarily followed by a collapse, and sinking of the vital powers below par. This is true of every form of drink of which alcohol is a constituent."[1]

There is no evidence that Wilson had an influence on soldiers, the target audience of his book. The slim volume was not mentioned by anyone, not even the handful of government officials charged with army health. Surg. Gen. Samuel P. Moore certainly understood sanitary principles and made efforts to promote them, but he experienced little success. As early as October 1861, Moore complained to Confederate Secretary of War Judah P. Benjamin that his instructions simply were not followed. He had tasked all medical directors of major commands to "insist that proper hygienic regulations be rigidly enforced" but came to see that many commanders either did so only in "a spasmodic character, and soon ceased," or did not attempt to do so at all. Moore blamed the regimental officers, not the medical directors. He convinced Adj. Gen. Samuel Cooper to issue an order on September 1, 1861, mandating the enforcement of sanitary principles. Only six weeks later Moore urged Benjamin to issue another order "that cleanliness of the men should be attended to. Daily ablutions should never be omitted especially of face, chest, and arms. Bathing should be used whenever the opportunity permits." Moore wanted bedding straw to be renewed frequently, tents struck every three or four days, and all kitchen garbage removed from camp on a daily basis. "Much attention should be paid to the food of the soldier," he told the war secretary. The men did not cook their rations well and needed fresh bread whenever that was feasible. If not, "biscuit or hard bread should form the common article of diet in camp life, as it is easily preserved."[2]

Issuing yet another order on these matters could not help much. Benjamin told Confederate President Jefferson Davis that the War Department could not compensate for lax compliance to regulations by officers in the field. "If colonels forget that they bear a parental relation toward their regiments and neglect the most obvious sanitary precaution," he could do little about it. "If generals deem the supervision of the hospital arrangements and treatment of the sick a task too irksome to be endured," the secretary could do little about that either. "It seems most impossible to obtain that regular, faithful, and systematic compliance with rules which can alone maintain the discipline and preserve the efficiency of large bodies of men," Benjamin told Davis in December 1861, "and I have been disappointed in more than one instance" in the highest-ranking generals of the army in those matters.[3]

The Confederate Congress became concerned about these issues as well. It had appointed a special committee to investigate the workings of the various War Department bureaus that supported the army; that committee submitted its report in January 1862. Its members recommended a thorough system of inspection to cover a variety of topics, including food preparation and clothing of volunteers. While this eventually was instituted, it hardly made a difference. Mostly, it simply produced a good deal of paperwork that was filed without leading to serious or widespread efforts to correct problems.[4]

Some civilians in the Confederacy understood these issues and offered advice to the government about how to address them. George G. Woodward, a physician of Louisville, Mississippi, suggested to Davis that a surgeon be assigned to each company in the army. He assumed they would be more keen on improving sanitary conditions in camp than the company officers and believed that voluntary enlistments would be spurred if families of enlistees knew that the army was doing all it could to care for their sons. Each company could choose its own surgeon. Davis passed this suggestion on to the War Department, but nothing was done about it. The parsimonious Congress would have balked at the huge expense of paying for ten additional surgeons for every regiment.[5]

From the beginning of the war, Confederate authorities developed a defeatist attitude about enforcing preventive healthcare regimens in the Southern army. As we have seen, enforcement of such principles was uneven at best in the Union army, but it proved to be worse in the Confederate force, even though we do not have a dataset of evidence to guide our understanding of this point. The scattered evidence, however, makes it clear that Southerners in general simply did not take sanitary principles very seriously.

CAMP SITUATION

Confederate army regulations concerning the layout of camps mirrored those of the Union forces. In some ways the actual settlement of camps also paralleled the way it came about among Federal units. Early in the war some Confederate camps were well situated and laid out. Two large Confederate winter camps have been investigated by archaeologists with interesting results. A cantonment consisting of four individual camps covering 193 acres for 3,500 troops supported the Confederate blockade of the Potomac River near Evansport, Virginia, during the winter of 1861–62. Two of the camps were laid out by naval personnel unfamiliar with army camp regulations and differed significantly in arrangement from the two camps laid out by army officers. But even within the army camps, the archaeologists found evidence of variations from the formula. The foundation remnants of 697 huts indicated that they varied widely in size and shape. But another large Confederate cantonment, established on the grounds of former President James Madison's Montpelier to house 4,600 men during the early months of 1864 indicated more regularity. There, an intense archaeological examination of one regimental site with 125 huts found them closely laid out according to regulations. Each hut site had a depression near it in the ground, which was assumed to be a borrow pit yielding clay for daubing the log structures.[6]

In general, regimental and brigade officers of Cheatham's Division near Murfreesboro, Tennessee, had selected healthy areas for their camps in December 1862. Division officers also selected good campsites near Shelbyville following the Stones River Campaign. Maj. Joseph Vaulx Jr., Frank Cheatham's assistant inspector general, praised the camp of Stewart's Brigade as occupying an "excellent location" where "wood and water are convenient and abundant." Maney's Brigade and Smith's Brigade also found "naturally a healthy" location, but the water was "not of the best quality." It came from "a wet weather branch & runs through a portion of the encampment & in rainy weather becomes somewhat impregnated with the filth around the encampment."[7]

But that was the main problem. While one can find plenty of dirty Union army camps identified in Sanitary Commission camp inspection returns, there can be no doubt that there were far more of them among Confederate forces. Vaulx frankly reported in his inspection of Cheatham's Division during late March 1863 that camp policing was in "a bad state. Trash, garbage & excrement in many instances in proximity to the tents,"

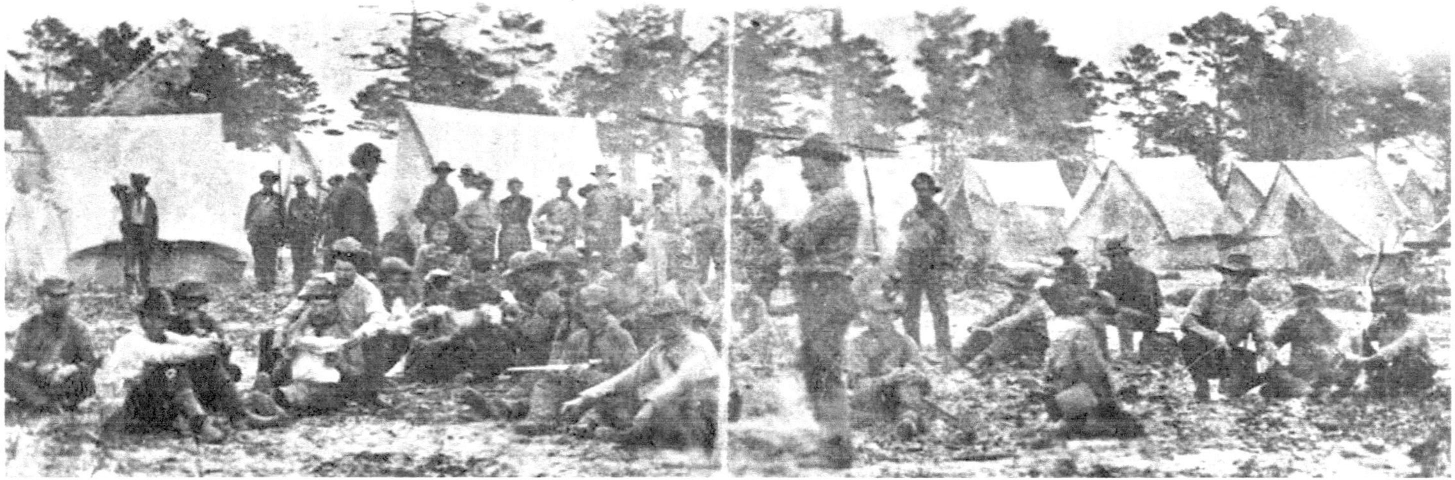

Confederate Camp. There was a debate during and after the Civil War about whether the Confederates kept dirtier camps than the Federals. One cannot judge simply from this photograph of an Alabama regiment's living space near Pensacola, Florida, but the weight of opinion in personal accounts by both Union and Confederate soldiers was that the Southerners' camps were worse. (Library of Congress, Prints & Photographs Division, Civil War Photographs, LCDIG-ppmsca-35462)

especially in the Twenty-Eighth Tennessee. But even in brigades where the problem was not so acute, it was still bad enough. In Maney's Brigade the grounds "also have been neglected and were not promptly put in order as they should have been. Sinks have been dug but are not exclusively used by the men, nor kept in good order."[8]

The problem was not confined to Cheatham's Division. A brief inspection of brigade-level camps among the forces defending Vicksburg soon after the onset of the siege in May 1863 revealed that only three of a dozen brigades qualified as maintaining good camp sanitation; the rest were vaguely classified as "tolerable" or "not very good." One can find a clean Confederate camp now and then, such as that maintained by Joshua K. Callaway, orderly sergeant of the Twenty-Eighth Alabama, who put his men "to cleaning up the camp, sweeping out the street." But one can also find many instances of real carelessness when it came to camp police among all formations in all branches of the Confederate service.[9]

One problem lay in the administration of inspections. The Confederate army never instituted a program designed to inspect the sanitary conditions of semipermanent camps. There was, in short nothing like the Fifteenth Corps medical inspection reports or the US Sanitary Commission camp inspection returns in the South. All Confederate inspectors were supposed to blend the topic of camp sanitation into a general inspection that covered many areas not associated with hygiene. A conscientious inspector paid attention to camp and personal cleanliness, but many others did not, focusing instead on drill, discipline, and the state of arms and ammunition in a regiment. The Confederate army did not create the position of medical inspector as had the Federal force in 1863, further limiting the high command's understanding of the true state of the camp environment.[10]

Perception of camp cleanliness in the Southern army depended to a degree on who was looking at the issue. Many Federal soldiers took notice when they entered an abandoned Confederate camp and made judgments on their enemy. During the Peninsula Campaign of 1862, when the Rebels retired many miles toward Richmond and gave up many unit camps, all Federals who commented on the captured sites found them filthy and disordered in comparison to their own. The same was true of abandoned Confederate campsites around Murfreesboro after the Battle of Stones River and around Chattanooga after Union soldiers secured control of that town in late 1863. It also was true of temporary campsites evacuated during the Atlanta Campaign in 1864. "The Rebels were awful dirty and the smell in their camps dreadful," commented Capt. Charles W. Wills of the 103rd Illinois. Rice C. Bull of the 123rd New York felt the same way but was a bit more understanding. After the fall of Atlanta in September 1864, his regiment pitched camp three hundred yards from an abandoned Confederate campsite, careful not to be too close to the place because it was "dirty and full of vermin. These conditions were found in all the enemy camps we passed through during the campaign. When we could avoid it we never camped on ground that had been used by them. They could make the same criticism about the ground we camped on, for we lived in conditions equally dirty."[11]

In fact, some Confederates who saw Union campsites did proclaim them to be dirty, but some Rebel soldiers did not. William L. Nugent, a cavalrymen serving during the Atlanta Campaign, found Union camps "filled with vermin of every description. Our infantry camps, it is true, are obnoxious to the same objection to a certain extent: but they are not near as bad as the Yankees." But Ellison Capers, commander of the Twenty-Fourth South Carolina, did not agree. He challenged anyone to look at an abandoned Union camp if they thought the South could boast of enjoying "a superior civilization to our foes. His offal is raked up and hauled off—his grounds are clean—his sinks are regularly dug & observed by *the men.* His dead are carefully buried & *every grave marked & fenced in!* Their Army is much superior to ours in *Discipline & Drill,* essential to success."[12]

Yet another perspective on this topic comes from a discerning civilian eye. H. V. Redfield, a resident of East Tennessee, had a unique opportunity to explore both Union and Confederate camps and had decided opinions about them. He found that the Federals always made themselves as comfortable as possible—improvising beds, for example—while the Confederates did not bother with such things. The Northerners seemed to be busy and industrious, while the Southerners were lazy. Federal camps were much cleaner overall. "In the Southern camp you could hardly go twenty steps without getting into filth of some sort, while in the camp of the other side all deposits of filth were carefully removed out of the way."[13]

SHELTER

When it came to shelter, the Confederates tended to prefer huts for semipermanent camps. During the first winter of the war, these crude structures were built by the thousands. In some cases this came about because of preferences for some sort of wooden structure over tents, but in many instances one suspects tent shortages led to it as well. Hut roofs usually were made of canvas. William Meade Dame of the Richmond Howitzers thought that any soldier satisfied with living in a tent when it was possible to build a hut was simply lazy. Dame and his messmates carefully marked out the perimeter of the hut they intended to build; then they excavated three or four feet to provide more vertical space in the structure. The next step was to cut trees for logs twelve to eighteen inches thick and twelve feet long, then to fashion a chimney of wood and finish with mud daubing the chinks. [14]

There was a real shortage of tents in the Confederacy. Even as early as June 1862, Joshua Callaway mentioned that there were only four tents in his company of the Twenty-Eighth Alabama. At war's midpoint the Twenty-Fourth Alabama had tents only for the officers, while the men slept in the open. Those Confederates who lived in tents for any length of time also tended to excavate the site to make more room for themselves, or they constructed a stockade to raise the tent above the natural level of ground. The men also expanded outward by fashioning a brush arbor under which they could sit and have their meals. When tents were available, they were of the same type as used in the Union army. Some were conical in shape, others were A tents, and still others were wall tents. Very few Confederate soldiers mentioned shelter tents. Inspection reports consistently indicated that when tents were available, they were in nothing more than tolerable condition and quantity.[15]

In settled winter quarters, the problem of safe heating came up. Henry Morton Stanley of the Sixth Arkansas suggested a good way to solve the problem. His mates shared a conical tent, but keeping an open fire under the tripod created much smoke and endangered their feet while sleeping. Stanley engineered a sunken hearth linked to a chimney located outside the tent by a flue, which warmed the interior without filling it with smoke. This was a system common in Union winter camps as well.[16]

Bedding in Confederate semipermanent camps consisted mostly of sleeping on the ground with a blanket, but some Rebel soldiers had bed ticks filled with leaves. Others described elaborate attempts to create elevated beds. For this they used forked sticks and long poles, spreading blankets over these makeshift structures to get away from the damp earth. The more fastidious among them did this even during campaigns whenever they had a chance, but mostly it was done in camps of some duration. "It is like lying on a fodder rack," confessed Callaway. This type of bedding served a useful purpose for health if not comfort. The Confederates relied much on donations from home for bed covering and advised the folks that only blankets would fill their needs. Old carpets were too heavy to carry and "too unpliable to keep" men warm, reported William Nelson Pendleton. Quilts made of cotton also were not good for use in the field because once moistened, they were "exceedingly difficult to dry."[17]

CLOTHING

Confederate army regulations detailed the prescribed uniform of the officers and the rank and file, mandating that all were to wear it. They "will not be permitted to keep in their possession any other clothing." But, of course, that did not happen. Shortages of material, weak manufacturing capability, and the terrible logistical arrangements of the Confederate war effort all conspired to force most Rebel soldiers to fend for themselves as far as clothing was concerned. Clothes from home, or articles taken from captured Union soldiers and even dead and wounded Federals on the battlefield, became more important sources of clothing for many Confederates than their own government. Cheatham's inspector found "a variety of styles colors & material" when he examined the troops in March 1863. "A great portion of it being homemade there is very little approach to Uniformity." As with virtually every other Confederate inspector, Vaulx concluded his discussion of clothing by noting how many and what type of article was needed. In his case that amounted to one thousand pairs of shoes for the division. Anderson's Brigade of Withers's Division needed three hundred coats, six hundred shirts and underwear, three hundred pants, six hundred pairs of socks, and two hundred pairs of shoes in the same month. Seven months later an unidentified inspector not only listed the clothing needed by Clayton's Brigade of Stewart's Division but also indicated how many men were already supplied with those articles. The brigade did not have 15.3 percent of the hats, jackets, and underwear; 50.4 percent of the socks; 39.1 percent of the shoes; and 40.9 percent of the blankets it required.[18]

Army regulations allowed for each company to employ up to four women laundresses, who received a wage, fixed by a regimental council of administration, plus a government ration each day. But there is little evidence that washerwomen in any appreciable numbers cleaned Confederate clothing. The majority of troops had to do this themselves or used slave labor. In this regard they were quite like their counterparts in the Federal army, except that Union soldiers relied on refugee Blacks rather than slaves and paid them.[19]

PERSONAL CLEANLINESS

Among both Union and Confederate commentators, there developed a strong tendency to view the Rebel soldier as particularly insensitive to personal cleanliness. John S. Wise, the son of former Virginia Governor Henry Wise and a member of his father's brigade during the war, expressed this strain of thought in the most frank manner. "To appreciate fully the truth that men are but children of a larger growth, one must have commanded soldiers. Without constant guardians and government and punishment, they become careless about clothes, food, ammunition, cleanliness, and even personal safety." He saw them give away their clothing, eat far too much or throw away their rations, and live for the day without a thought of tomorrow. Officers had to be "nurse, monitor, and purveyor for grownup children, in whom the bumps of improvidence and destructiveness are abnormally developed."[20]

Wise might have exaggerated a bit, but he also identified a truth. Many young men–turned–volunteer soldier readily fell into his characterization. Lt. Albert Theodore Goodloe of the Thirty-Fifth Alabama put it more gently when he wrote, "there were some soldiers who were not as careful of cleanliness, in person and clothing, as they might have been." But Goodloe admitted that even those who were careful had to contend with using only one change of clothing, marching and living in dust and mud, riding in filthy railroad cars, and sleeping on the ground. For everyone in the army, "there was the barest possibility oftentimes of an approach to cleanliness." These conditions applied to Union soldiers as well, and Confederate staff member William L. Nugent found Federals captured during the Atlanta Campaign to be in poor shape as far as personal hygiene was concerned. "Their clothes are filthy, torn & greasy and their persons are very offensive."[21]

Of course, one can find Confederate soldiers who tried to keep clean. It was easier to do so in semipermanent camps, but during an active campaign, it was almost impossible. One could go for days on end with no opportunity to wash his face and hands, much less take a real bath. "We are the dirteyest set [of] men you ever saw," wrote Andrew J. White of the Thirtieth Georgia during the Atlanta Campaign, "it has bin so dirty & we have had no time to wash hardly time to wash our faces & hands a clean Suit of close [*sic*] would go well with me now." As White indicated, shortages of clothing were a worse problem for the Confederates than for the Federals. Goodloe noted that many of his men did not have underwear.

Moreover, body lice, a natural consequence of failure to keep clean, became a serious problem by the early summer of 1862.[22]

The Confederate government tried to instill a sense of cleanliness among the troops. Its regulations for the army stipulated that "where conveniences for bathing are to be had, the men should bathe once a week. The feet to be washed at least twice a week. The hair *kept short,* and beard neatly trimmed." But the problem, as always, was compliance with regulations. Noncommissioned officers were the vanguard of enforcement efforts, charged with the duty of making sure the privates would "wash their hands and faces daily; that they brush or comb their heads." Yet most of them failed to fulfill their duties. Lt. Col. Alfred Roman of Pierre G. T. Beauregard's staff inspected Joseph Wheeler's cavalry early in 1865 and found that "camp itch prevails pretty extensively in several brigades. This is due, no doubt, to the uncleanliness of some of the men, who neglect their persons to a shameful extent. The Chief Commissary should be made to furnish soap to the Corps, and to make regular issues of it. Washing of some sort must be encouraged."[23]

By the latter part of the war, a large accumulation of Confederate prisoners in Northern prison camps offered the Federals an opportunity to judge their enemy's habits of personal cleanliness. Sanitary Commission inspector William F. Swalm closely surveyed the prisoners held at Point Lookout, Maryland, in November 1863. He found unacceptable levels of filth. The prisoners kept their tent areas littered with "pieces of cracker, meat, [and] ashes" both inside and outside their sleeping quarters. "I even heard their own men say that they never saw such a dirty set in their lives, fully convincing me that it is their element, and they roll into it as a hog will wallow in the mire." Confederate officers in the camp seemed to be indifferent to the dirt. Army surgeons responsible for the prisoners confirmed Swalm's report, and the Union commander responsible for the camp agreed. "That they are a dirty, lousy set is true enough," wrote Brig. Gen. Gilman Marston, pointing out that his subordinates had given the prisoners everything they needed to clean up, but they did not want to do so. He thought Confederate officers were the chief problem; they did not think it important to maintain camp police.[24]

Another Sanitary Commission inspector had an opportunity of seeing Confederate soldiers up close. Lewis H. Steiner happened to be in Frederick, Maryland, when elements of the Army of Northern Virginia moved through the place in September 1862. "A dirtier, filthier, more unsavory set of human beings never *strolled* through a town," he recalled. "All were alike dirty and repulsive." Officers and men occupied the same level in that regard. "Faces looked as if they had not been acquainted with water for weeks: hair, shaggy and unkempt, seemed entirely a stranger to the operations of brush or comb." In fact, Steiner watched these men for a week before the failure of Lee's incursion into Maryland resulted in their retreat south. "All of them show a lack of energy and spirit, a want of thrift and cleanliness, which are altogether paradoxical to our men."[25]

Of course, Steiner observed Confederate soldiers on campaign, when it was very difficult to properly tend to matters of personal cleanliness. But Swalm observed them in a settled prison camp with more than enough time on their hands to wash their clothes, bathe, and clean up their tent areas. Those men simply did not want to keep clean and their officers allowed it. To be fair one could find enough Union soldiers who also did not take personal cleanliness seriously, but the proportion was far greater in Confederate ranks.

SINKS

There is little evidence concerning the use of latrines in the Confederate service, probably because of the private nature of the subject. Our understanding of sinks in the Union force comes mostly from the Sanitary Commission camp inspection returns; no such cache of information exists for the Confederate army. We know that sinks were used, but we do not know what proportion of regiments regularly dug them. All indications suggest that their use was at a lower level than in the Union army, especially given the lower level of officer supervision of the men's personal cleanliness.

We can point to a handful of references to sinks in official communications. Confederate army regulations spelled out the location for them compared to the camp and stipulated that a screen of bushes should provide privacy, much as did Union army regulations. Confederate regulations, however, only casually mentioned that dirt should be shoveled onto the contents "occasionally." Gen. Braxton Bragg issued a general order requiring all regiments in the Army of the Mississippi, the major Confederate field force in the western theater, to dig sinks and police them regularly. Officers were required to inspect them daily. How well units obeyed this order is an open question. An inspection report covering local defense troops cooperating with Lee's Army of Northern Virginia in the defense of Richmond during

November 1864 noted that a full array of sinks had been dug and the men were ordered to use them. It is worth noting that references to sinks do not appear in the documents generated by such high-level units as field armies and geographic departments in the Union force as they do in the Confederate army. This suggests an extremely lax enforcement of this basic camp-sanitation measure on the lower levels of the Confederate force. If most regiments had been digging sinks and policing them, there would have been no need for a field army or department commander to mention it.[26]

FOOD

There can be no doubt that the Confederate soldier ate far less well than his Union counterpart. This has always been a highly prominent theme of soldier life in the Civil War, and in general it was an accurate perception. The fact that short rations were an endemic problem in the Rebel army was due mostly to the inadequacies of the Confederate logistical system. But other important issues are whether Southern observers understood that a balanced diet was important; that an overabundance of meat in the army ration and a shortage of vegetables, for example, led to scurvy; and whether efforts were made to correct dietary abuses in the system of army rations. With nothing like the Sanitary Commission camp inspection reports to go on, answers to these questions must be gleaned from other sources.

But those sources really do not help very much. They mostly discuss the shortages of various aspects of the army diet rather than assessing the relative health value of them. An inspection report for Cheatham's Division in December 1862 listed the ration items issued to the troops that month. They included flour, meal, bacon, fresh beef or pork, salt, sugar at times, and rice. Items that were needed, according to the inspector, were vinegar, candles, and soap. What was not issued, or listed as needed by the inspector, were vegetables of any kind, fresh or preserved. Beef and pork were in increasingly short supply as the war continued. By 1863, some commentators suggested substituting fish for meat in the army ration, an idea that was rejected by the commissaries because of the cost and problems associated with preserving it.[27]

Ironically, the Confederate soldier may have eaten a more balanced diet in some ways than his Union counterpart simply because of this shortage of meat. Osteoarchaeologists who have examined the remains of Confederate soldiers and historical archaeologists who have investigated Rebel campsites picture Southern soldiers as having to live on a diet of corn and vegetables mostly taken from the countryside, with only a modest amount of beef and pork in their diet. But the main problem for the troops was getting enough of the vegetables through the strained logistical system. They were among the most perishable of food items and, even in a well-ordered supply chain, were not easy to transport long distances. There was no issuing of desiccated vegetables in the Confederate army because no Southern manufacturing establishment focused on producing this type of food. Scouring the countryside for provisions was a common practice, but it soon stripped any given region of available food for soldier and civilian alike.[28]

Problems of sheer hunger afflicted Confederate soldiers by the thousands. Lt. Simeon R. Martin of the Forty-Sixth Mississippi recalled the habit of making a cake of water and sugar, frying it in a pan, "warming it till it dissolved and then allowing it to cool and harden." He admitted it was not healthy, but the dish staved off the worst hunger for a while. Shortages were one thing, but the issue of inedible rations was another problem that should have been solvable. When the Third Texas consistently received cornmeal that was obviously unfit for human consumption while stationed at Galveston, the men reacted by staging a mutiny. They refused to drill on August 10, 1863, and reliable troops had to be called out to threaten them with arrest and worse until the men relented. Lt. Col. E. F. Gray, the regimental commander, admitted that the cornmeal was "sour, dirty, weevil-eaten, and filled with ants and worms, and not bolted." That such fare had been allowed to be issued even once, much less many times, stands as a testament to the inefficiency of the Confederate food system.[29]

COOKING

Confederate soldiers shared with their Federal counterparts an abysmal lack of knowledge about how to prepare their rations for healthy eating. As young men, they had not been taught how to cook while living with their families and now were expected to fend for themselves in the army. Regulations did not provide any help in this regard, stipulating, in fact, that soldiers were solely responsible for their cooking and forbidding the hiring of civilians to do that necessary task. The army was supposed to provide all cooking utensils, and the troops were ordered to be careful "in washing and scouring" them. Regulations assumed that cooking would be done on the mess system and stipulated that individuals in each mess should take their turn preparing the food rather than have one man as a permanent cook.[30]

As in so many other areas, the army regulations failed to spur the creation of an effective system of cooking. The special committee sent by the Confederate Congress to investigate the quartermaster, commissary, and medical departments visited many camps and hospitals and concluded that bad cooking was a fundamental cause of health problems in the Confederate army. In fact it focused on the lack of good, healthy soft bread for the men while in semipermanent camps and hospitals. "Until good bread is furnished to the Army we look in vain for a permanent restoration of health." Where made available, fresh bread had worked wonders, according to the committee.[31]

Many Confederate soldiers would have agreed with the committee conclusions. Henry Morton Stanley pointedly criticized the Rebel army for allowing its recruits to endure a painful period of adjustment to the reality of camp life, a period that lasted several months and tested their constitutions and stamina until they came to learn, through trial and error, an acceptable way to prepare their rations. A master cook, or "chef," hired to teach company cooks the proper way to prepare army rations "would have been useful for the *prevention*" of disease "in fifty per cent of the cases; but the age was not advanced enough to recognise this," Stanley wrote in his memoirs. Joshua Callaway also mentioned this problem in a wartime letter. "Our victuals are generally cooked hastily, our biscuits without soda, our beef hash without seasoning, & of course we can scarcely eat it."[32]

The men tried hard to find a way to prepare rations in a way that saved time and trouble and still produce edible food. In some cases they were helped by others. Callaway's mess utilized the services of a slave brought into the army by one of its members; this Black man turned out to be a good cook. But most Confederate soldiers entered into a crash course in culinary arts that more or less turned them into acceptably competent cooks.[33]

The government faltered in its commitment to provide cooking utensils for the troops. No matter which unit was inspected, no matter the date or the location, every inspection report indicated a shortage of cooking utensils. In some units the need was great, in others mild, but no Confederate unit had enough camp kettles or mess pans. In Anderson's Brigade, for example, there were only two-thirds the number of cooking utensils needed by the men during March 1863.[34]

WATER

When it came to the quality of water, everything depended on the locality. Semipermanent camps located near good sources of water allowed for healthy drinking, but many areas of the South offered few sources of potable water. The concentration of regiments around Corinth, Mississippi, during the spring of 1862 produced terrible health problems associated with bad water, including diarrhea. The men used "branch water or just any that we can get out of a creek or hollow, or anything but Springs and wells as they are scarce here," reported William N. Mattison of the Nineteenth South Carolina. A few months later Mattison's regiment moved to near Harrison, Tennessee, where it found spring water of much better quality for drinking, cooking, and washing. Confederate soldiers prized water from a spring above all other sources and often were amazed at the purity and volume a good one could provide. After the Battle of Stones River, Rebel soldiers noticed a significant decrease in the quality of water near Shelbyville compared to Murfreesboro after they retreated from the latter town. But those assigned to central Mississippi during Grant's operations against Vicksburg found themselves in one of the worst areas as far as good water was concerned. The dry climate and the nature of the soil led to scarce sources of readily available water for large concentrations of troops. "This is the worst place for water," wrote W. B. Lance to his family, "we can't hardly drink it we Just have to get it out of old ponds wherar [*sic*] it stands it looks like tarr I don't see how we can stand it."[35]

Substituting brewed beverages for poor local water was not much of an option. Coffee, for example, was in critically short supply in the Confederacy. All of it had to be imported, and the Union naval blockade largely cut off such imports. Confederate soldiers tried a variety of substitutes such as rye but generally did not like them. Genuine coffee was so scarce that the Confederate surgeon general restricted its use to hospitals, where it was used "solely for its medicinal effects as a stimulant."[36]

ALCOHOL

But another prepared liquid, alcohol, was in ample supply in the Confederacy. In fact, it became a major problem. The army tried to restrict its use by prohibiting any issue of whiskey except "in cases of extraordinary fatigue and exposure." Bragg in particular attempted to curb liquor with strict regulations within his command, which were adopted by the Confederate Adjutant and Inspector General's Office in January 1862. A general order identified intoxication as "the cause of nearly every evil from which we suffer" because it filled the guardhouse and led to sickness, inefficiency, and courts-martial. As in the Union army, alcohol was to be issued by the authorities only on the recommendation of medical officers and approved by unit commanders. A few months later efforts were made to prohibit the distillation of grain into alcohol except by government license in order to limit soldier drunkenness and save grain as food for the troops.[37]

It proved impossible to literally divorce all soldiers from sources of liquor. They managed to obtain it somehow, and problems of drunkenness continued to a greater or lesser degree. Moreover, the military system was willing to allow official issues of whiskey. The Battle of Stones River produced many official issues because it took place early in winter, with terribly cold temperatures for troops exposed day and night to the elements. It was the first and only time, according to T. J. Walker of the Ninth Tennessee, that his division received an official issue of whiskey. This issue was pretty general throughout the Army of Tennessee, but according to P. R. Jones of the Tenth Texas Cavalry (dismounted), more than half his company refused to accept it. Those who imbibed reported varying amounts, from a small drink to a good, hearty swig, indicating that the measure of the ration tended to vary from unit to unit. The standard issue was one gill, which was equivalent to four ounces, or one-fourth of a pint. But N. J. Hampton of the Eighteenth Tennessee managed to fill his canteen with whiskey and took it onto the field to aid the wounded. The issue of liquor was so widespread that even Union soldiers noticed it. When they conversed with captured Confederates and the subject cropped up, many Federals insisted that a tincture of gunpowder was mixed in with the alcohol the Confederates drank.[38] But there is no supporting evidence for such a conclusion.

MORALE

Confederate authorities paid no attention of any kind to amusements or morale of the troops in semipermanent camps. Still, they were concerned about the men's commitment to the cause and tried in feeble ways to bolster it by instituting a system of rewards for heroism in battle. But that system, consisting of the creation of a Roll of Honor to identify men in each regiment who had performed conspicuous deeds in combat, never fully developed because of the time, effort, and expense of creating it. At any rate, rewarding men for combat service was not part of the Northern sanitarian effort to sustain morale on a daily basis in camp. The Confederate soldier was even more on his own than his Union counterpart in dealing with idle time.

According to most accounts, the men did not mind creating their own amusements. "The social intercourse among the soldiers, aside from any other form of recreation, was a very agreeable manner of spending our time," asserted Goodloe. "Members of different messes would visit each other in an informal way, and we would often cluster about in camp, as we fell in with each other by accident or otherwise, and talk over the affairs of the day." When socializing grew stale, soldiers often improvised some sort of sport. Snowball fights after a winter storm mixed recreation with an odd sort of replication of combat. They often developed from small affairs into events wherein entire brigades or divisions massed to pelt each other with vigor, resulting in minor injuries. This also was not exactly what Northern sanitarians meant when they discussed camp amusements. Another idea for passing time was put forward by a civilian named G. W. Culpepper of Grantville, Georgia, who advised Jefferson Davis to encourage more observance of Sunday religious services as a way to occupy the soldiers' attention. Culpepper believed that would not only keep them on the straight and narrow but also avert much camp illness.[39]

RECRUIT EXAMINATION

The Confederate army deliberately watered down its recruit examination policy to bring as many men into service as possible. Surgeon General Moore instructed his subordinates not to pay attention to "trivial defects" and to pass all recruits who were "capable of bearing arms." This directive was issued in July 1862, soon after conscription had been instituted. Surgeons' examinations of recruits probably had been just as lax before that date when the core of the Confederate army was created through state-government action prior to conscription. Moore persisted in encouraging surgeons to be lax about this matter. In February 1863 the Adjutant and Inspector General's Office issued a general order denouncing "trivial disability" as an exemption from the draft. If a man could do "various occupations of civil life," then he could be a soldier. This meant that neither "slight deformity," deafness, speech impediment, functional disturbance of the heart, myopia, or hemorrhoids could be considered causes of disqualification for military service, unless they were exhibited in extreme forms. Even the loss of one eye or of several fingers did not excuse a man from army service, with authorities noting that he could be useful as a hospital worker or a quartermaster. Except for weeding out the most obvious physical problems, examining surgeons had no role to play in screening recruits and draftees.[40]

VACCINATION

Confederate authorities paid much more attention to smallpox vaccination than they did to recruit examination. As in the Union army, periodic outbreaks of this horrible disease caused alarm. The Confederate reaction was consistent with Federal efforts to curb its spread, which was inoculation of everyone within reach of the outbreak. In the end, the Confederate army did about as good a job of containing these occurrences as did the Federal army.

Although the Richmond government required smallpox vaccination for all enlistees in the army, there is no evidence that it took place during the first year of the war, when volunteer regiments were raised by state authority. If it did take place, the event failed to raise any notice in soldier accounts or in official reports. There is equally no evidence that draftees were regularly if ever vaccinated on induction into the army.[41]

But as noted, Confederate surgeons reacted in the same way as Union surgeons when smallpox broke out in their units. When it appeared in the Army of Northern Virginia during the winter of 1862–63, the entire army was vaccinated. That large-scale inoculation produced elevated levels of spurious results. The authors of the *Medical and Surgical History of the War of the Rebellion,* on examining evidence of this, noted that Robert E. Lee reportedly had five thousand men not fit for service when the Battle of Chancellorsville took place (May 1–4, 1863), and they implied this was due to the unusually high rate of spurious vaccination. They believed that taking vaccine matter from other adults was the cause of this problem and that using matter secured from children was safer. Southern physician Joseph Jones conducted extensive research into the incidence of spurious vaccinations in the Rebel army, noting that it was at a high level even in the civilian population during the war years. Jones concluded that the causes of spurious vaccination included the generally poor health caused by the bad diet of most Confederate soldiers, taking vaccine matter from poor sources, and allowing the matter to become dried and thus losing potency before applying it.[42]

The forces serving in the Department of Mississippi and East Louisiana also experienced an outbreak of smallpox late in 1862, which called forth an effort to inoculate everyone in the field force of that department. "I vaccinated every man in the Regiment as a preventative against Small Pox," wrote Surg. Thomas J. Blackwell of the Thirty-First Mississippi. When it appeared in the Thirteenth Tennessee in the Army of Tennessee, the regiment was separated from its brigade and "prompt measures were taken to secure the vaccination of all its members." The Forty-Fourth Mississippi missed the Battle of Stones River because of being quarantined due to an outbreak of smallpox before the engagement. There were no unusually elevated levels of spurious vaccination in this outbreak occurring within the Army of Tennessee late in 1862, but some regiments received bad vaccine matter. James Robert Maxwell recalled that it was tainted with some "very virulent disease" that was "worse than smallpox." He avoided this problem because a previous vaccination had produced a "good scar." The prevailing thought of the day was that "as long as an old scar showed up plainly that person was immune."[43]

Cases of smallpox continued to pop up in both the Army of Tennessee and the Army of Northern Virginia throughout the rest of the war. Abner Embry McGarity, surgeon of the Twenty-First Georgia, reported that cases in the latter army typically were brought to camp by furloughed men returning to duty and "scarcely ever spreads. It has been in almost every Regt. I know of and has never spread any yet." Surg. Urban G. Owen inoculated himself when a case of smallpox appeared in his Fourth Tennessee in the Army of Tennessee. "It took well with me," he told his wife. "It took well on me when a boy, & I was with the Smallpox a great deal while in New-York."[44]

REGIMENTAL HOSPITALS

The Confederate army created a hospital system similar to that of the Union army, but there is far less information about the most basic level of that system, the regimental hospital, than on the Federal regimental healthcare system. James M. Williams described pretty bad conditions in the hospital of his Twenty-First Alabama right after the Battle of Shiloh. "Our sick have a hard time in camp—insufficient medical attendance—lack of proper medicines—bad weather—improper food—and hospital tents—are carrying off men whose lives might be saved: two died in our regimental hospital tent last night; and another one will soon follow."[45]

The terrible conditions described by Williams may not have been typical of all Confederate regiments, and bad health situations could be found among Union regiments as well. But the evidence indicates that regimental hospitals in the Southern forces were much less endowed with equipment and supplies than was average among Northern units. Cheatham's Division, for example, had no more than three ambulances to serve the entire command, although surgeons utilized thirty-one two-horse wagons as makeshift ambulances. Elevated levels of illness among the rank and file in some Confederate regiments persisted even into 1864, long after those units had undergone their initiation into army life. Lt. Marcus Ely, for example, believed that more than a third of the men in his company of the Fifty-Fourth Georgia were sick in May 1864.[46]

OFFICER SUPERVISION

As in the Union force, Confederate officers were required to supervise all aspects of their unit's health. Army regulations mandated that regimental commanders inspect their men the last day of every month, while company commanders were to inspect each Sunday morning in addition to making "frequent visits" to their men's living quarters and food-preparation areas. The army placed special emphasis on officer supervision of rations to see that the proper items and amounts were actually issued. They were to "visit the kitchen daily, and inspect the kettles, and at all times carefully attend to the messing and economy" of the company, regiment, or post. The regulations often were reflected in unit administration. For example, in the Fifth Company, Washington Artillery, orders mandated that chiefs of sections and of messes were to observe their men "as to persons, clothing, arms, accoutrements, and equipments," blending sanitary concerns with the state of equipment and the overall readiness of the battery for combat.[47]

And that, really, was part of the problem. The Confederate military system did not press the need for preventive healthcare measures or the officers responsible for it as a separate, special duty. There are a number of inspection reports generated by Rebel officers, but they overwhelmingly tended to deal with equipment, discipline, and drill rather than with the many aspects of camp sanitation. The strong tendency was for inspectors to pay attention to everything but camp police, personal cleanliness, food preparation, and water quality in favor of things that related to combat readiness.

Most of the blame for the limited exercise of military effectiveness in Confederate camps has to be laid on regimental and company officers. Alfred Roman spared no criticism of them after inspecting Wheeler's cavalry early in 1865. "When officers are not personally acquainted with the affairs of their commands; when Colonels have to question their Captains, and Captains their Orderly sergeants, to answer to most of the questions that are asked of them in relation to their regiments and companies; when they so forget the difference between them and their subordinates, as to destroy the very semblance of rank and authority; when they seem ashamed to appear soldier like in their bearing, in their tone of command, and in their daily official intercourse with their men," it was time to get rid of them, he told Beauregard. But, of course, that was not an option. Once that veneer of authority was broken, it could not be replaced, and there were few if any replacements for failed unit officers at this stage of the conflict.[48]

CONCLUSION

There were far too few sanitarians in the South, and not many of them served in the army. Regimental and company commanders had too little administrative hold on their troops to have much of an effect on preventive healthcare. Even in the North, which had a healthy sanitarian movement in civilian society that was reflected in many ways by army policy, the results were at best mixed. But in the Confederate army, the few efforts to enforce sanitary principles were abject failures but for a few exceptions, as in reacting to smallpox outbreaks.

Joseph Jones, the well-known Southern physician who compiled massive amounts of statistics on Confederate soldier health during the war, wrote bluntly of this problem in the years following Appomattox. "There is no doubt but that in the recent struggle an immense number of valuable lives were sacrificed to bad police and sanitary regulations and to foul badly ventilated hospitals established in the center of crowded cities." The authors of the *Medical and Surgical History of the War of the Rebellion* concluded, based largely on Jones's data, that the Confederate army suffered a sickness rate about double that of the Federal army. They also concluded that disease was more fatal among Rebel soldiers than among Union troops. If that was true, much of it has to be ascribed, as did Jones, to the ignorance with which the Confederates approached the many aspects of preventive healthcare, from camp situation to officer supervision, espoused by Civil War–era sanitarians.[49]

11

After the Civil War

The result of all the work performed by the inspectors of the US Sanitary Commission, along with surgeons in the army, to reduce the challenges to soldier health became a matter of importance after the fighting ended. In the best-case scenario, Civil War–era sanitarians hoped to see evidence that preventive healthcare measures had been effective in curbing illness and mortality. Even better would have been evidence that their work served as a shining example to be followed by succeeding generations compelled to conduct a major war effort. In other words, they hoped that their work in the Civil War would have the same effect on the United States as the sufferings of the Crimean War had spurred major reforms in the British way of safeguarding soldier health. There was no quick or easy way for sanitarians to come to this desired conclusion because the Civil War had been so much longer, bigger, and more involved than the Crimean conflict. Its lessons were hard to find.

For example, the US Army tried to come to grips with the health history of the huge volunteer force that had won the war by publishing a massive amount of data on illness and mortality in the multivolume *Medical and Surgical History of the War of the Rebellion.* The compilers and authors relied heavily on evaluating data to come up with a positive picture of their own work at reducing the debilitating effects of camp life. They noted that the British Army had suffered a death rate of 94.9 men per 1,000 due to disease in January 1855, its worst rate during the Crimean War. In comparison, the Union army suffered on average the death of 53.4 men per 1,000 during the Civil War. Its worst rate, during the winter of 1862–63, was 63 men per 1,000. The compilers also compared the Civil War rate with the US Army death rate from disease before 1861, which was 18.98 per 1,000. They concluded that this was too high for peacetime and compared badly to the German peacetime death rate before the outbreak of the Franco-Prussian War (1870–71), which was around 5 men per 1,000. The German disease-related death rate greatly increased when the war with France broke out in 1870, reaching an average of 24.51 men per 1,000. In other words, it was normal for all national armies to see a huge increase in mortality due to disease in wartime compared to peacetime situations. In the United States the disease-related death rate dramatically dropped to 9.51 per 1,000 from 1866 to 1883, not only much lower than the wartime rates but also only half of what it had been before the Civil War.[1]

Brig. Gen. James B. Fry, the provost marshal general, also compiled statistics based on the extensive records his office maintained. He concluded that region, environment, and logistical power had a lot to do with death rates from disease. Troops serving in the Gulf region, in the lowlands of the Mississippi Valley, and in the Atlantic coastal regions suffered higher rates. He placed the general rate of death from disease at 59.22 men per 1,000; in comparison, the rates rose to 70.45 in the Gulf region and 71.55 in the Mississippi Valley. Troops serving in Virginia experienced a much lower rate, 37.88 men per 1,000. Fry ascribed this to a healthier region combined with a stronger, more reliable supply system feeding the Army of the Potomac.[2]

Statistical evidence such as this helps a good deal to set disease and healthcare in the Civil War within its proper context. One can conclude that massing huge numbers of troops for active operations inevitably raised the health challenges and required a correspondingly higher level of efforts at preventive healthcare measures of all kinds. The Union army succeeded in meeting that challenge better than did the British and French armies of the Crimean War but less well than the German army during the Franco-Prussian War. The American force apparently learned from the Civil War experience to cut its disease-related death rate in half after 1865 compared to its prewar experience. Fry's careful analysis indicated that much depended on circumstances; environmental factors played a huge role, for example, increasing the health challenges in some areas and decreasing them in others.

It also bears repeating that the bulk of the Union army consisted of volunteers fresh from civilian life, hastily organized largely by state governments, and existing as a separate military force of the central government. Although the regulations of the regular army were largely applied to this volunteer force, the extent to which they were obeyed remained problematic. Volunteer officers as a group simply did not uniformly share the same commitment to professional standards of conduct in their chosen field. As temporary soldiers, they had less interest in thoroughly learning the profession of arms.

SPANISH-AMERICAN WAR

Unfortunately, this problem resurfaced with dire consequences in the next US war, highlighting the problem of applying regular army rules to a hastily organized volunteer force. Only thirty-three years after Appomattox, the Spanish-American War (1898) called forth the mobilization of 200,000 volunteer troops by state governments to cooperate with the regular army. Although representing only 6.6 percent of the nearly 3 million volunteers who served the Federal government in the Civil War, the administration of preventive healthcare measures was atrocious during the conflict with Spain. This problem did not stem from a lack of information on the part of the army establishment, but rather from the very poor application of measures by volunteer officers, who seemed to have taken camp-police responsibilities even more lightly than did their predecessors of 1861.[3] Apparently, no lessons from the harsh experience of the Civil War had been learned about transferring sanitary knowledge from the regular to the volunteer force after 1865.

Spanish-American War officers had the Civil War as an example and, even more importantly, could draw on advances in civilian healthcare that had occurred between the two conflicts. By 1873, Englishman William Budd had built on earlier findings by Pierre Louis in France in 1829 to argue for the necessity of thorough cleansing of clothing, bed linen, and lavatories to contain the spread of typhoid fever, which produced severe diarrhea, abdominal pain, rashes, and delirium and had been a major problem during the Civil War.[4] Whatever progress in sanitary precautions that took place in civilian society do not seem to have seeped much into the thinking of the young men who joined the army in 1898, enlisted men and officers alike.

The common fly was the agent that primarily transmitted typhoid bacillus throughout army camps. It alighted on open deposits of feces and thereafter carried the bacillus everywhere it went. In short, camp sanitation was the best way to avert this awful disease. Because this bacillus was widespread in civilian society, it was inevitable that a certain proportion of volunteers would bring it with them in milder forms into the army. The Typhoid Board, created by the army in 1898, concluded that a typical

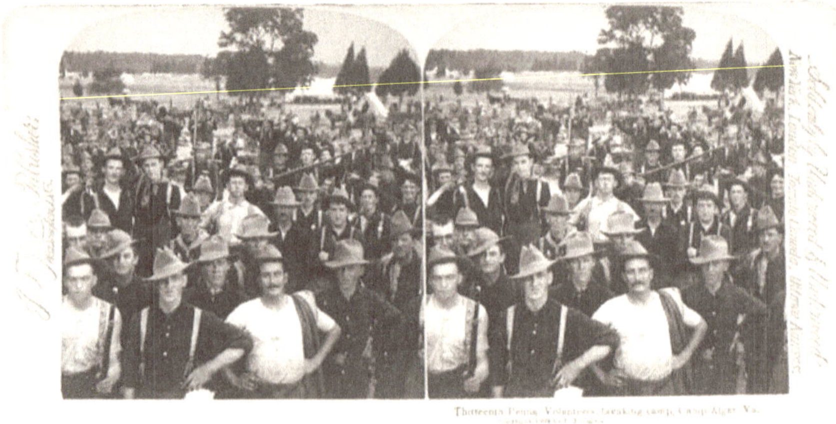

Spanish-American War Soldiers in Camp. These men of the Thirteenth Pennsylvania at Camp Alger, Virginia, shared the camping experience of all the other hastily mobilized volunteer regiments of the Spanish-American War. As with the early Union regiments of the Civil War, camp sanitation was dreadfully neglected by these men, which produced far more disease than should have been expected, considering the experience of the Civil War. But few Spanish-American War volunteer officers knew of that experience or of current sanitary science, all to their men's detriment. John Fillis Jarvis published this photograph in 1899. (Library of Congress, Prints & Photographs Division, LCDIG-stereo-1s49449)

regiment probably had at least one to four men already infected with it, and many of them seemed healthy. Poorly maintained latrines were the most common nodes of the vector that spread the bacillus in congested army camps. Flies, which were attracted by smell rather than sight, flitted between the latrine and the dinner table and even crawled in the open mouths of fever patients. Flies laid their eggs preferably on horse manure, one pound of which supported one thousand larvae and pupae, but they also laid eggs on human feces and decaying fruits and vegetables.[5]

The three-member Typhoid Board thoroughly investigated this problem in the Spanish-American War, examining the medical records of 108,000 men. When it filed its report in 1901, the board blamed typhoid on poor camp sanitation. It found latrines filled to overflowing, fecal matter scattered on the surface of the ground, soiled paper around the sinks, and flies swarming everywhere. The board found that medical officers repeatedly warned line officers of this problem to little avail. The volunteer officers were unusually lax, motivated by a desire to curry popularity with the rank and file, or they dismissed medical-officer recommendations as unimportant or an intrusion on their prerogatives. Some officers also looked upon camp fever as an inevitable fact of army life to be endured rather than attacked. Surg. Gen. George

M. Sternberg had issued orders for strict camp hygiene at the start of the war, but he was largely ignored by the volunteer officers. His subordinates in the field had complete control of soldiers who were admitted to regimental and all other army hospitals, but they could only advise unit commanders as to preventive healthcare measures for all the other troops.[6]

Neglecting basic camp sanitation produced a military environment that encouraged the fly population to explode and severely damaged the health and readiness of volunteer regiments. An unacceptably high 7.5 percent of all soldiers during the Spanish-American War contracted typhoid fever, and 7.7 percent of those who caught the disease died from its effects. It could be little comfort to know that in the Second Boer War (1899–1902) a total of 27.7 percent of the 208,226 British soldiers involved contracted typhoid fever, with 13.9 percent of them perishing from it. A few years later the Japanese Army took a lesson from the Spanish-American War and instituted better sanitary training into its ranks. As a result it suffered a very low rate of the disease during the Russo-Japanese War (1904–5). In a single field army of 599,617 men, only 1.6 percent contracted typhoid fever, but the death rate among those affected was very high, 32.5 percent.[7]

Another perspective on the camp crisis of the Spanish-American War is to highlight the very short duration of that conflict. War was declared in April and a peace arrangement was made in August 1898. A comparable period in the Civil War would have been from April to August 1861, which was the worst period for camp-sanitation problems in the Union army. The hastily organized regiments of the early months of that conflict produced the terrible camp conditions that prompted the US Sanitary Commission to institute its massive camp inspection program. As the Civil War lengthened, camp conditions improved greatly from those terrible first four months. In the Spanish-American War, however, the conflict ended before the volunteer officers and surgeons had a chance to learn on the job how to take care of their men.

THE FIGHT FOR CAMP SANITATION IN THE TWENTIETH CENTURY

The experience of the Spanish-American War finally created what the Civil War should have been: a watershed event in the history of the US Army's fight against camp diseases. The war of 1898 highlighted the same problems that had bedeviled the Civil War military force—the lax attention to hygiene among volunteer officers, the division of authority between medical officers and regimental commanders, and the difficulty of enforcing well-established rules in a force that was temporary and separate from the regulars. As the awful truth sank in, army officers raised the alarm, fearful that a future war could be even worse than the 1898 conflict. Capt. Peter E. Traub of the Thirteenth US Cavalry won a Gold Medal for an essay published in the *Journal of the Military Service Institution of the United States* in 1905 in which he argued that military hygiene needed to be taught to all army officers as part of their training. He pointed out what Civil War sanitarians had known—that prevention of disease was far better than treatment of it. The death rate from illness in 1898 was nothing less than "disgraceful" to the army, and something had to be done to prevent it from ever happening again.[8]

Alfred A. Woodhull had already retired from the army when the fourth edition of his *Military Hygiene for Officers of the Line* appeared in 1909. He had served as a Union army surgeon during the Civil War and was the medical inspector for the Army of the James during the last year of that conflict. From 1886 to 1890, Woodhull had taught military hygiene at the Infantry and Cavalry School, Fort Leavenworth, Kansas, and wrote his lectures for initial publication in 1890. The effort failed, of course, to avert the medical problems of the Spanish-American War despite the fact that a second edition appeared the year of that conflict. By the time of the fourth edition, more than six years after the war, the army was more attuned to its message, which would have sounded familiar to Civil War sanitarians. "The very first element in the efficiency of an army is its health," Woodhull stated. He called it "a serious and constant duty" that could not be shirked. Like Traub, he urged full education for all line officers in the significance of sanitary principles.[9]

Woodhull discussed camp situation, housing (conical and shelter tents were still common), proper ventilation of living quarters, proper military clothing, food, disposal of kitchen waste, and careful recruit examination, and he strongly stressed officer supervision of all elements relating to the health of the men. Like the Civil War sanitarians, Woodhull urged officers to encourage efforts "to amuse the men," including dramatic entertainment by the troops, games, and educational programs. He emphasized the importance of military music, arguing that "good bands are . . . good hygienic agents." Water purifiers and filters were needed, especially when on campaign. Woodhull warned that smallpox had not yet been eradicated and believed there was still a need to vaccinate all recruits. Inspections to gauge the level of personal cleanliness should not be confined to looking at the outward appearance of the man. Woodhull wanted officers to make their troops remove shoes and one sock as well as open their coats and shirts for a closer look.[10]

Toilet facilities and practices received special attention from the former Civil War surgeon. In semipermanent camps sinks need not be offensive to sight or smell if they were dug and placed properly and then maintained daily with fresh dirt and disinfectant. On the march Woodhull offered advice about how to deal with individual calls of nature. He urged officers to plan a halt in the march a half hour after starting in the morning to allow the men to attend to their need. Officers should designate which side of the road to be used, downwind if possible, and order the men to cover the deposit. A detail of a few men with shovels would follow up in case some troops failed to obey that order. All of this was very sound advice, but one wonders how fully officers would follow it. By this time, the army was issuing soluble toilet paper, and Woodhull wanted its use to be mandatory, especially for water closets on army posts, which "ignorant recruits are so liable to derange with newspaper, bits of cloth, and sometimes with more unsuitable objects."[11]

The US Army came off looking rather shabby in the way it approached camp sanitation in Woodhull's book. His early experience in the Civil War had imbued a lifelong devotion to the concept, and he viewed it with relatively little change over his long army career. "Military hygiene has been practiced in a rule-of-thumb and imperfect way for a long time," he wrote. But judging by reports emanating from the Russo-Japanese War, the new army of Japan had achieved a far higher level of sanitary fitness than the Americans. That conflict had shown that, "the claims of theorists are not futile, and that there is such a science as military hygiene and such an art as applied sanitation."[12]

In addition to Woodhull's strong commentary, Surgeon General Sternberg weighed in on the public debate with a scathing analysis published as a book in 1912. He noted that of the 6,406 regulars and volunteers who had died in service from May 1, 1898, to April 30, 1899, disease had claimed 5,438. That represented 84.8 percent of American deaths in that war; by comparison, in the Union army about 66 percent of those who died perished from disease. The death rate in the army caused by typhoid fever during the Spanish-American War, Sternberg noted, was about equal to the same rate in the largest US cities of that time. Ironically, the army had been making progress in reducing typhoid fever as a health problem before the war with Spain. Sternberg reported that the rate had been cut in half during the ten-year period ending 1897 compared to the previous ten-year period ending in 1887 (55 deaths per 100,000 versus 108 per 100,000). But the Spanish-American War mobilization had caused the typhoid-fever death rate to soar by twenty-two times compared to the prior decade record, and that was due entirely to the influx of raw volunteers and the shortage of regular army medical staff to help them acclimate to camp life. Sternberg documented his attempts to avert this calamity, reproducing his directions for camp sanitation issued on April 25, 1898, and supplementing it with clear advice in his book about the proper way to police and arrange army camps with preventive healthcare measures in mind.[13]

Sternberg laid the blame for the war's sad history of camp sanitation squarely on the volunteer officers. They came from a civilian culture that in many ways was still largely indifferent to preventive healthcare principles and took that limiting view with them into the army. "The officers and enlisted men of our volunteer regiments were as a rule intelligent, patriotic and brave, but they were not disciplined. Each man was in the habit of judging for himself and of acting in accordance with his individual judgment." They placed sanitary principles low on their list of priorities. Many volunteer surgeons were not able to meet the challenge of converting quickly from a civilian to a military mode of thinking about healthcare.[14]

Traub, Woodhull, and Sternberg were writing in a postwar period during which the army establishment and the federal government finally realized that the root problem lay in the volunteer system of manpower mobilization. It was an inefficient way of preparing for war. The result was a dramatic alteration in the mobilization policy of the nation. After more than a century of relying on the action of state governments to raise troops, the most successful example of which had occurred during the Civil War, the federal government began to organize a system for direct mobilization by the central authority. This change, coupled with an enlarged and multivaried program of basic training for officers and men, gave the US Army far more control over the mobilization process along with more control over shaping the attitudes and practices of newly raised personnel. The army adopted a more modern approach to creating a large war machine that would produce good results in a variety of areas, including healthcare for the troops.[15]

FROM VOLUNTEER TO CONSCRIPT

The only way the central authority could gain true control of manpower mobilization was to institute a full-fledged conscription system. That was done with the Selective Service Act, signed on May 18, 1917, soon after the United States entered World War I. Although resisted by some, this first modern draft in the country's history brought 2,758,542 men into military service. An additional 2,000,000 men volunteered directly to the federal government, not through state-government authorities. All of them, draftees and volunteers alike, went through the same induction process, which inculcated the principles of camp sanitation. Those principles had, for the most part, not really changed since the Civil War, but their enforcement certainly changed for the better.[16]

One area in which huge strides had been made by 1917 lay in soldier morale. Little of an institutional nature had been implemented to amuse the Civil War soldier except regimental bands. But by the era of World War I, corporate culture in the United States had encouraged the shaping of morale by the army establishment. The federal government cooperated closely with several private organizations to provide amusement for American troops while in camp. Efforts ranged across the board, but the most attention was given to the proliferation of reading material and encouraging boxing as a sport. The War Department created the Commission on Training Camp Activities, which worked with the Young Men's Christian Association, the American Library Association, and the Knights of Columbus. Surveys were taken to see what inductees most wanted to do, as these organizations blended those preferences with their own vision of shaping the morality, minds, and philosophies of millions of young American men while they were in service. Much of the motivation was not only to prevent them from drifting into vice but also to indoctrinate them into the developing mass consumer culture of the country through providing a range of items they could purchase after returning to civilian life—"forging the soldier-consumer," as historian Mark T. Hauser has put it.[17]

Half a century after the Civil War, the American army had largely solved the problem of poor application of sanitary principles by eliminating the volunteer system and substituting the draft to obtain tighter control over fresh recruits and their officers. The results were shown in late 1918, when the fighting came to an end in World War I. That conflict proved to be the first in American history during which about as many men died of disease as of combat-related causes. While 50,280 succumbed to battle, 57,460 died of illness, mostly due to the Spanish Influenza pandemic. This compared with the 84.8 percent of deaths due to illness in the Spanish-American War and the two-thirds who died of illness in the Civil War.[18]

As a case study, the British Army's performance in healthcare during World War II (1939–45) illustrates what was possible if the right attitudes and administrative systems came together. A recent study by historian Mark Harrison argued that the key was close cooperation between medical officers and line commanders. Most of that had to come from the line officers, who had to become "medically minded" to reap the full benefits of healthcare for their men. British Eighth Army officers took sanitary precautions seriously during the North African campaigns, which resulted in a much lower sickness rate than among their opponents in the Afrika Korps during the key battle of El Alamein in October 1942. The Germans suffered from a sickness rate almost three times higher than the British at that time because Erwin Rommel and his subordinates placed low priority on preventive healthcare measures. In Bernard L. Montgomery's command, in contrast, "specialist hygiene sections" cleaned up refuse and constructed and maintained privies. They also inoculated soldiers and local civilians alike for a variety of diseases and pursued fly-control policies with vigor. These sections also educated and indoctrinated the troops to drill home the importance of sanitary principles.[19]

As in every war, environment played a huge role in soldier health. World War II, which spanned the globe, was conducted in a wide variety of climates and landscapes, some of which were more threatening to the troops than others. Statistics show that disease remained a bigger threat to the troops than combat on the whole. For example, in Southeast Asia, one of the most health-threatening environments of the war, 418 British soldiers were affected by disease compared to 32 affected by combat during 1945. In contrast, the ratio was 163 compared to 64 in northwestern Europe during the same year. But far fewer men who contracted any disease died from it than in any previous conflict. In World War II "fewer than one in one hundred deaths in the British Army" were due to illness. Officers finally understood that medicine "could maximize the potential of manpower."[20]

The Civil War took place near the end of a historic period wherein medical care failed to curb the most dangerous problem faced by soldiers—disease. Most of that disease threat emerged from the rapid gathering of large numbers of men into congested military communities with inadequate ideas about how to arrange their living spaces. Even after medical personnel became aware of the dangers of those spaces by the early nineteenth century, they had great difficulty convincing officers of the need to manage the camp environment to reduce illness, winning that struggle only in the twentieth century. At best, one can only see partial success on the part of medical officers during the Civil War in creating a fit atmosphere for the implementation of preventive healthcare measures in the Union and Confederate armies.

THE LONG VIEW

An interesting assemblage of statistics on death due to disease compared to combat has been put together by historian John Landers. It covers several major armies from the early seventeenth century to the late nineteenth century and indicates that relatively little changed during this time period as far as averting the problem of disease in large military forces. The highest proportion of disease-related deaths compared to overall deaths ran up to 88 percent for Swedish forces from 1620 to 1719 and 81.3 percent for the British Army during the French Revolutionary and Napoleonic Wars. The French army during the Napoleonic period (77.6 percent), the British force in the Crimean War (79.3 percent), the French army in the Crimea (78.8 percent), and the Russian army during the Russo-Turkish War (78.4 percent) constituted the next-highest category of rates. Slightly lower were the rates for all forces involved in the Iberian campaigns of the Napoleonic Wars (69.2 percent), the Russian force in the Crimean War (68.6 percent), the Union army in the American Civil War (69.4 percent, according to Landers's figures), the Austrian army (68.1 percent) and the Prussian force (62.4 percent) in the Austro-Prussian War, and the German force in the Franco-Prussian War (69.4 percent). These long-view statistics indicate fluctuation over time, but they remain within brackets that extend from 62.4 percent to 88 percent. In short, the overwhelming majority of all soldier deaths in war for nearly three hundred years had been due to illness rather than combat. The Civil War fit well within those brackets, although closer to the lower end than the higher.[21]

Historian Vincent J. Cirillo compiled his own long view of American military deaths due to disease from the Revolutionary War to the occupation of Iraq in the early twenty-first century. He divided that time period into a "Disease Era" (1775 to 1918), during which illness accounted for more soldier deaths than did combat, and a "Trauma Era" (1941 to the present), in which battle accounted for more deaths than illness. In fact, during the Trauma Era, accidents led to most of the noncombat deaths in the US armed forces. Cirillo identified the Mexican War (1846–48) as a prominent example of the Disease Era. Volunteer troops suffered twice the disease mortality rate of the regulars "because the latter had a better grasp of the importance of personal hygiene and camp sanitation." According to his figures, camp disease accounted for 96.8 percent of the 11,347 noncombat deaths in that conflict. Although the problem was greatly reduced during World War I, Cirillo argued that the US disease death rate of that conflict was higher than the rate for many of the other belligerents of the Great War.[22]

World War II, the first conflict in which US forces suffered more combat deaths than disease deaths, began the Trauma Era. The army strove to gain a handle on the camp environment not only through sanitary procedures but also by inoculating the men for a wide variety of diseases, including smallpox and typhoid fever. Because of the wide array of climates and environments, American servicemen suffered high levels of disease-related ailments, but only a small percentage of them perished. Using Cirillo's data and combining only the deaths caused by disease with those caused by combat (excluding accidental and other types of fatalities), only 6 percent of the total American deaths in World War II were caused by disease. The ratio reduced further during the Korean War (1.8 percent) and the Vietnam War (1.9 percent). In the latter conflict 8.7 percent of the 10,700 noncombat deaths were due to disease, the rest mostly due to accidents. Because combat deaths were so low in the Persian Gulf War of 1991, the thirty Americans who perished of disease represented 16 percent of noncombat deaths. But during the occupation of Iraq from 2003 to 2008, the percentage slipped down to 2.1 percent.[23]

The Civil War took place near the end of the Disease Era, too early for Union soldiers to have the benefit of widespread acceptance of camp-sanitation procedures, improved inoculation technology, and an expanded medical staff charged with covering all aspects of preventive healthcare. It is interesting, however, that even the best preventive healthcare programs of the Trauma Era could not eliminate disease threats from the military environment. They could and did tremendously reduce those threats and offered generally effective healthcare when disease struck, thus greatly reducing mortality. But even in the country's most recent conflicts, some American soldiers have died of disease. Control rather than elimination of illness was the key to the reduction of fatalities during the past eighty years.

THE CIVIL WAR CAMP ENVIRONMENT IN RETROSPECT

During the Civil War, the camp environment was not by any means the only health threat to Union soldiers. On campaign they were exposed to a variety of environments that challenged their well-being and consequently reduced their effectiveness as soldiers. The US Sanitary Commission could offer very little in the way of helping men endure the rigors of campaign and battle, but it tried mightily to help them while in semipermanent camps between campaigns. The first step was its program of inspection and advice; the second step was shipping needed supplies to the camps to supplement army issue. The commission worked quite loosely with the military establishment in this endeavor that, as we have seen in the previous chapters, had at best a limited effect on improving the camp environment in order to prevent disease.

Civil War soldiers were aware of the fact that camp diseases were a major threat to their health, but few of them dwelt too much on it. They filled their letters and diaries with details about camp life, often complaining of its problems but also dwelling on its delights and even its charms. After the war their memoirs were filled with nostalgic images of camp life, especially the camaraderie, or the bonding of fellow soldiers. As historian Phoebe S. K. Young has pointed out, Civil War soldiers were not the first large group of Americans to live outdoors for a certain purpose, but they certainly became the most famous such group after 1865. Their postwar writings publicized camp life far more extensively than any previous group of American campers, probably more so than any subsequent group as well. Camp diseases became muted in this postwar memory. Time and distance brought out the comforting aspects of camp life and softened the disturbing awareness of disease, dirt, and bad food that had been major elements of army life during the Civil War.[24]

Conclusion

The best source of information on how Union soldiers lived while occupying semipermanent camps during the Civil War comes not from their letters, diaries, or memoirs but from the camp inspection returns compiled by the US Sanitary Commission. While personal accounts offer much colorful commentary on soldier life, they are individual, impressionistic sources of information that are sporadic in nature. Personal accounts offer pungent commentary but do not cover all aspects of camp life, nor do they cover the entire Union force in a systematic way. In the absence of any better sources of information, they must be relied upon, but their limitations should be kept in mind.

In contrast, the camp inspection returns are voluminous, with 1,465 returns residing in the archive of the US Sanitary Commission at the New York Public Library. They cover fifteen subject areas connected with camp life, not concerned only about cleanliness but also a host of other factors, including hospitals, supervision, and morale. In spanning the entire Union army over the whole war zone from 1861 to early 1864, they cover all geographic regions as well as a long duration of time. The returns systematically examine those fifteen subject areas to present a mass of detailed information in a far more balanced and comprehensive way than any collection of personal accounts by soldiers. The returns also provide us with the opportunity to compile statistical data, something virtually impossible by consulting personal accounts. Sanitarians in the commission, as well as in civilian life and in the military, described the principles that guided their thinking about camp life; the returns give us the information to gauge how far the Union army managed to put those principles into action. An added benefit of using the information on these returns is to gauge how well the volunteer units of the Federal army acted to fulfill regulations and orders concerning camp sanitation. Thus, the inspection returns are a wonderful source of information on army administration as well as on camp life and soldier health in the Civil War.

As indicated in the introduction, I selected 280 returns to serve as a balanced cross-section of the whole. The camp inspectors filled out these returns primarily with yes and no answers to questions posed about the fifteen subject areas on the commission's standard camp-inspection form. They also often made qualitative remarks on any issue for further clarification. To add statistical power to the returns, I categorized the answers as "Good," "Fair," and "Bad." After completing the classification, I went back to the returns I examined at the beginning of the process and recategorized them to see if my second round coincided with my first evaluation. It did so, adding credence to my methodology.

My sample was selected across geographic theaters of operations and included all the three branches of service as well as engineers and Black regiments. No statistically significant differences were found by geographic location of the army or by type of units. These findings suggest that rather than separate subcultures existing in the Union army regarding sanitation issues, there was an overall camp-sanitation culture. Even though there were significant differences across units, these were not caused by geographic location or branch of service but simply by idiosyncratic differences among soldiers (or officers) across units.

Throughout chapters 2–9, I have referred to what percentages of the inspected units were evaluated as good, fair, and bad in each of the fifteen subject areas. This allowed a view of each topic in terms of how well health standards were met. In the following pages, however, I apply a different level of analysis to rank the subject areas to see which ones the Federal units performed well in and which presented the most problems.

The first two columns of the table, "Good" and "Fair," represent success in meeting sanitary principles, with a good rating indicating greater success than a fair rating. For this reason, the ranking for success (third column) is weighted to reflect that greater success for the good classification in each of the fifteen subject areas. The weighting is achieved by multiplying the percentage under "Good" by 1.5 and adding the percentage under "Fair." After that, the subject areas are ranked, with the highest score for success (denoted as 1) to the lowest, (denoted as 15) shown in column 3. For example, the units

Success and Failure Rankings

Subject Areas	Success			Failure	
	"Good" (Highly Successful)	"Fair" (Moderately Successful)	Weighted Ranking Based on Success*	"Bad" (Failure)	Ranking Based on Failure (where least failure is ranked as best=1)
Camp Situation	39.6%	41.5%	100.9 (6)	18.9%	6
Shelter	50.0%	45.4%	120.4 (2)	4.6%	1 (best)
Clothing	47.5%	42.2%	113.5 (3)	10.3%	3
Personal Cleanliness	28.9%	52.5%	95.9 (8)	18.6%	5
Slops	57.8%	22.1%	108.8 (5)	20.1%	7
Sinks	36.7%	30.0%	85.1 (9)	33.3%	12
Food	25.0%	32.2%	69.7 (14)	42.8%	14
Cooking	51.7%	33.6%	111.2 (4)	14.7%	4
Water	72.5%	20.0%	128.8 (1, best)	7.5%	2
Alcohol	41.4%	38.5%	100.6 (7)	20.1%	7
Morale	26.7%	38.6%	78.7 (11)	34.7%	11
Recruit Examination	18.5%	57.2%	85.0 (10)	24.3%	9
Vaccination	29.3%	34.3%	78.3 (12)	36.4%	13
Regimental Hospitals	18.2%	36.1%	63.4 (15, worst)	45.7%	15 (worst)
Officer Supervision	15.3%	52.5%	75.5 (13)	32.2%	10

* 1.5 times Good Rating + Fair Rating = Weighted Ranking (e.g., 1.5 x 39.6 + 41.5 = 100.9)

represented by the 280 returns performed the best in securing a good water supply and worst in maintaining a regimental hospital.

Failure in meeting sanitary principles is directly based on the rating under "Bad," the fourth column, which clearly denotes an inability to meet what the sanitarians believed was necessary for an effective military force. In some subject areas the failure was relatively less than in others. Here, the subject areas are ranked in column 5, with the least failure denoted as 1 (best) and the worst failure as 15. For example, the units had the lowest failure rating in the subject area of shelter while failing most miserably in the area of regimental hospitals.

In eleven of the subject areas, the ranking for success was either the same or just one point different than the subject area's ranking for failure. In the other four subject areas—personal cleanliness, slops, sinks, and officer supervision—the difference was two to three points. Overall, the rankings in columns 3 and 5 are highly consistent. Here is what the ranking of each subject area implies.

1. Water was first in the success ranking. It came in second on the failure ranking, meaning that its bad rating was the second lowest of all subject areas. In other words, water ranked at or near the top either way. Officers and enlisted men needed little encouragement to understand how important potable water was to their well-being. Given that sites for semipermanent camps were typically selected with some time and care, officers considered how readily good sources of water could be accessed in the area. Only 7.5 percent of the units failed to do so.

2. Shelter rated second in the success ranking and first in the failure ranking (meaning least failure of all subject areas). That does not mean there were no problems with soldier housing; the returns fully document those shortcomings. It is just that only 4.6 percent of the regiments had severe issues. The high overall rating resulted from the fact that there was time in semipermanent camps for officers and men to make the best accommodations they could, and camp inspectors realized it. Even though tents may have been old and moldy, they provided a modicum of shelter for the men, enough for them to get by with a hardy attitude. Sanitary principles stressed that tents and huts were better than barracks and civilian housing. Union regiments rarely used either of the latter two types while mostly living in tents and huts, so they came close to meeting sanitary principles.

3. Clothing represented the third most successful subject area by either ranking. The Federal uniform, woolen with innocuous colors, loose fitting, and with reasonably effective caps and hats, complied well with the principles enunciated by Civil War sanitarians for practical military clothing. Camp inspectors therefore had no reason to criticize the uniform on sanitary grounds. Their only concern lay in the realm of army logistics and administration. If the regiments received the items due them in a timely manner, they received good evaluations. The fact that clothing ranked third in the success rating indicates that in this area the army system worked pretty well. Only 10.3 percent of the units did poorly in getting uniforms to their men.

4. Cooking was the fourth-most-successful subject area by either ranking. That is surprising given the lack of effective education as to how the men should prepare their rations. Camp inspectors did not take that into account for this subject area. They also did not consistently give bad ratings to regiments that allowed individual cooking, a mode of food preparation that sanitarians uniformly frowned upon. Inspectors took into account soldier satisfaction, which was highest when they cooked individually, and

gave credit when regiments had even the semblance of officer supervision. In these ways cooking eked out a high ranking for success contrary to what a strict sanitarian view of the subject area might have elicited.

5. Slops rated fifth on the success ranking and seventh using the failure ranking. Much attention was paid to getting food waste out of the camps by setting up barrels to dump it into and emptying the contents outside the perimeter on a daily basis. Camp inspectors found much to praise in this way, even though they also found poor slop-disposal routines in one-fifth (20.1 percent) of the units.

6. Camp situation placed sixth by either ranking. One could expect it to rank higher because unit officers usually had opportunities to carefully select the sites for their semipermanent camps. But there were many sanitary principles involved that made that choice difficult. For example, sanitarians preferred slopes so that rainwater would drain away quickly. They also wanted a soil type that would facilitate drainage, favoring a sandy mix rather than pure clay. Sanitarians advised not to situate within woods because the trees inhibited the free flow of fresh air through the camp. And they wanted to have a supply of good water nearby, which was one of the easier principles to fulfill. But to find a site with all these advantages restricted the officers' options. Camp inspectors tended to adhere strictly to their principles in evaluating this subject area.

7. Alcohol rated seventh on both the success and failure rankings. That may come as a surprise to historians, who have relied heavily on personal accounts to assess the role of liquor in Civil War soldier life. If one relied solely on those accounts, it would give the impression that the Union army was awash in liquor. But camp inspectors found otherwise. Regimental officers and regimental surgeons overwhelmingly stated that problems related to alcohol were limited to a small minority of addicted men in the ranks who constantly sought to find and consume it. They admitted that most of the men placed in the guardhouse for infractions of discipline were put there by drunkenness. Camp inspectors were instructed to document how many men occupied the guardhouse, and it always was a small fraction of the total manpower in the regiment. The impression one gets from these camp inspection returns is that of prevailing sobriety rather than endemic drunkenness. The Union force was not such a hard-drinking army as previously thought. This reflects well on army administration for keeping liquor out of the camps, except for those individuals who were so addicted to it that they could not be stopped. It also reflects well on the influence of the prewar temperance and prohibition movement in helping keep Union troops sober.

8. Personal cleanliness placed eighth in the success ranking and fifth on the failure ranking. Most of the units (52.5 percent) were evaluated as fair, while the rest received assessments somewhat evenly divided between good and bad. The fact is that habits of personal cleanliness were heavily dependent on the individual. No matter how much officers urged their men to wash their faces, hands, and necks every day and to bathe and wash their underwear every week, it all depended on each individual to take up that responsibility. Most regiments did this in a reasonable way, and some went beyond expectations. But some units simply did not do so well in this area. Officers could go only so far in inspecting personal cleanliness and were reluctant to supervise the men's bathing.

9. Sinks rated ninth on the success ranking and twelfth on the failure ranking. It would seem to have been an easy job to achieve a much higher ranking; after all, everyone should have seen the importance of putting human waste far from their quarters, where it belonged. But the regiments did a surprisingly mediocre job of this necessary chore. Most of them had sinks but failed to maintain them by adding a layer of dirt or disinfectant on a daily basis. A surprising number of units had no sinks at all. Moreover, sanitarians agreed that the men should not urinate within the boundaries of the camp at night, but soldiers did so on a widespread basis, most likely because they did not want to venture far in the darkness. There was little effort by the officers to correct that abuse because it was not easy to do so.

10. Recruit examination ranked tenth in success and ninth in failure. This must have been a disappointment to sanitarians. They stressed the importance of a thorough physical examination to cull men with health conditions that reduced their ability to perform military duties. The army administration had thoroughly understood this importance for decades before the Civil War. The only people who did not understand it were the volunteer regimental officers and many of their volunteer surgeons. Camp inspectors gave the regiments bad ratings in this subject area because many factors led volunteer officers to forego a thorough recruit examination despite army regulations to do so. This subject area goes directly to the topic of military effectiveness, with devastating results for the volunteer force. Only when recruit examination was under the control of the US Army, as during the prewar years and when the provost marshal general was in charge of it from 1863 to 1865, were the regulations followed.

11. Morale rated as eleventh by either ranking. Ironically, specific questions on the returns clearly indicate that morale was quite high among the units visited. Inspectors usually answered "yes" to the question of whether

the men were in good spirits. But they responded "no" to the question of whether the army did anything to encourage high morale. The fact is that the men amused themselves, using their own devices to keep up their spirits. The army itself invested little in any administrative effort to shape their morale. Because sanitarians thought the army had a responsibility to do more to keep spirits high, they reacted negatively. For example, the government was supposed to maintain regimental bands, which it initially did but then reneged on that commitment in July 1862. Camp inspectors held the units to strict accountability on that score, and thus the army administration came off pretty badly in terms of trying to keep the men occupied in a positive way instead of idling away their time in the semipermanent camps.

12. Vaccination placed twelfth on the success ranking and thirteenth on the failure ranking. The requirement to inoculate all recruits against smallpox was combined with recruit examinations as an entry-level process, to be conducted when the regiment was being organized. That organizational review usually was hasty, hectic, and filled with pressure to keep recruit numbers high so everyone could be quickly mustered into service. There was precious little time allowed to properly vaccinate or examine recruits, and thus both requirements were shortchanged by the mobilization policy of state volunteers. On the positive side the returns provided evidence that most of the recruits had been vaccinated against smallpox earlier in their lives, although medical theory argued that revaccination should be conducted about every five years.

13. Officer supervision stood thirteenth in the success ranking and tenth in the failure ranking. Camp inspectors documented widespread ignorance of preventive healthcare responsibilities among regimental and company commanders as well as among regimental surgeons. They also documented widespread indifference to enforcing sanitary principles. This subject area was one that goes directly and deeply to the topic of military effectiveness. The low evaluation must have distressed commission officials. If volunteer officers could not understand that they bore an important responsibility for supervising the men's health, then there was relatively little the administrative structure could do about enforcing sanitary principles.

14. Food placed low (fourteenth) in both rankings, which demands some explanation. Although the Union army was generally well supplied with food, the diet was unbalanced, with too much emphasis on meat. This was the result of a perceived preference for beef among the soldiers and the desire of commissaries to feed that hunger. The official ration allowed for a balanced diet but did not mandate it. Commissaries could select among op-

tions, and too many of them exercised that degree of latitude to give the majority of meat-hungry men what they wanted. Many Union soldiers wanted more vegetables and fruits but did not receive them as a result. Sanitarians supported meat as a major part of the army diet, but they equally stressed the need for a corresponding amount of plant food to create balance in nutrients. The low ranking for food therefore came from a strict adherence to sanitarian principles among the camp inspectors. They noted that vegetables were lacking and fruit was almost nonexistent in the regiments they visited.

15. Regimental hospitals rated as the worst of all fifteen subject areas by either ranking. Camp inspectors were appalled at the sorry state of most regimental hospitals in terms of inadequate equipment and supplies as well as in terms of the organization of the hospitals and the competence level of the regimental surgeons. In contrast to some other subject areas such as cooking, they held regimental hospitals to a strict evaluation, perhaps because many of those inspectors were themselves physicians. Their dismal assessments reflect poorly on some aspects of army support and logistics, lowering our view of military effectiveness in the volunteer force. But the sorry state of most regimental hospitals was due as much to incompetent medical staff as to the limitations of army supply, which also reflects poorly on the efficiency of the volunteer force.

A careful reading of the contents of these camp inspection returns presents a mixed picture of effectiveness in fulfilling sanitary principles for healthy camp living during the Civil War. In some areas the volunteers did well, while in others they did very poorly, and every gradation between can be documented. Much of the reason for this lies in the nature of the Union force called up to fight the war. It was raised directly from the populace by state governments, led by officers with as little military training and experience as the rank and file, and tended to by civilian physicians who were as ignorant of military healthcare as everyone else in the regiments. A huge learning curve faced these officers and surgeons, and it is not surprising that they achieved limited success in adapting to military regulations.

But many sanitarians of the Civil War era, who were eager to praise their own efforts, did not see it this way. They adopted the most positive viewpoint in an effort to convince themselves that, like the example of the Crimean War on British and French sanitary practices, the Civil War would be the beginning of a new era in military hygiene in the United States. "During the war there were immense strides made in public hygiene," declared Dr. Henry I. Bowditch as he spoke to the International Medical Congress in Philadelphia in September 1876. A Massachusetts abolitionist, professor of clinical medicine at Harvard University during the war years, and a contributor to the science of public health, Bowditch was certain that the efforts of fellow sanitarians had made a large difference in the conflict. "We cannot doubt that every surgeon who served during the war . . . became more practically versed in the advantages of the prevention of disease over the cure of it, than he ever was before." Bowditch believed that this awareness spilled over into the postwar civilian life of the nation to propel sanitary principles to the forefront of public-health concerns.[1]

A similarly positive view of the war experience was expressed by Dr. George Derby, who had served as an army surgeon and worked at Boston City Hospital after the conflict. In an address to the Massachusetts Medical Society in 1867, he was certain that "our most sanguine hopes were fulfilled" for preventive healthcare measures. With "a little care and discretion," army doctors could foster the cooperative relationship between officer and surgeon that was essential for the implementation of "the rules of hygienic science as applied to war." Derby firmly believed there was a connection between a clean camp and elevated levels of health among the men. "Good and sufficient clothing, clean and well drained camps, abundant food and plenty of coffee, unlimited exposure to sun and air, and hospitals perfectly ventilated" had produced good results. Derby cited statistics from the Mexican War, wherein 10–11 percent of American soldiers died annually of disease, and from the Crimean conflict, in which 25 percent of allied soldiers had suffered the same fate, compared to the Civil War, with about 6 percent of Union soldiers perishing from disease-related causes, to prove his point.[2]

Derby positioned the Civil War as a turning point in the history of military medicine. It was the first time that sanitary principles current in the great cities of Europe, and to a much more limited degree in the urban centers of the United States, had been largely applied to soldiers. He believed that the Union army could serve as a model for larger application of those principles in America. "The neatness of our camps might indeed give a useful hint to Massachusetts farmers whose sinks, house drains, privies and adjacent premises would often be the better for such 'policing' as a Medical Inspector would require for a soldier's quarters."[3]

This positive view has been echoed by recent historians, who see in the Civil War an important watershed in the development of preventive healthcare principles as applied to civilian society. They have noted that many army surgeons became active in the public-healthcare movement after 1865 and, like Derby, have pointed to the Union army's camp policing as the proper way to attack elevated levels of disease, especially in urban settings. "The Civil War experience unquestionably shaped the sanitary reform movement in the critical decades of the late nineteenth century," concluded historian Suellen Hoy.[4]

But we have seen enough in the previous chapters to call into question this triumphalist view of sanitary care in Union army camps during the Civil War. It is quite possible that the conflict was a watershed in public acceptance of sanitary principles in the civilian life of the nation, and that physicians gained new respect generally as scientists capable of engineering health in society at large. But the results of the US Sanitary Commission camp inspection program provide ample evidence that the principles of preventive healthcare were not so widely accepted or implemented in the army infrastructure as to justify such sweeping conclusions about the conflict's positive role in military healthcare. As far as the Union army was concerned, sanitary measures had some effect, but not by any means of a revolutionary nature. At best one could say that they curbed what undoubtedly would have been a worse situation without eliminating the major threats posed by army camps to the health of the men.

Samuel Gridley Howe noticed this problem from the beginning of the war. Sent to inspect the camps of three Massachusetts regiments in the Washington, DC, area early in May 1861, he thoughtfully reported his findings to Gov. John A. Andrew. Howe used his experience as a volunteer in the Greek War for Independence forty years earlier as a comparison. He noted that there were two great objects in view when corralling soldiers into army camps: the first was to train them for war, and the second was to "raise their physical powers to a maximum." Training was attended to with vigor; all officers seemed attuned to the need for drill and tactical preparation. Soldier health, unfortunately, received far from universal attention. There was a "lamentable distinction" here, in that the tactical preparation was the province of the officers and the sanitary condition the province of the surgeons. Howe argued that "a really good officer will also be a good sanitarian," but those responsibilities were "almost everywhere overlooked" by the volunteer commanders. Boxers were not only trained how to hit well but also fed properly; in contrast, soldiers were well drilled but fed "on salt junk" and housed in stuffy quarters "with foul air."[5]

Still, Howe was willing to give the Union army at this early stage of the war fairly high marks. "Compared with European armies in the field, ours is healthy; compared with the rebel army it is probably very healthy; but compared with a half million men at home, it is fearfully unhealthy." He was hopeful of improvement in the near future, but it had to be based on a fruitful melding of medical advice by unit surgeons and administrative control by unit commanders, which he could not yet see in action. Howe wanted Union soldiers to be lifted above "the common and low standard of armies" to a level not yet demonstrated in military service.[6]

The best hope for the accomplishment of this lofty goal was the camp inspection program of the US Sanitary Commission. As a nongovernmental organization, the commission gained the approval of the Federal government but achieved no power to enforce its views in the army. It could only investigate, which the government welcomed, and offer advice to unit commanders and surgeons alike. Whether that advice was received gratefully and acted upon was up to the receivers. But at least the commission was trying to spread the news of sanitary principles to the men most responsible for acting on them and, in the process, compiling a massive source of information on the actual state of camp sanitation during the war.

Camp inspectors were fully aware of the challenges they faced from the beginning of the inspection program. The "great difficulty" of the first year of the war "was the want on the part of the officers and men, of a due appreciation of the importance of sanitary precautions," wrote A. N. Read of regiments he inspected in Kentucky in the fall of 1861. "They could not understand the necessity of thoroughly policing a camp," especially if it was to be occupied for only a short while. Read visited twenty-four regiments during three weeks and summarized the problems as poor camp location, bad tents, horrible cooking, and inattention to establishing and maintaining sinks. He drew the officers' attention to these problems and found some limited improvement when paying a second visit. Read focused attention on one regiment in particular while refusing to name it. "The cooking bad. The men dirty. In short, by want of cleanliness and attention to the requirements of civilized life, the men were in danger of losing all self-respect." But when revisiting a few days after he wrote this report, he found much improvement.[7]

It is good that Read believed he had made a difference in that regiment's case, but Henry W. Warriner was not sure of his own efforts. While at Benton Barracks near St. Louis, he found the Third Michigan Cavalry in poor shape. Its commander, Col. Robert H. G. Minty—"an Irishman, slight in stature, amiable, elegant in manners, about 30 years of age and apparently a scholar"—did not have a good attitude toward sanitary principles. "A fundamental notion of discipline with him is, that not much can be done with *volunteers* in the way of controlling their personal habits." Warriner felt that the men were not as healthy as they needed to be for active service and that the cause stemmed from "over-crowded Barracks. I have to-day made eloquent complaint to the Post Commander. He was moved. Will the *men* be?"[8]

Indeed, the volunteer nature of the Union army was the key to the commission's decision to organize the camp inspection program in the first place. The inspectors were charged with the diagnostic task not only of discovering sanitary problems but also of trying to correct them by urging changes on the regimental officers and surgeons. "Their position was not an enviable one," concluded Alex McDonald right after the war. "Their duties compelled a close scrutiny of all excesses, abuses, incompetency, carelessness or negligence, and immediate action for the removal of all causes of complaint." The inspectors gained friends in some camps but made enemies in others. In the latter case it might have been that the inspector "failed to approach the official with due deference to his rank, or he [the officer] may have been opposed to 'permitting civilians to interfere with military matters,'" as McDonald put it. Yet he noted that when open to advice, some officers used the camp visit as a turning point in the sanitary condition of the unit. John H. Douglas felt that the mere act of asking questions had an influence on regimental officers because it indirectly gave them an idea of exactly what to think about when planning camp routine. He usually talked not only to the commander and the surgeon but also to the adjutant of the regiment.[9]

But talking did not always work. Some army officers resented a civilian who offered criticism of their work, and one can understand that in some cases this might be justified. A case in point bears on the sanitary condition of Camp Douglas (near Chicago), which housed many Confederate prisoners when Dr. Henry W. Bellows, the president of the US Sanitary Commission, visited in June 1862. "The amount of standing water, of unpoliced grounds, of foul sinks, of unventilated and crowded barracks, of general disorder, of soil reeking with miasmatic accretions, of rotten bones and the empytings of camp-kettles, is enough to drive a sanitarian to despair." Bellows considered it nearly impossible to clean up "soil loaded with accumulated filth" or barracks "with two stories of vermin and animal exhalations." He proposed moving the entire camp to a new bit of ground and offered to provide plans for the accommodation of 10,000 men in the new location. William Hoffman, the commissary general of prisoners, rejected Bellows's view. He did not think Camp Douglas was in such bad shape nor did it need to be moved. Hoffman believed it could be renovated at little cost, mostly by using the prisoners as laborers, and that policy was approved. But prisoner exchanges drained Hoffman's potential labor source, and even the prison guards left because they had been enlisted for only a few months of service. As a result, when more prisoners arrived early in 1863, conditions at the camp quickly worsened, and Bellows dispatched two commission inspectors to look into them in May.[10] There is no evidence that this additional inspection produced results.

A similar situation developed for another prison pen, Camp Lookout in Maryland. William F. Swalm inspected the sixteen-acre compound, which housed 8,000 prisoners, when he visited in November 1863. He found virtually every sanitary rule violated. Swalm noted that sinks were not conveniently located or well maintained, the men were allowed to relieve themselves wherever they wished, the tent areas and interiors were filthy, rations were short, the hospital was in bad shape, the surgeon in charge was not energetic, and the camp generally was very dirty.[11]

Unlike Bellows's view of conditions at Camp Douglas, which Hoffman admitted was valid, responsible army officers reacted very negatively when Swalm's report was made known to them. Gilman Marston, commander of Saint Mary's District, which included the location of Camp Lookout, called Swalm's report "disingenuous and false. It is surprising that the commission should employ agents so stupid or dishonest as the author of this report." Marston admitted that the prisoners had terrible habits of personal cleanliness, but the Union army had provided them with everything they needed for camp life. He urged Hoffman to see the camp for himself or to send "a soldier or army surgeon, who knows what camp life is and who has sufficient ability to apprehend the facts and integrity enough to state them." Hoffman did send an army surgeon named Augustus M. Clark to inspect Camp Lookout. Clark reported that the tents were crowded and the drainage was poor, the sinks were in bad shape and the personal cleanliness of the prisoners was quite bad. He admitted that the officer in charge of the prison hospital was incompetent. Yet, being a practical man, he also admitted that conditions were not likely to improve as long as the prisoners themselves did not take sanitary principles seriously.[12]

Army administration decided to leave things as they were at Camp Lookout. Hoffman told the Sanitary Commission that Swalm's report was erroneous and asked that it not be made public. Word of conditions at the camp reached Secretary of War Edwin M. Stanton, who sent Maj. Gen. Benjamin F. Butler to inspect it. Butler went much further than Marston in reporting that the camp was in admirable shape. While lower-level army officers admitted the problem but could see no real chance of improvement, higher-level officers whitewashed the incident to show that no problem existed.[13]

The interesting point about Camp Lookout is Marston's initial reaction to Swalm's report, which reeked of irritation toward an outsider judging army standards. While the conditions at Camp Lookout obviously were terrible, one can understand to a degree Marston's frustration. Army officers dealt with such problems at hundreds of posts and often had little effect on forcing changes to improve them. Most of them knew about sanitary principles but were practical men who understood how limited their efforts could be. Thus, their standard was much lower than the civilians who worked for the Sanitary Commission. Those inspectors made quick evaluations based on short visits and gauged army camps according to the highest expectations. Inevitably, there would be clashes of opinion, hurt feelings, and resentment growing out of the delicate relationship between commission inspector and commanding officer.

Yet generally speaking, in trying to educate army officers about their responsibilities concerning "*Preventive* or *Hygienic*" medical care, camp inspectors found most of them polite, attentive, and gracious. How well they absorbed these lessons was difficult for the inspectors to tell, but at least the visitor only occasionally met overt hostility. They could more readily assess the reception of their advice when consulting with medical officers than with unit commanders. But inspectors noted that with many volunteer surgeons, they had a long way to go. "It is difficult for medical men to shake off the habits of civil practice in which there is not much demand for attention to preventive measures," wrote Dr. James P. Prince of the Twenty-Second Massachusetts and later of the Thirty-Sixth Massachusetts. He admitted of his fellow volunteer surgeons that they "were for the most part ignorant of the true conditions of military hygiene, and nearly all the information imparted on this subject came through the agents of the Sanitary Commission."[14]

Prince was wrong to state that the commission inspectors were the main source of information about sanitary principles. The volunteer surgeons had a relationship not only with the camp inspectors but with regular army physicians as well. Surg. Alonzo J. Phelps of the Thirty-Third Ohio complained after the war that those regular army doctors did little to help him and other volunteers learn the ropes of military healthcare. "We naturally looked to them as directors and instructors," he wrote.

> We were disappointed to find that they had no instructions to give other than those which were to be found in the Army Regulations. These "Regulations" embraced but little more than directions how to procure medical

> supplies by requisition and to prescribe the forms for certain reports; and howsoever well they might have answered the requirements of the army in time of peace, they were totally inadequate now with an army of hundreds of thousands in active service. The new medical officer therefore, was thrown from the first upon his own resources; and whatever of excellence characterized the medical department of the army at the close of the war was the result of the aptitude of the American mind to adapt itself to any emergency that calls forth its action.[15]

Phelps made an important point, and the key was the intersection between the small regular army structure and the separate organization adopted for the huge and hastily created volunteer army. The relationship between the two forces charged with fighting the Civil War was tenuous at best. Regular officers filled most of the higher levels of command, those on the corps, field army, and military department levels. But from the division down to the company, command positions were overwhelmingly filled by volunteer officers. Even within the established bureaus that supported both army structures, most of the officers were volunteers temporarily serving in those bureau assignments. There were two ways that the regular army could have exerted more influence on the volunteer army. One was to staff important positions within the volunteer units with regular officers. That was utterly impossible considering the relative sizes of the two forces. There were far too few regulars to go around. The second was to establish schools of instruction so that regular army personnel could teach the volunteer officers how to conduct their military business not only in terms of preventive healthcare but also for literally all their many duties. This was a feasible course of action, but it was never attempted. Again, there were very few regular personnel capable of teaching; more importantly, there simply was no precedent in the American army for such schools. The major European forces had long before 1861 understood the need for schools of instruction in many areas of army life and had complex and thriving military educational systems operating in peacetime. But beyond the US Military Academy at West Point, Americans had nothing comparable to those European systems for training personnel on all levels about how to fulfill their duties.[16]

The volunteers were largely on their own, with their only guide being the army regulations. Phelps correctly noted that those instructions only offered a bare-bones approach to the duties of the army surgeon, providing little more than statements of responsibilities with no advice on how to fulfill them. Phelps cited one particular example, the subject area relating to recruit examination, to support his point. He thought that volunteer surgeons operated under "the prevailing impression that for the volunteer service it was not necessary to be as severe as if examining for the regular army. This was a great error to commence with" and led to significant problems that could have been averted if a tighter relationship between the volunteer and regular surgeons had been established.[17]

Left largely on their own, volunteer surgeons turned in a mixed record of success in acclimating themselves to military duties. Some camp inspectors praised surgeons for their readiness to learn. Godfrey Aigner felt that they were "getting gradually alive to their own preventive duties" the more he talked with them early in the war. But Marvin M. Marsh found a wall separating him from both the officers and the surgeons of a regular artillery battery at Hilton Head, South Carolina, in 1863. They resented the shipment of supplies and food sent by the Sanitary Commission to units in the field as intrusions on their territory. Expectations of such articles from outside the army system bred irresponsibility on the part of the men and weakened their reliance on their own officers. This was a slap against the commission that Marsh could not help but notice.[18]

In this way as in all others, the work of the camp inspectors was riven with evidence of limited effectiveness at imparting the message of preventive healthcare. The main message was that keeping clean promoted health, a mantra repeated by many inspectors and regimental surgeons alike. Evidence to be found in regimental histories and personal accounts prove that this message sank in for many volunteers but not others. Maj. Henry Lee Higginson worked assiduously to implement key sanitary principles in the First Massachusetts Cavalry. "If we never see a fight," he wrote of its officers, "we all have nevertheless learned to care for and manage men: you'd be surprised to find how little our intelligent Yankees know of caring for their own health. They eat and drink all sorts of things." Brig. Gen. John J. Peck also imbibed the lessons as he managed a brigade of infantry. "Camps have been changed frequently. Tents have been often struck; the ground cleared and aired. Side hills and high ground have been preferred. Much attention has been paid to drainage. Troops were not allowed to go below the surface in their tents. Vaccination has been general." Peck praised the medical staff, calling his chief surgeon "skillful, intelligent, and faithful." Many volunteer officers acknowledged that they had experienced a learning curve from the war's beginning to its end as far as camp sanitation was concerned. "At this stage of the war," Thomas W. Hyde wrote of the Petersburg Campaign, "we had . . . learned the value of hygiene, and paid as much attention to the health of the men as to their drill and discipline. If we had known how to look after their health earlier, it might have shortened the war."[19]

That there should be a tight connection between camp cleanliness and good health seemed obvious to those men who listened to Sanitary Commission inspectors. But inspectors themselves now and then came across examples of regiments that practiced good camp hygiene and yet suffered elevated levels of sickness. F. U. Johnston admitted this in his report of the 148th Pennsylvania. "The whole camp is clean and airy," yet typhoid fever was a persistent problem that could only be explained by theorizing that some men had contracted it elsewhere and brought it to the camp. Alfred L. Castleman found the reverse when he visited the Thirty-Sixth Illinois. "I have scarcely met in this Army a regiment so badly policed. The insides of the tents are very dirty, the men sleep on rubber blankets on the damp ground, or on straw, damp & foul, which has been used for 6 to 8 weeks. The streets and drains clogged with rubbish in a State of decay. Yet there is not a regiment here which presents so clean a record of health." Castleman offered no explanation for this contradiction of theoretical expectations.[20]

The Sanitary Commission downplayed the sporadic evidence that clean camps did not necessarily lead to healthy regiments or that dirty camps inevitably produced a lot of illness. It assumed, not without cause, that the connection between camp condition and soldier health was real in most cases. In fact, after a year and a half of camp inspections, the commission tried to push these views further onto the army. Soon after Lincoln called for 300,000 additional volunteers early in July 1862, its executive committee assured the president that the results of the camp inspection program had yielded "definite conclusion as to measures necessary to protect these new levies against certain of the dangers which threaten them." The committee mostly focused on the "careless and superficial medical inspection of recruits" as the chief problem. It pointed out that, despite army regulations, no real examination had taken place in 1861. As a result, it estimated that 25 percent of the recruits were physically and medically unfit for service. "Some regiments left 10 per cent. of their men in hospitals on the road before they reached the seat of war," the committee informed the president.[21]

The Sanitary Commission tried to position itself as the chief authority in the nation when it came to preventive healthcare in the army, based largely on the results of its camp inspection program. Those returns revealed enough information about camp hygiene to prove the validity of sanitary science. In this way the committee sought to add weight to its recommendations that only regular army surgeons completely unconnected with volunteer regiments should be in charge of recruit examination. It also urged Lincoln to institute some control measures that could force volunteer officers to obey sanitary rules. Camp inspectors had tried to do this through personal interaction with surgeons, but some sort of institutional compulsion was also needed. The committee urged Lincoln to put the additional 300,000 volunteers into older regiments; creating entirely new volunteer units would merely duplicate the problems experienced in 1861 and lead to another round of starting from scratch as far as sanitary education was concerned. It even went so far as to urge the consolidation of all volunteer regiments into the regular army structure to better ensure that regulations were followed.[22]

This effort to influence policy at the top of the Union military system failed to produce results. Lincoln was not willing to institute changes in the mobilization process, which was heavily based on the spirit of voluntarism and relied on state governments to organize regiments and commission their officers before transferring them to the Federal government. Sanitary Commission inspectors remained only an advisory corps—their advice could be taken or not by volunteer officers and surgeons for the duration of the war.

But the proper perspective on this important topic is to recognize that the Sanitary Commission did not have a monopoly on information about preventive healthcare. The army had long known about sanitary science and had a good set of policies on the books for promoting it. At the start of the war, Robert C. Wood, the acting surgeon general, urged Secretary of War Simon Cameron to set up "preliminary arrangements for the preservation of the health of the troops." Before the commission came into being, Wood suggested the creation of an advisory board to help the army develop the most up-to-date policies for camp sanitation. He named several men, including Henry Bellows, who would soon become involved in the commission, as possible members of this board. Apparently, that board was never created, but very soon the commission began operating and started advising the army. George B. McClellan agreed with its recommendation that a medical director be appointed for the Army of the Potomac, that an ambulance corps be organized for the army, and that male and female nurses be hired for work in its hospitals. These ideas soon spread to other field armies across the nation.[23]

Apparently, there was no Sanitary Commission contribution to the army's creation of a new position in its medical system, that of medical inspector.

Congressional action had authorized the creation of a corps of medical inspectors through legislation on April 16 and December 27, 1862, but it was not until early in 1863 that the army implemented the change. This was a potentially significant step in promoting camp hygiene because it mandated regular and thorough inspections of all army camps and posts, with special reference to the most important elements of camp cleanliness and levels of sickness among regiments. The medical inspector was charged with "supervision of all that relates to the sanitary condition of the Army." He was to work with unit commanders to effect improvement when needed.[24]

The work of these medical inspectors provided much detailed information about camp conditions—the Fifteenth Corps reports are a prime example—but whether their work led to significant improvement in those conditions is not clear. Judging from Fifteenth Corps reports, there was uneven improvement over time, if any at all. One must keep in mind that these inspectors were mostly drawn from volunteer regiments, and they in turn inspected volunteer regiments.

When Congress passed the Enrollment Act on March 3, 1863, creating the first national draft in the Northern states, it also vested control of conscription to the provost marshal general of the army, Col. James B. Fry. His bureau also was given control over the process of voluntary enlistments and instituted a thorough program of recruit examination that would have made the Sanitary Commission proud. Close to one-third of enlistees and draftees were rejected for a variety of physical and mental conditions by surgeons hired by the bureau in these recruit examinations.[25]

Under Fry's direction, the Provost Marshal General Bureau kept tabs on losses to better fulfill its job of recruiting new soldiers. Using information from muster and pay rolls, Fry saw a sharp distinction between the losses of officers and enlisted men. While one officer was lost for every eighteen enlisted men due to combat, only one officer died of disease for every ninety enlisted men who died of illness. "Officers are better sheltered than men," Fry concluded, "and their food is generally better in quality and more varied in kind, so that they suffer less from diseases of the digestive organs. They are not so much crowded together in tents and quarters, and are therefore less subject to contagious and epidemic maladies. They have superior advantages in regard to personal cleanliness."[26]

Fry's interesting statistics and conclusions highlighted the role of sanitary science. Officers had far more opportunities to avoid camp diseases precisely because their situation within the army system allowed for more individual choice in everything from housing to bathing. But the system could not be expected to allow enlisted men a similar latitude of choice. Entry into the army took away most of those choices, and the soldiers did not regain them until discharge. While in service, enlisted men were the charges of the government. The army has to be given good marks in its willingness to understand the principles of camp sanitation and its attempts to promote them as much as it was feasible to do so.

The US Sanitary Commission also deserves good marks for trying hard to support and implement those principles, largely through the camp inspection program. It was a "laborious inspection system" as Bellows told General-in-Chief Henry W. Halleck in September 1862, but it had resulted in much information of "scientific value." The inspection program declined, however, by late 1863. Alex McDonald noted that "this inspection work was not so necessary as previously," and therefore the number of inspectors was greatly reduced. Very few camp inspection returns were filed in 1864 and none in 1865.[27]

As a whole, the returns do not provide proof that the camp inspection program had a marked effect on improving health in the Union army. While many of them indicate that advice to regimental officers was well taken, the returns do not necessarily follow through in a systematic way to gauge improvement over time. Of the 280 returns used in this study, 103 represent repeat visits to regiments that had earlier been inspected, usually by a different inspector. Among those 103 returns are represented thirty-six regiments with from two to five returns each. Although this apparently was the result of circumstance rather than design, these multiple inspections offer some insight into the question of improvement over time based on an inspector's advice. But an examination of their results clearly shows that there was no consistent improvement in the camp conditions of these thirty-six regiments. Instead, the returns indicate wild fluctuation over time.

This suggests a real limitation of the camp inspection program as an agent of change, even though the returns are extremely valuable as diagnostic tools to identify unit sanitation problems. The visits provided snapshots of camp sanitation for one regiment on one day of its service. That day cannot be taken as fully representative of the unit's history, for a week later its camp sanitation may have been much better or much worse, only to change again a month later. So much depended on circumstances because all the elements that came together to produce the camp environment made for a very complicated mix that changed a good deal from day to day, week to week. Even conscientious officers and surgeons would have had their hands full in trying to control all those elements; consequently, there were good results on some days and poor results on others even in well-managed units.

As we have seen, whatever the faults of the Union army system in terms of sanitary care, the situation was much worse for the Confederates. No sanitary movement supported education among their officers, no significant Confederate army program pushed sanitary principles, and most observers agreed that Rebel camps tended to be filthy. Henry Morton Stanley brought to this question an outsider's view, having been born in Wales. "The fault of the American generalship was that it devoted itself solely to strategy and fighting, and providing commissariat supplies; but seldom, or never, to the kindly science of health-preservation." Stanley could not recall during his service as a soldier in the Sixth Arkansas that any officer "examined the state of our messes, or stooped to show that, though he was our military superior, he could take a friendly and neighbourly interest in our well-being." Once sick, a man was cared for, but there seemed to be no idea that illness could be averted by preventive care.[28]

Ironically, the volunteer nature of recruitment for the US Navy did not prevent important strides forward in naval hygiene. The environment of naval service differed remarkably from service in land forces, but the need for sanitary care was just as important. The key to shipboard service was in maintaining a clean, dry, and well-ventilated living and working space for the sailor. Preventive healthcare on warships had been a major focus of reform in the Royal Navy during the later eighteenth century, still the age of sail, and it continued to be important in the early stages of the age of ironclad vessels. In fact, steam and iron construction posed new health hazards plus new advantages in managing sailor healthcare. Overall, the Royal Navy had far more advantages administratively than did the British Army. Warships were self-contained little communities under the full authority of the captain, who had enormous power to institute change in shipboard life. Given the overriding need to conserve manpower, the navy also had an overriding incentive to take preventive healthcare seriously.[29]

Efforts to improve sanitary measures on board Union warships during the Civil War were much more successful than in the Union army. A committee of the US Sanitary Commission investigated life aboard ironclad monitors early in 1864 and recommended improvements in cleanliness, dryness, and ventilation. These measures were implemented and contributed to a dramatic reduction in the sick rate among monitor sailors, from over 25 percent in 1863 to a little over 5 percent in 1865. Once pointed in the right direction, naval officers quickly instituted the kind of sanitary changes that would have pleased any sanitarian. Even on the gunboat fleet operating on the Mississippi River, naval officers maintained far higher standards of personal cleanliness among crewmembers than did the army for its soldiers. When several hundred soldiers were detailed to help man river gunboats early in 1863, Rear Adm. David Dixon Porter instructed his boat commanders that their first priority was to train those men in how to operate the vessel's heavy guns and their second priority was to "tend to getting them cleaned up, having their hair cut, beards trimmed, etc."[30]

In both the Union and Confederate armies and in the Union navy, the key factor was the officer in charge of his men. In the navy he tended to be careful and strict concerning preventive health measures. This attitude was worked into his professional culture, and commanding a small group of men living in close proximity with each other in a small space, it also was easier for him to accomplish the best in preventive healthcare. But in the land forces of both belligerents, the volunteer nature of the troops raised to fight the war produced too many officers with no training and little incentive to learn more about war than each felt was necessary to get by. Drawn straight from civilian life with no preparation for military duties, no desire to be a soldier except as part of their answer to a governmental call for temporary service, volunteer officers shared with the enlisted men a sheer ignorance of camp sanitation that posed a major threat to their well-being. All the efforts of the prewar regular army to impose its knowledge and standards on that massive volunteer force, which stood at a million men at peak strength, failed to thoroughly deal with the many problems of camp sanitation. The supplemental work of the US Sanitary Commission through its camp inspection program helped a good deal, but it failed to thoroughly instill those important principles.

Considerations of how well volunteer officers learned their jobs has mostly focused on combat-related issues and the personal relationships between them and the enlisted men. The historical literature has portrayed the officers as mostly learning how to perform in these areas reasonably well.[31] But the area of camp sanitation has not been studied by historians who have focused on midlevel officers in the Civil War. Here, the situation was much more mixed, with a strong tendency toward the lower end of the effectiveness scale.

But that was not the view of US Surg. Gen. William A. Hammond, who adopted a very strident view of camp sanitation. Motivated to put the best face on the issue, he argued in 1863 that unspecified reports "show[ed] the excellent sanitary condition which has generally prevailed. There have been some exceptions," Hammond admitted, but he thought these were few. As the results of the Sanitary Commission camp inspection returns clearly indicate, that was a highly unrealistic assessment by the surgeon general.[32]

In his history of the Sanitary Commission, Charles J. Stillé was careful not to go too far in praising either the level of camp hygiene in the Civil War or his commission's camp inspection program. He noted the "very extraordinary" ignorance of many officers concerning sanitary care and admitted that they were indignant when told about it by camp inspectors. "Their surprise was almost ludicrous," he noted, but most officers took the advice seriously, in his view, and tried to improve their camps. "The Inspectors were almost universally received with courtesy by the officers, and their suggestions were listened to with the greatest interest and attention."[33]

Compared to Hammond's evaluation of the army's sanitary level, Stillé's assessments of that level and of the Sanitary Commission's inspection efforts were closer to the truth. The commission's efforts were highly commendable, highly unprecedented, and no doubt resulted in improvement in the camp environment in many cases. How widespread that improvement happened to be, how lasting it was, and whether it resulted in any postwar advance in sanitary progress for civilian society is not easy to determine. The only conclusion one can make on that score is that glowing assessments that fail to acknowledge limitations are not convincing. Greater strides toward preventive healthcare goals took place in the decades after 1865, but whether they had a direct connection with the Civil War experience is questionable. The horrible episodes of typhoid fever that Spanish-American War soldiers endured cast a huge shadow over any triumphalist appraisal of lessons learned by the US Army from the Civil War. If the military administration could not learn how to make volunteers obey sanitary rules during the Civil War, it is no surprise that similar problems cropped up in the next conflict.

Moreover, the limited effect of preventive healthcare measures in the Civil War contributed to the elevated levels of illness in the Union army. From the start of the war until December 31, 1862, the army treated 1,661,602 cases of disease in a force that averaged about 600,000 men. Of that number, 482,764 cases (29.05 percent) were due to diarrhea and dysentery, conditions directly linked to camp sanitation and diet.[34]

Camp sanitation was not a major problem in World War II, but interestingly, the US Army encountered somewhat similar problems of incorporating a huge mass of men into a relatively small prewar force to fight that expansive conflict. The men were draftees rather than volunteers, and they were inducted directly by the central government, not by the state governments. Despite being in control of the mobilization process, the army found that it was not easy to make the draftees understand and respect regulations. These men were better educated, enjoyed higher intellectual levels than the pre–World War II soldiers, and questioned, complained, and criticized military procedure far more. In fact, the army had to invest much time and effort into finding out what the draftees wanted and how to help them acclimate to military life without changing proven regulations too much. It succeeded pretty well, considering that troop strength went from 250,000 men in 1940 to 8,000,000 at peak strength in a relatively short time.[35]

Civil War army officials could not conduct surveys to find out what volunteer enlisted men wanted or bend their rules to accommodate the lack of interest among volunteer officers in learning how to care for their men in camp. All they could do was tell those officers they needed to take responsibility for that care and create a system to determine how well it was being done. It is surprising to find so little follow up to medical inspection reports and to Sanitary Commission returns with the intention of correcting abuses in the area of camp sanitation. Civil War armies had gone a short distance toward effectiveness when they created rules and added inspections, but they did not follow through on the next step—taking action to clean things up in a thorough and consistent way.

The relative lack of a lasting influence on army culture does not make the US Sanitary Commission camp inspection program a cypher in Civil War history. The fact that there was such a commission at all, that it strove so eagerly to evaluate camp living conditions and educate volunteer officers and surgeons about the camp environment, and that the US Army also tried to improve that environment all represented dramatic departures from the past. All these efforts could not overcome the many obstacles to sanitary progress, chief among which was ignorance and lack of receptivity among the men most important in cleaning up the campsites. Nevertheless, some regimental camps became cleaner, a certain percentage of soldiers became healthier, and the effectiveness level of the Union army became better to some degree by the efforts of the commission's camp inspectors and the army's medical inspectors. That alone justified the effort—and it justifies modern study of camp sanitation in the Civil War.

Notes

ABBREVIATIONS

In citing works in the notes, short titles are generally used. Frequently cited sources are identified by the following abbreviations:

ADAH	Alabama Department of Archives and History, Montgomery
AHC	Atlanta History Center, Atlanta, GA
ALPL	Abraham Lincoln Presidential Library, Springfield, IL
AU	Auburn University, Special Collections and Archives, Auburn, AL
HL	Huntington Library, San Marino, CA
IHS	Indiana Historical Society, Indianapolis
LC	Library of Congress, Manuscripts Division, Washington, DC
LSU	Louisiana State University, Louisiana and Lower Mississippi Valley Collection, Baton Rouge
NARA	National Archives and Records Administration, Washington, DC
NLM	National Library of Medicine, Bethesda, MD
NYPL	New York Public Library, Rare Books and Manuscripts, Astor, Lenox, and Tilden Foundations, New York City
NYSL	New York State Library, Albany
OR	*The War of the Rebellion: A Compilation of the Official Records of the Union and Confederate Armies,* 70 vols. in 128 pts. (US Government Printing Office, 1880–1901). Citations to series 1 unless otherwise stated.
ORN	*Official Records of the Union and Confederate Navies in the War of the Rebellion,* 30 vols. (US Government Printing Office, 1894–1922)
TU	Tulane University, Special Collections, New Orleans, LA
UM	University of Michigan, William L. Clements Library, Ann Arbor
USSC	US Sanitary Commission
VNMP	Vicksburg National Military Park, Vicksburg, MS
WHS	Wisconsin Historical Society, Madison

INTRODUCTION

1. *OR*, ser. 3, 5:115.

2. Wiley, *Life of Billy Yank*, 125–28; Maxwell, *Lincoln's Fifth Wheel*, 31–49.

3. Hoy, *Chasing Dirt*, 43–44; Humphreys, *Marrow of Tragedy*, 127–28, 132; Meier, "Organic Armies," 41–44; Meier, *Nature's Civil War*, 75–77; Browning and Silver, *Environmental History of the Civil War*, 20–21.

4. See, for example, Murray, *War, Strategy, and Military Effectiveness*.

5. Meier, "Organic Armies," 37–52; Meier, *Nature's Civil War*, 16–22, 35–64; Meier, "U.S. Sanitary Commission Physicians," 20. For a discussion of how Americans in general viewed the link between health and environment in pre–Civil War America, see also Valenčius, *Health of the Country*.

1. WAR AND SOLDIER HEALTH

1. Landers, "Destructiveness of Pre-Industrial Warfare," 458.

2. Landers, "Destructiveness of Pre-Industrial Warfare," 458; Hodge, "On the Mortality Arising from Military Operations," 247, 251; Macleod, *Notes on the Surgery of the War in the Crimea*, 38–39.

3. Peterson, "Insects, Disease, and Military History," 148, 150–51, 153–54, 158.

4. Jackson, *Formation, Discipline, and Economy of Armies*, xviii, xxxiv, xxxviii, lvi.

5. Jackson, *Formation, Discipline, and Economy of Armies*, 6–10, 12, 25–26, 27–237 (quote, 222–23).

6. Jackson, *Formation, Discipline, and Economy of Armies*, 255–56, 266, 270, 358.

7. Jackson, *Formation, Discipline, and Economy of Armies*, 360, 362–63, 369–70.

8. Jackson, *Formation, Discipline, and Economy of Armies*, 341, 343–44, 350, 359.

9. Jackson, *Formation, Discipline, and Economy of Armies*, 351, 359.

10. Jackson, *Formation, Discipline, and Economy of Armies*, 329–35.

11. Gillett, *Army Medical Department*, 124.

12. Gillett, *Army Medical Department*, 124.

13. [Shattuck], *General Plan for the Promotion of Public and Personal Health*, 13, 24, 28, 102. See also Warren, *Preservation of Health*.

14. Stillé, *United States Sanitary Commission*, 27; Macleod, *Notes on the Surgery of the War in the Crimea*, 27; Farr, "Health of the British Army," 474, 479.

15. Baudens, *On Military and Camp Hospitals*, 36, 45–49.

16. Baudens, *On Military and Camp Hospitals*, 32–34.

17. De Fonblanque, *Treatise on the Administration and Organization of the British Army*, 418–20.

18. Stillé, *United States Sanitary Commission*, 30–32.

19. McClellan, *Armies of Europe*, 63; Delafield, *Art of War in Europe*, 90; Mordecai, *Military Commission to Europe*, 80.

20. Humphreys, *Marrow of Tragedy*, 46; Nightingale, *Notes on Hospitals*, 56.

21. Smith and Stillé, "Report . . . on the Value of Vaccination in Armies," 18–19, 22; Humphreys, *Marrow of Tragedy*, 272.

22. "John Ordronaux (doctor)," https://en.wikipedia.org/wiki/John_Ordronaux_(doctor); Ordronaux, *Hints on Health in Armies,* 5, 7.

23. Ordronaux, *Hints on Health in Armies,* 10–11, 13, 15–16.

24. Ordronaux, *Hints on Health in Armies,* 14, 22–23, 28–29.

25. Ordronaux, *Hints on Health in Armies,* 14, 24–29, 32.

26. Ordronaux, *Hints on Health in Armies,* 13, 90.

27. Hammond, *Treatise on Hygiene,* vii, 14–15.

28. Hammond, *Treatise on Hygiene,* 452.

29. Hammond, *Treatise on Hygiene,* ix-x, 65–72, 75–76, 296.

30. Roemer, *Cavalry,* 387–89; Congdon, *Congdon's Cavalry Compendium,* 29–33; Butterfield, *Camp and Outpost Duty,* 103–9.

31. Maxwell, *Lincoln's Fifth Wheel,* 2–8; Humphreys, *Marrow of Tragedy,* 103–4.

32. Maxwell, *Lincoln's Fifth Wheel,* 4–13; Humphreys, *Marrow of Tragedy,* 104.

33. Stillé, *United States Sanitary Commission,* 83.

34. Stillé, *United States Sanitary Commission,* 79–80, 119.

35. Bellows, "Notes of a Preliminary Sanitary Survey of the Forces of the United States, in the Ohio and Mississippi Valleys," 2; Stillé, *United States Sanitary Commission,* 85, 87.

36. Alex McDonald, "Notes on Sanitation in the Field," Feb. 20, 1866, Ser. 1, Folder 1107, Roll 8, USSC Records, NYPL; Stillé, *United States Sanitary Commission,* 96–97; Humphreys, *Marrow of Tragedy,* 127; Van Buren, *Rules for Preserving the Health of the Soldier,* 2–4; Post and Van Buren, *Report on Military Hygiene and Therapeutics,* 9.

37. Stillé, *United States Sanitary Commission,* 99–100; Humphreys, "'This Place of Death,'" 16–17.

38. Stillé, *United States Sanitary Commission,* 97; Humphreys, *Marrow of Tragedy,* 128; "General Instructions to Sanitary Inspectors," 1–7, 11.

39. Newberry, "Report on the Condition of the Troops and the Operations of the Sanitary Commission," 17–18.

40. Guide to Collection, Box 118 and 119, USSC Records, NYPL.

41. Guide to Collection, Box 118 and 119, USSC Records, NYPL.

42. George L. Andrews return, 5th Vermont, Oct. 16, 1861; and F. U. Johnston return, 26th New Jersey, Feb. 9, 1862, both Ser. 7, Folder 1107, Roll 8, USSC Records, NYPL; McDonald, "Notes on Sanitation in the Field," Feb. 20, 1866.

43. Guide to Collection, Box 118 and 119, USSC Records, NYPL.

44. See Fifteenth Corps camp inspection reports, Ser. 1, Folder 1, Roll 1; and Folder 451, Roll 3, USSC Records, NYPL.

45. *New York Times,* Feb. 14, 1860; *ORN,* 22:660; "Dr. Aigner's Report on the Sanitary Conditions of the U.S. Forces in the District of Cairo during the months of December & January," Feb. 11, 1862, Ser. 1, Folder "Writings Re. Civil War, 1861–1865," Roll 12, USSC Records, NYPL.

46. "Bernard Jean Bettelheim," *Wikipedia;* B. J. Bettelheim return, 57th Indiana, Mar. 17, 1863, Ser. 7, USSC Records, NYPL; Vance, *Report of the Adjutant General of the State of Illinois,* 6:3.

47. McNeil, "Dr. Alfred L. Castleman," 291–95; Alfred L. Castleman return, 79th Pennsylvania, Mar. 19, 1863, Ser. 7, USSC Records, NYPL.

48. "Dr. Robert Collyer Dead Following Illness"; Holmes, *Life and Letters of Robert Collyer,* 1:241, 250, 255–56, 258.

49. Bentz et al., "Magnanimous Professional Life and Tragic Demise of J. H. Douglas," 1499–1501.

50. *History of the Fifteenth Regiment, Iowa Veteran Volunteer Infantry,* 44, 612; *OR,* 10(1):290; Boyd, *Civil War Diary,* 14.

51. *Morning Call* (Paterson, NJ), Feb. 19, 1910.

52. Jacobsen, "Franklin B. Hough," 311–15; Biographical Note and "Sketches of the Field and Camp in a Series of Letters from a Sanitary Inspector to the Little Folks at Home, Vol. 1, Washington, Feb. 1862," 13, Franklin Benjamin Hough Papers, NYSL; Baudens, *On Military and Camp Hospitals,* ix; Hall, *Ninety-Seventh Regiment New York Volunteers,* 346; Hough, *Duryée's Brigade,* iii, 131.

53. Estilow, "Clara Barton's Network," https://www.civilwarmed.org/surgeons-call/barton-network/.

54. "Lewis Henry Steiner," https://en.wikipedia.org/wiki/Lewis_Henry_Steiner; [Steiner], *Report of Lewis H. Steiner,* 1–43.

55. William F. Swalm, https://www.findagrave.com/memorial/153103427/william-f-swalm; *Roster of All Regimental Surgeons,* 153, 169; "Muster-In Roll of Field, Staff and Non-Commissioned Staff in the 84th Regt. N.Y.S.V.," https://dmna.ny.gov/historic/reghist/civil/MusterRolls/Infantry/84thInf_NYSV_MusterRoll.pdf.

56. "Robert Ware—Union Surgeon," https://civilwarmed.org/robert-ware/; *Record of the Service of the Forty-Fourth Massachusetts,* 234; *Harvard Memorial Biographies,* 1:238–40.

57. *Harvard Memorial Biographies,* 1:241–44, 246–49; *Record of the Service of the Forty-Fourth Massachusetts,* 236, 256–57; [Haines], *Letters from the Forty-Fourth Regiment M.V.M.,* 19, 98.

58. *Harvard Memorial Biographies,* 1:250–51; *Record of the Service of the Forty-Fourth Massachusetts,* 177, 245; [Haines], *Letters from the Forty-Fourth Regiment M.V.M.,* 106; Wyeth, *Leaves from a Diary,* 48, 52; unidentified newspaper clipping, extract of letter by S. Storrow, Apr. 29, [1863]; extract of letter from Col. Francis L. Lee to Mrs. Charles Lee, Apr. 10, 1863; and Henry W. Bellows to Dr. John Ware, May 8, 1863, all Robert Ware Scrapbook, Center for the History of Medicine, Harvard University, Boston, MA.

59. *Springfield (MA) Union,* Nov. 24, 1871.

60. "Gordon H. Winslow (1805–1864)," https://www.wikitree.com/wiki/winslow-1751; Phisterer, *New York in the War of the Rebellion,* 2:1768.

61. *OR,* ser. 3, 2:298.

2. CAMP SITUATION

1. McClellan, *Regulations and Instructions,* 57n.

2. Nolan, *Cavalry,* 258, 260.

3. Grafton, *Treatise on the Camp and March,* 8; Whitehorne, "Blueprint for Nineteenth-Century Camps," 30–31, 33, 37.

4. Ordronaux, *Hints on Health in Armies,* 52, 54; Hammond, *Treatise on Hygiene,* 251–53, 460; Van Buren, *Rules for Preserving the Health of the Soldier,* 5–6.

5. *Revised Regulations,* 74; *OR,* ser. 3, 1:216; *OR,* 25(2):491, 46(1):619, 692, 703, 47(3):260, 42(1):451–52.

6. Lapham, *My Recollections,* 111; Opdycke, *To Battle for God and the Right,* 145: Simmons, *History of the 84th Reg't Ill. Vols.,* 48, 52; Bull, *Soldiering,* 13; Rhodes, *Battery B, First Regiment Rhode Island Light Artillery,* 309; Whittaker, *Volunteer Cavalry,* 60–63.

7. Billings, *Hardtack and Coffee,* 73–74; Morhous, *Reminiscences of the 123d Regiment, N.Y.S.V.,* 128; Newberry, "Report on the Condition of the Troops and the Operations of the Sanitary Commission," 26; Jackson and O'Donnell, *Back Home in Oneida,* 93; George Ditto Diary, May 21, 1863, ALPL; Stormont, *Fifty-Eighth Regiment of Indiana Volunteer Infantry,* 332; *OR,* 47(3):45; Whitehorne, "Blueprint for Nineteenth-Century Camps," 28, 42; Thompson, *Thirteenth Regiment of New Hampshire Volunteer Infantry,* 89, 94.

8. Babcock, *Selections from the Letters and Diaries,* 27–28; Copp, *Reminiscences,* 22–23.

9. Bentz and Kim, "Sevierville Hill Site," 1, 44; Winter, "Civil War Fortifications and Campgrounds on Maryland Heights," 119, 122; Jones, "'Our Brigade Has Never Been in Winter Quarters,'" 30; Bies, "Guarding the Junction," 74, 84; Balicki, "Fall 1863 Bivouac of the 14th Connecticut," 159, 167, 173.

10. Wilder, *Practicing Medicine,* 125; Wilder memoir, 40, William Frank Wilder Collection, LC; Osborn, *No Middle Ground,* 143–44; Perry, *Letters from a Surgeon,* 124.

11. Whitman, *Civil War Letters,* 108; Simmons, *History of the 84th Reg't Ill. Vols.,* 160; *OR,* 35(2):112; Neuman to Mr. and Mrs. Tripp, Sept. 16, 1864, James Neuman and Tripp Family Civil War Correspondence, AHC; General Order No. 27, 1st Division, Seventeenth Corps, June 26, 1865, M. F. Force Papers, University of Washington, Special Collections, Seattle; Williams, *General Reub Williams's Memories,* 131–32.

12. Hammond et al., "Scurvy," 24; Wainwright, *Diary of Battle,* 296–97; Chamberlain to not stated, Jan. 29, 1863, Joseph Wright Chamberlain Papers, IHS; Davidson to Annie, Feb. 1, 1862 [1863], James Innes Davidson Papers, ADAH; Bull, *Soldiering,* 30, 32; Scherneckau, *Marching with the First Nebraska,* 181; *OR,* 24(1):92; J. A. Spielman diary, June 24, 1863, 17th Iowa Folder, VNMP, copy.

13. Castleman, *Army of the Potomac,* 7, 9, 18–19.

14. Castleman, *Army of the Potomac,* 19, 44, 48.

15. Castleman, *Army of the Potomac,* 50–51, 56–57, 60, 75.

16. Castleman, *Army of the Potomac,* 68, 122–23, 227–29.

17. Castleman, *Army of the Potomac,* 275, 280–88.

18. [Olmsted], "Report of a Preliminary Survey of the Camps," 2–5.

19. George W. Avery, "Report of the Sanitary Management of U.S. Forces at Ship Island Miss in 1861 & 62," Ser. 1, Folder 1293, Roll 9, USSC Records, NYPL; "Sketches of the Field and Camp in a Series of Letters from a Sanitary Inspector to the Little Folks at Home, Vol. 1, Washington, Feb. 1862," 64–67, Franklin Benjamin Hough Papers, NYSL.

20. Orpheus Everts, "Medical History of the 20th Ind Vol Infy July 1861 to Au-

gust 1862," 3–4, 8–9, Ser. 1, Folder 35, Roll 1, USSC Records, NYPL; [Marsh], "Report on the Sanitary State of the Troops at Charleston," 79.

21. "Report of Acting Med. Inspector Edward D. Kittoe, for the 15th Army Corps, Dept. of the Tennessee, for the week ending April 12th 1863," Ser. 1, Folder 1; and "Report of Acting Med. Inspector E. O. F. Roler, for the 15th Army Corps, Dept of the Tennessee, for the week ending Sept. 12th 1863," Ser. 1, Folder 4, both Roll 1, USSC Records, NYPL.

22. "Remarks to accompany Tabular Report, Act. Med. Inspector E. O. F. Roler, 15th Army Corps 2nd Div. for the week ending Sept. 19th 1863," Ser. 1, Folder 5, Roll 1, USSC Records, NYPL.

23. "Remarks to accompany Report of Act. Med. Inspector of the 15th Army Corps, Dept. and Army of the Tennessee, for the month of Feb. 1864," Ser. 1, Folder 305; "Remarks to accompany Report of Actg. Med. Inspector of the 15th Army Corps, Army and Dept. of the Tennessee for the month of March 1864," Ser. 1, Folder 296; and John M. Woodworth to L. D. Huntington, June 21, 1865, Ser. 1, Folder 301, all Roll 2, USSC Records, NYPL; *Supplement to the Official Records,* pt. 1, 7:633.

24. Edward A. Crane return, 2nd Vermont, Feb. 26, 1862; Edward A. Crane return, 3rd Vermont, Jan. 3, Mar. 4, 1862; Robert Ware return, 50th New York Engineers, Feb. 7, 1862; George L. Andrews return, 2nd Vermont, Nov. 27, 1861; George L. Andrews return, 5th Wisconsin, Nov. 25, 1861; and Edward A. Crane return, 5th Vermont, Jan. 6, 1862, all Ser. 7, USSC Records, NYPL.

25. Franklin B. Hough return, 2nd New Jersey, Feb. 12, 1862; and Franklin B. Hough return, 32nd New York, Feb. 18, 1862, both Ser. 7, USSC Records, NYPL.

26. Edward A. Crane return, 128th New York, Jan. 22, 1863, and 162nd New York, Jan. 28, 1863; and George A. Blake return, 1st Louisiana Heavy Artillery Colored, Nov. 7, 1863, all Ser. 7, USSC Records, NYPL.

27. F. U. Johnston return, 17th Maine, Feb. 10, 1863, and 72nd Pennsylvania, Apr. 3, 1863; William M. Chamberlain return, 4th New York Heavy Artillery, Mar. 29, 1862; and Alex McDonald return, 119th Pennsylvania, Mar. 27, 1863, all Ser. 7, USSC Records, NYPL.

28. Edward A. Crane return, 7th Vermont, May 9, 1863, and 38th Iowa, Feb. 10, 1864; unsigned return, 2nd Iowa, Aug. 13, 1861; Robert Jones return, 36th New York, July 19, 1861; and James Gall return, 1st US Colored Troops, Sept. 24, 1863, all Ser. 7, USSC Records, NYPL.

29. T. B. Smith return, 9th New York Artillery, Jan. 2, 1863; and Edward A. Crane return, 24th Connecticut, Dec. 24, 1862, both Ser. 7, USSC Records, NYPL.

30. William F. Swalm return, 26th Wisconsin, Mar. 17, 1863; and F. U. Johnston return, 69th Pennsylvania, Apr. 3, 1863, both Ser. 7, USSC Records, NYPL.

31. F. U. Johnston return, 9th New Hampshire, Jan. 7–29, 1863; Robert Collyer return, 5th Wisconsin, Aug. 20, 1861; W. M. Prentice return, 2nd Tennessee, May 4, 1863; Robert Jones return, 36th New York, July 19, 1861; and Robert Jones returns, 40th New York, July 15, Sept. 2, 1861, all Ser. 7, USSC Records, NYPL.

32. Bernard J. Bettelheim return, 79th Illinois and 30th Indiana, May 14–15, 1863; Robert Collyer return, 5th Wisconsin, Aug. 20, 1861; George L. Andrews return, 5th Vermont, Nov. 27, 1861; Franklin B. Hough return, 3rd New York Cavalry, Apr. 10,

1862; and Alex McDonald return, 30th New York, Mar. 9, 1863, all Ser. 7, USSC Records, NYPL.

33. George A. Blake return, 40th New York, Dec. 17, 1861, Ser. 7, USSC Records, NYPL.

34. Godfrey Aigner return, 12th Illinois, Aug. 23, 1861; William M. Chamberlain return, 2nd US Sharpshooters, Nov. 30, 1861; George L. Andrews returns, 1st Massachusetts Cavalry, Feb. 25, Apr. 4, 1862; Marvin M. Marsh return, 8th Maine, Mar. 6, 1863; Alex McDonald return, 7th Wisconsin, Mar. 25, 1863; Alex McDonald return, 147th New York, Mar. 25, 1863; and Jesse W. Page return, 3rd Massachusetts, June 9, 1863, all Ser. 7, USSC Records, NYPL.

35. Bernard J. Bettelheim returns, 1st Kentucky and 2nd Kentucky, Apr. 3–4, 1863; Bernard J. Bettelheim returns, 110th Illinois and 9th Indiana, Apr. 1, 3, 1863; William F. Swalm return, 26th Wisconsin, Mar. 17, 1863; and Bernard J. Bettelheim return, 57th Indiana, Mar. 17, 1863, all Ser. 7, USSC Records, NYPL.

36. Julius Nichols return, 13th Massachusetts Battery, Mar. 14, 1863; and Julius Nichols return, 3rd Pennsylvania Heavy Artillery, Mar. 13, 1863, both Ser. 7, USSC Records, NYPL.

37. George G. Edgerly return, 10th Corps d'Afrique, Oct. 26, 1863, Ser. 7, USSC Records, NYPL.

3. SHELTER

1. Macleod, *Notes on the Surgery of the War in the Crimea,* 31.

2. Mordecai, *Military Commission to Europe,* 78–79, 83.

3. McClellan, *Armies of Europe,* 81, 84, 109; Delafield, *Art of War in Europe,* 86–87.

4. Nelson, "'Right Nice Little House[s],'" 177–93.

5. Ordronaux, *Hints on Health in Armies,* 55–58, 94, 135–36.

6. Ordronaux, *Hints on Health in Armies,* 36, 38–39, 129–32.

7. Hammond, *Treatise on Hygiene,* 151–52, 397–98, 448, 450.

8. *Revised Regulations,* 76; Morhous, *Reminiscences of the 123d Regiment, N.Y.S.V.,* 128; Tuttle, *Civil War Journal,* 52; Sargent, "For Our Beloved Country," 73; Bull, *Soldiering,* 11; Jones, *Artilleryman's Diary,* 208; Hough note in Baudens, *On Military and Camp Hospitals,* 46n.

9. Nelson, "'Right Nice Little House[s],'" 183; Hough note in Baudens, *On Military and Camp Hospitals,* 47–48n; Billings, *Hardtack and Coffee,* 46–47.

10. Hammond, *Treatise on Hygiene,* 449–50; Newberry, "Report on the Condition of the Troops and the Operations of the Sanitary Commission," 25–27.

11. Billings, *Hardtack and Coffee,* 49, 54; Jackson and O'Donnell, *Back Home in Oneida,* 47–48.

12. Floyd, *Fortieth(Mozart) Regiment New York Volunteers,* 55–57; *OR,* 25(2):491; Stanley, *Personal Memoirs,* 103; Bull, *Soldiering,* 10; Beecham, *As If It Were Glory,* 5; Sargent, "For Our Beloved Country," 76; Evans to sister, June 11, 1863, Thomas Evans Letters and Diary, Eastern Washington University, Archives and Special Collections, Cheney.

13. Hough note in Baudens, *On Military and Camp Hospitals,* 46n; "Dr. Aigner's Report on the Sanitary Conditions of the U.S. Forces in the District of Cairo during the months of December & January," Feb. 11, 1862, Ser. 1, Folder "Writings Re. Civil War, 1861–1865," Roll 12, USSC Records, NYPL; Williams, *From the Cannon's Mouth,* 30; Hard, *Eighth Cavalry Regiment Illinois Volunteers,* 43.

14. Sargent, "For Our Beloved Country," 46, 49; Ferguson, *On to Atlanta,* 60; Billings, *Hardtack and Coffee,* 78.

15. Bull, *Soldiering,* 16, 22.

16. Wainwright, *Diary of Battle,* 317; Muffly, *Story of Our Regiment,* 70–72; Thompson, *Thirteenth Regiment of New Hampshire Volunteer Infantry,* 209–11.

17. Sargent, "For Our Beloved Country," 67–68.

18. Billings, *Hardtack and Coffee,* 45–46; Jackson and O'Donnell, *Back Home in Oneida,* 25; [Haines], *Letters from the Forty-Fourth Regiment M.V.M.,* 19; Regimental Order No. 14, 14th Maine, June 11, 1862; and circular, 14th Maine, June 13, 1862, both Ser. 1, Folder 1206, Roll 8, USSC Records, NYPL.

19. Hard, *Eighth Cavalry Regiment Illinois Volunteers,* 69.

20. Boughton to Friends at Home, May 21, 1863, Clement Abner Boughton Papers, UM; Whittaker, *Volunteer Cavalry,* 53; Williams, *From the Cannon's Mouth,* 30, 36; Sheldon, *"Twenty-Seventh,"* 35–36; Wild, *Memoirs and History of Capt. F. W. Alexander's Baltimore Battery,* 29–30; *OR,* 36(1):211–12, 42(1):195, 622–23; Sargent, "For Our Beloved Country," 63–64; Edwin Witherby Brown, "Under a Poncho with Grant and Sherman," 64, Miami University, Special Collections, Oxford, OH; Roemer, *Reminiscences,* 156, 255–56.

21. Williams, *From the Cannon's Mouth,* 165.

22. Scherneckau, *Marching with the First Nebraska,* 170–71, 174; Wild, *Memoirs and History of Capt. F. W. Alexander's Baltimore Battery,* 24; Orpheus Everts, "Medical History of the 20th Ind Vol Infy July 1861 to August 1862," 9–10, Ser. 1, Folder 35, Roll 1, USSC Records, NYPL; Billings, *Hardtack and Coffee,* 48; "Report of Lewis H. Steiner, Sanitary Inspector attached to the Division Commanded by Maj. Genl. N. P. Banks, made Feb. 18, 1862, to the Sanitary Commission," 12–13, 16, Lewis H. Steiner Papers, NLM.

23. Stewart, "Battle of Stone River," 10; Billings, *Hardtack and Coffee,* 47, 300; Wild, *Memoirs and History of Capt. F. W. Alexander's Baltimore Battery,* 25.

24. Billings, *Hardtack and Coffee,* 48; Simmons, *History of the 84th Reg't. Ill. Vols.,* 40; Webster and Cameron, *First Wisconsin Battery,* 31.

25. Wilder memoir, 2, William Frank Wilder Collection, LC; Billings, *Hardtack and Coffee,* 48–50; [Marsh], "Report on the Sanitary State of the Troops at Charleston," 78–79; Grant, *Papers,* 11:451; Williams, *General Reub Williams's Memories,* 131; Hough note in Baudens, *On Military and Camp Hospitals,* 48n.

26. Baudens, *On Military and Camp Hospitals,* 47; Ordronaux, *Hints on Health in Armies,* 136–39; McClellan, *European Cavalry,* 182–83; Roemer, *Cavalry,* 205.

27. Ordronaux, *Hints on Health in Armies,* 138; Williams, *From the Cannon's Mouth,* 73.

28. *OR,* 17(2):485; Bull, *Soldiering,* 10; Billings, *Hardtack and Coffee,* 51–53; Wells A. Bushnell Memoirs, 63, Western Reserve Historical Society, Cleveland, OH;

Stewart, "Battle of Stone River," 10–11; Stevenson, *78th Regiment O.V.V.I.*, 193–94; Howe, *Civil War Times*, 57.

29. Scherneckau, *Marching with the First Nebraska*, 177; Beecham, *As If It Were Glory*, 18; George Ditto Diary, May 21, 1863, ALPL; Stewart, "Battle of Stone River," 11; Beatty, *Memoirs of a Volunteer*, 173–74.

30. *OR*, ser. 3, 4:253; *OR*, 34(3):399; Wilson, "Extensive Side of Nineteenth-Century Military Economy," 315–16, 318.

31. Simmons, *History of the 84th Reg't. Ill. Vols.*, 49; Stewart, "Battle of Stone River," 11; Widney, *Campaigning with "Uncle Billy,"* 127–28; Sylvester Strong to father, Aug. 7, 1863, Sylvester and Albert Strong Civil War Letters, WHS; Williams, *From the Cannon's Mouth*, 140; Lovel Newton Parker Diary, Jan. 14, 1863, HL; Bull, *Soldiering*, 10–11.

32. Wright, *Eighth Regiment Kentucky Vol. Inf.*, 136–38; *History of the Seventy-Third Indiana Volunteers*, 151; John S. Hedges Report, 30, UM; *OR*, 32(3):435.

33. Wilson, "Extensive Side of Nineteenth-Century Military Economy," 299, 302, 305, 310–11, 317, 319, 330.

34. Stanley, *Personal Memoirs*, 119; *OR*, 14:458, 15:525, 35(2):113; Wilder, *Practicing Medicine*, 88.

35. Babcock, *Selections from the Letters and Diaries*, 29; Castleman, *Army of the Potomac*, 60; *OR*, 5:720, 25(2):491–92; Orpheus Everts, "Medical History of the 20th Ind Vol Infy July 1861 to August 1862," 3, Ser. 1, Folder 35, Roll 1, USSC Records, NYPL.

36. Bull, *Soldiering*, 11.

37. "Remarks to accompany Report of Acting Med. Inspector of the 15th Army Corps, Dept. of the Tennessee, for the week ending April 12th 1863," Ser. 1, Folder 1; "Remarks to accompany the weekly report of the acting Medical Inspector of the 15th Army Corps, Dept. of the Tennessee, for the week ending April 19th 1863," Ser. 1, Folder 1; "Remarks to accompany (Tabular) Report of Acting Med. Inspector of 15th Army Corps, Dept. of the Tennessee, for the week ending September 12th 1863," Ser. 1, Folder 4; "Remarks to accompany Tabular Report, Act. Med. Inspector E. O. F. Roler, 15th Corps 2nd Div. for the week ending Sept. 19th 1863," Ser. 1, Folder 5; and "Remarks to accompany the Tabular Report of Act. Med. Inspector E. O. F. Roler, 15th Army Corps, for the week ending Sept. 27th 1863, Camp near Black River, Miss.," Ser. 1, Folder 5, all Roll 1, USSC Records, NYPL.

38. "Remarks to accompany Report of Acting Medical Inspector of the 15th Army Corps, Dept. and Army of the Tennessee, for the month of Feb. 1864," Ser. 1, Folders 302–5; and "Remarks to accompany Report of Act. Med. Inspector of the 15th Army Corps, Dept. and Army of the Tennessee, for the month of March 1864," Ser. 1, Folder 298, both Roll 2, USSC Records, NYPL.

39. William M. Chamberlain return, 36th New York, Oct. 9, 1861; William M. Chamberlain return, 2nd Rhode Island, Nov. 28, 1861; and William M. Chamberlain return, 8th New York, Nov. 7, 1861, all Ser. 7, USSC Records, NYPL.

40. James Gall return, 2nd North Carolina (US), Sept. 16, 1863; Henry Oliver return, 4th New York Battery, Feb. 1, 1862; and Alex McDonald return, 30th New York, Mar. 9, 1863, all Ser. 7, USSC Records, NYPL.

41. E. J. Dunning return, 20th New York, July 17, 1861, Ser. 7, USSC Records, NYPL.

42. Marvin M. Marsh return, 8th Maine, Mar. 6, 1863; James Gall return, 2nd North Carolina (US), Sept. 16, 1863; and James Gall return, 1st US Colored Troops, Sept. 24, 1863, all Ser. 7, USSC Records, NYPL.

43. Lewis H. Steiner return, Zouaves d'Afrique, Dec. 1861; Robert Ware return, 20th Massachusetts, Dec. 29, 1861; William M. Chamberlain return, 2nd US Sharpshooters, Nov. 30, 1861; and Edward A. Crane return, Battery D, 5th US Artillery, Feb. 11, 1862, all Ser. 7, USSC Records, NYPL.

44. Robert Jones return, 40th New York, July 15, 1861; and E. J. Dunning return, 1st Vermont, July 21, 1861, both Ser. 7, USSC Records, NYPL.

45. James P. Prince, "The Peninsula Campaign, 1862," Ser. 1, Folder 511, Roll 4, USSC Records, NYPL.

46. Jesse W. Page return, 5th Massachusetts, June 19, 1863; and Bernard J. Bettelheim return, 58th Indiana, Mar. 25, 1863, both Ser. 7, USSC Records, NYPL.

47. James Gall return, 4th US Colored Troops, Nov. 7, 1863, Ser. 7, USSC Records, NYPL.

48. Bernard J. Bettelheim return, 57th Indiana, Mar. 17, 1863; Bettelheim returns, 9th Kentucky, 79th Indiana, and 19th Ohio, Mar. 26–27, 1863; and Bettelheim returns, 74th Illinois and 75th Illinois, Apr. 24–25, 1863, all Ser. 7, USSC Records, NYPL.

49. George G. Edgerly return, 11th Regiment Corps d'Afrique, Oct. 22, 1863; Edgerly return, 3rd Regiment Corps d'Afrique, Oct. 23, 1863; Edgerly return, 6th Michigan, Oct. 24, 1863; and Edgerly return, 2nd Vermont Battery, Oct. 30, 1863, all Ser. 7, USSC Records, NYPL.

50. Lewis H. Steiner return, 3rd Wisconsin, Jan. 31, 1862; and Gordon H. Winslow return, 5th New York, Jan. 22, 1862, both Ser. 7, USSC Records, NYPL.

51. J. H. Douglas return, 4th Iowa, Dec. 28, 1861; and Henry W. Warriner return, Battalion, 1st Nebraska Cavalry, Dec. 24, 1861, both Ser. 7, USSC Records, NYPL.

52. *Harvard Memorial Biographies,* 1:248; Robert Ware return, 7th New York, Feb. 2, 1862, Ser. 7, USSC Records, NYPL; *Record of the Service of the Forty-Fourth Massachusetts,* 242–43.

53. F. U. Johnston return, 69th Pennsylvania, Apr. 3, 1863; Henry Oliver return, 1st Massachusetts, Dec. 13, 1861; Robert Ware return, 11th Pennsylvania Cavalry, Dec. 11, 1861; Alex McDonald return, 7th Wisconsin, Mar. 25, 1863; Robert Ware return, 1st Minnesota, Feb. 20, 1862; and Alex McDonald return, 147th New York, Mar. 25, 1863, all Ser. 7, USSC Records, NYPL.

54. Henry Oliver return, 8th Illinois Cavalry, Mar. 8, 1862, Ser. 7, USSC Records, NYPL.

55. Julius Nichols return, 19th Wisconsin, Mar. 27, 1863, Ser. 7, USSC Records, NYPL.

4. CLOTHING AND PERSONAL CLEANLINESS

1. Ordronaux, *Hints on Health in Armies,* 77.

2. For a full discussion of the origin and cultural history of Zouave military clothing, see Harrison and Brown, *Zouave Theaters.*

3. Billings, *Hardtack and Coffee,* 316–18; *OR,* 52(1):197–98, 23(2):317.

4. Ordronaux, *Hints on Health in Armies,* 77–78; Hammond, *Treatise on Hygiene,* 579–80, 592; "Soldiers' Health," attached to Franklin B. Hough return, 2nd DC, Apr. 8, 1862, Ser. 7, USSC Records, NYPL.

5. Ordronaux, *Hints on Health in Armies,* 80; Hammond, *Treatise on Hygiene,* 589–90.

6. Hammond, *Treatise on Hygiene,* 590–92.

7. *OR,* ser. 3, 4:886; *OR,* 14:458; Ordronaux, *Hints on Health in Armies,* 80; Billings, *Hardtack and Coffee,* 276; Sherman, *Sherman's Civil War,* 106; "Soldiers' Health," attached to Franklin B. Hough return, 2nd DC, Apr. 8, 1862, Ser. 7, USSC Records, NYPL.

8. Hammond, *Treatise on Hygiene,* 596.

9. Billings, *Hardtack and Coffee,* 54–55.

10. Van Buren, *Rules for Preserving the Health of the Soldier,* 6–7; Ordronaux, *Hints on Health in Armies,* 92–93; Butterfield, *Camp and Outpost Duty,* 109; Billings, *Hardtack and Coffee,* 78; Sherman, *Sherman's Civil War,* 501.

11. E. J. Dunning return, 20th New York, July 17, 1861; W. M. Chamberlain return, 15th New York Engineers, Feb. 7, 1862; and Edward Mead return, 2nd West Virginia, Mar. 27, 1862, all Ser. 7, USSC Records, NYPL.

12. George L. Andrews return, 3rd Vermont, Oct. 17, 1861; Andrews return, 19th Indiana, Oct. 9, 1861; Andrews return, 6th Wisconsin, Nov. 21, 1861; Robert Jones return, 2nd Rhode Island, July 16, 1861; Jones return, 36th New York, July 19, 1861; J. H. Douglas return, 12th Missouri, Dec. 24, 1861; and Edward A. Crane return, 2nd Vermont, Feb. 26, 1862, all Ser. 7, USSC Records, NYPL.

13. G. G. Edgerly return, 3rd Regiment Corps d'Afrique, Oct. 23, 1861; George A. Blake return, 9th Connecticut, Feb. 13, 1862; Robert Ware return, 71st Pennsylvania, Feb. 17, 1862; Henry Oliver return, 8th Illinois Cavalry, Mar. 8, 1862; J. H. Douglas return, 2nd Ohio Battery, Dec. 26, 1861; and James Gall return, 4th US Colored Troops, Nov. 7, 1863, all Ser. 7, USSC Records, NYPL.

14. Robert Jones return, 40th New York, July 15, 1862; and William F. Swalm return, Battery I, 1st New York Light Artillery, Mar. 5, 1863, both Ser. 7, USSC Records, NYPL.

15. Lewis H. Steiner return, Zouaves d'Afrique, Dec. 1861; Gordon H. Winslow return, 5th New York, Jan. 22, 1862; W. S. Hough return, 1st and 2nd US Sharpshooters, Feb. 6, 1862; and Edward A. Crane return, 2nd Vermont, Jan. 2, 1862, all Ser. 7, USSC Records, NYPL.

16. See, for example, Edward Mead return, Simmond's Kentucky Battery, Apr. 26, 1862, Ser. 7, USSC Records, NYPL.

17. M. P. Buel return, 1st Nebraska, Sept. 7, 1861; Lewis H. Steiner return, 3rd New York Artillery, Feb. 8, 1862; Franklin B. Hough return, 32nd New York, Feb. 18, 1862; and Bernard J. Bettelheim return, 57th Indiana, Mar. 17, 1863, all Ser. 7, USSC Records, NYPL.

18. Bushman and Bushman, "Early History of Cleanliness in America," 1214, 1222, 1225, 1233–36; Brown, *Foul Bodies,* 362; Hoy, *Chasing Dirt,* 7.

19. Luscombe, *Practical Observations,* 111–12; Warren, *Preservation of Health,* 100–101, 105.

20. Ordronaux, *Hints on Health in Armies,* 33–34, 58, 92.

21. Hammond, *Treatise on Hygiene,* 233–34, 238–39.

22. Butterfield, *Camp and Outpost Duty,* 106; Congdon, *Congdon's Cavalry Compendium,* 29.

23. Van Buren, *Rules for Preserving the Health of the Soldier,* 7.

24. Howe, *Letters and Journals,* 481.

25. Howe, *Letters and Journals,* 490.

26. Howe, *Letters and Journals,* 491.

27. [Olmsted], "Report of a Preliminary Survey of the Camps," 4–5.

28. Newberry, "Report on the Condition of the Troops and the Operations of the Sanitary Commission," 25, 28.

29. *Revised Regulations,* 21; *OR,* ser. 3, 4:886.

30. Belknap, "Obedience and Courage of the Private Soldier," 160–61; Wildcat to editors, Feb. 26, 1863, *Tuscarawas Advocate* (New Philadelphia, OH), Mar. 20, 1863; Billings, *Hardtack and Coffee,* 79, 83.

31. [Marsh], "Report on the Sanitary State of the Troops at Charleston," 79; *OR,* 14:458, 25(2):492, 35(2):113.

32. William H. Raynor Diary, June 7, 1863, 56th Ohio Folder, VNMP, copy; Regimental Order No. 14, 14th Maine, June 11, 1862, Ser. 1, Folder 1206, Roll 8, USSC Records, NYPL.

33. Whittaker, *Volunteer Cavalry,* 49–50.

34. Sargent, "For Our Beloved Country," 64; Bull, *Soldiering,* 112–13; Wild, *Memoirs and History of Capt. F. W. Alexander's Baltimore Battery,* 180–81; Billings, *Hardtack and Coffee,* 85; J. H. Douglas return, 1st Minnesota, Nov. 3, 1861, USSC Records, NYPL; *OR,* 42(1):195.

35. Hess, "Wildlife and the Civil War," 106; Humphreys, "Stranger to Our Camps," 269–72; Raoult et al., "Evidence for Louse-Transmitted Diseases," 112, 118, 120; Johnson, *Muskets and Medicine,* 166; Congdon, *Congdon's Cavalry Compendium,* 29–30.

36. "Report of Acting Med. Inspector Edward D. Kittoe, for the 15th Army Corps, Dept of the Tennessee, for the week ending April 12th 1863," Ser. 1, Folder 1; and "Report of Acting Med. Inspector E. O. F. Roler, for the 15th Army Corps, Dept. of the Tennessee, for the week ending Sept. 12th 1863," Ser. 1, Folder 4, both Roll 1, USSC Records, NYPL; *OR,* 47(3):10, 45.

37. Robert Jones return, 36th New York, July 19, 1861; W. M. Prentice return, 2nd Tennessee, May 4, 1863; C. W. Brink return, 2nd US Colored Troops, Oct. 31, 1863; Robert Jones return, 40th New York, July 15, 1861; Bernard J. Bettelheim returns, 36th Indiana, 23rd Kentucky, 84th Illinois, Apr. 22–23, 1863; and Bettelheim returns, 110th Illinois, 9th Indiana, Apr. 1, 3, 1863, all Ser. 7, USSC Records, NYPL.

38. Robert Ware return, 20th Massachusetts, Feb. 20, 1862; Bernard J. Bettelheim return, 6th Ohio, Mar. 31, 1863; and George G. Edgerly return, 10th Regiment Corps d'Afrique, Oct. 26, 1863, all Ser. 7, USSC Records, NYPL.

39. W. S. Hough return, 1st and 2nd US Sharpshooters, Feb. 6, 1862; and Edward A. Crane return, 161st New York, Dec. 25, 1862, both Ser. 7, USSC Records, NYPL.

40. Robert Jones return, 40th New York, Sept. 2, 1861; William M. Chamberlain, return 2nd US Sharpshooters, Nov. 30, 1861; Robert Ware return, 72nd Pennsylvania, Dec. 20, 1861; C. W. Brink return, 130th Pennsylvania, Aug. 27, 1862; Henry Oliver return, Battery B, 1st New York Light Artillery, Jan. 17, 1862; T. B. Smith return, 2nd Pennsylvania Artillery, Jan. 7, 1863; T. B. Smith return, 7th New York Artillery, Dec. 30, 1862; William M. Chamberlain return, 6th Wisconsin, Feb. 10, 1862; Robert Ware return, 69th Pennsylvania, Dec. 23, 1861; and William M. Chamberlain return, 36th New York, Jan. 17, 1862, all Ser. 7, USSC Records, NYPL.

41. George L. Andrews return, 5th Vermont, Oct. 16, 1861; George A. Blake return, 40th New York, Nov. 14, 1861; George L. Andrews return, 2nd Vermont, Nov. 27, 1862; Franklin B. Hough return, 11th and 12th New York Batteries, Feb. 26, 1862; William M. Chamberlain return, 1st New Hampshire Battery, Battery D, 1st Rhode Island Light Artillery, Battery B, 4th US Artillery, Mar. 4, 1862; Edward Meade return, Battery K, 1st Ohio Light Artillery, Mar. 19, 1862; Henry W. Warriner return, 55th Illinois, Jan. 2, 1862; Godfrey Aigner return, 10th Iowa, Jan. 5, 1862; and Bernard J. Bettelheim return, 57th Indiana, Mar. 17, 1863, all Ser. 7, USSC Records, NYPL.

42. Robert Ware return, 71st Pennsylvania, Dec. 21, 1861; William M. Chamberlain return, 39th New York, Dec. 27, 1861; Chamberlain return, 6th Wisconsin, Feb. 10, 1862; Robert Ware return, 2nd and 4th Battalions, 1st Wisconsin Artillery, Feb. 2, 1862; Franklin B. Hough return, 1st Connecticut Artillery, Feb. 5, 1862; and Henry W. Warriner return, Battalion, 1st Nebraska Cavalry, Dec. 24, 1861, all Ser. 7, USSC Records, NYPL.

43. T. B. Smith return, 7th New York Artillery, Dec. 30, 1862; J. W. Page return, 45th Massachusetts, June 23, 1863; George A. Blake return, 15th Maine, June 14, 1862; and Bernard J. Bettelheim return, Pioneer Corps, [1863], all Ser. 7, USSC Records, NYPL.

44. E. J. Dunning return, 20th New York, July 17, 1861; and F. U. Johnston return, 9th New Hampshire, Jan. 7–29, 1862, both Ser. 7, USSC Records, NYPL.

45. Henry W. Warriner return, Battalion, 1st Nebraska Cavalry, Dec. 24, 1861, Ser. 7, USSC Records, NYPL.

5. SLOPS AND SINKS

1. *OR,* 25(2):492, 14:458.

2. Baker, *Ninth Mass. Battery,* 133–34.

3. "Remarks to accompany the Tabular Report of Act. Med. Inspector E. O. F. Roler, 15th Army Corps, for the week ending Sept. 27th 1863, Camp near Black River, Miss.," Ser. 1, Folder 5, Roll 1; "Remarks to accompany Report of Act. Med. Inspector of the 15th Army Corps, Dept. and Army of the Tennessee, for the month of Feb. 1864, Ser. 1, Folder 305, Roll 2; and John M. Woodworth to L. D. Huntington, June 21, 1865, Ser. 1, Folder 301, Roll 2, all USSC Records, NYPL.

4. Robert Jones return, 40th New York, July 15, 1861; George L. Andrews return, 2nd Vermont, Nov. 27, 1861; and Henry Oliver return, Battery B, 1st New York Light Artillery, Jan. 17, 1862, all Ser. 7, USSC Records, NYPL.

5. William W. Estabrook return, 12th Illinois, Apr. 15, 1863; E. J. Dunning return, 20th New York, July 17, 1861; William M. Chamberlain return, Battery A, 1st New York Light Artillery, Nov. 9, 1861; Henry Oliver return, Battery G, 1st New York Light Artillery, Jan. 14, 1862; and Edward A. Crane return, 128th New York, Jan. 22, 1863, all Ser. 7, USSC Records, NYPL; Thompson, *Thirteenth Regiment of New Hampshire Volunteer Infantry*, 94.

6. George L. Andrews return, 5th Wisconsin, Nov. 25, 1861; W. M. Prentice return, 2nd Tennessee, Nov. 27, 1861; and Henry W. Warriner return, Battalion, 1st Nebraska Cavalry, Dec. 24, 1861, all Ser. 7, USSC Records, NYPL.

7. Franklin B. Hough return, 19th Indiana, Feb. 10, 1862; Robert Ware return, 72nd Pennsylvania, Feb. 15, 1862; Godfrey Aigner return, 29th Illinois, Oct. 12, 1861; and William W. Estabrook return, 2nd Iowa, Apr. 11, 1863, all Ser. 7, USSC Records, NYPL.

8. Alfred L. Castleman return, 42nd Indiana, Apr. 6, 1863; Bernard J. Bettelheim returns, 79th Illinois and 30th Indiana, May 14–15, 1863; Jesse W. Page return, 3rd Massachusetts, June 9, 1863; and James Gall return, 1st US Colored Troops, Sept. 24, 1863, all Ser. 7, USSC Records, NYPL; Phelps, "Remarks on Various Circumstances," 58–59.

9. Amos York to William T. Rigby, Jan. 12, 1903, 8th Indiana Folder, VNMP; Bowen, *First New York Dragoons*, 304–5.

10. Macleod, *Notes on the Surgery of the War in the Crimea*, 24–25; McClellan, *European Cavalry*, 132.

11. Ordronaux, *Hints on Health in Armies*, 39–40, 58, 132; Hammond, *Treatise on Hygiene*, 459–60; Van Buren, *Rules for Preserving the Health of the Soldier*, 5.

12. *Revised Regulations*, 76.

13. Circular, Medical Inspector's Office, Army of Kentucky, Sept. 25, 1862, Ser. 1, Folder 917, Roll 7, USSC Records, NYPL.

14. Circular, Medical Inspector's Office, Army of Kentucky, Sept. 25, 1862.

15. General Orders No. 3, Headquarters, 1st Brigade, Grover's Division, Jan. 5, 1863, Box 3a, Simon G. Jerrard Papers, LSU; *OR*, 25(2):492, 35(2):113; Baker, *Ninth Mass. Battery*, 134; Small, *Road to Richmond*, 198; Howe, *Civil War Times*, 150.

16. [Olmsted], "Report of a Preliminary Survey of the Camps," 4; Howe, *Letter on the Sanitary Condition of the Troops in the Neighborhood of Boston*, 12.

17. Newberry, "Report on the Condition of the Troops and the Operations of the Sanitary Commission," 25, 19–21.

18. Newberry, "Report on the Condition of the Troops and the Operations of the Sanitary Commission," 28–29.

19. Stanley, *Personal Memoirs*, 103.

20. "Report of Acting Med. Inspector Edward D. Kittoe, for the 15th Army Corps, Dept. of the Tennessee, for the week ending April 12th 1863," Ser. 1, Folder 1; "Report of Acting Med. Inspector E. O. F. Roler, for the 15th Army Corps, Dept. of the Tennessee, for the week ending Sept. 12th 1863," Ser. 1, Folder 4; and "Remarks to accompany the Tabular Report of Act. Med. Inspector E. O. F. Roler, 15th Army Corps, for the week ending Sept. 27th 1863, Camp near Black River, Miss.," Ser. 1, Folder 5, all Roll 1; and John M. Woodworth to L. D. Huntington, June 21, 1865, Ser. 1, Folder 301, Roll 2, all USSC Records, NYPL.

21. Robert Jones return, 40th New York, Sept. 2, 1861; Robert Ware return, 72nd Pennsylvania, Dec. 20, 1861; William M. Chamberlain return, Battery A, 1st New York Light Artillery, Nov. 9, 1861; Franklin B. Hough return, 4th Maine Battery, Apr. 10, 1862; John H. Douglas return, 24th Missouri, Dec. 28, 1861; and T. B. Smith return, 1st Michigan Mounted Rifles, Jan. 4, 1863, all Ser. 7, USSC Records, NYPL.

22. Robert Jones return, 40th New York, July 15, 1861; Robert Collyer return, 5th Wisconsin, Aug. 20, 1861; and A. N. Read return, 18th Ohio, Nov. 13, 1861, all Ser. 7, USSC Records, NYPL.

23. William M. Chamberlain return, 15th New York Engineers, Oct. 10, 1861; and Robert Ware return, 11th Pennsylvania Cavalry, Dec. 11, 1861, both Ser. 7, USSC Records, NYPL.

24. George L. Andrews return, Brickel's 1st New York Artillery Battalion, Dec. 3, 1861; Henry Oliver return, Battery B, 1st New York Light Artillery, Jan. 17, 1862; Robert Ware return, 2nd Battalion and 4th Battalion, 1st Wisconsin Artillery, Feb. 2, 1862; and Franklin B. Hough return, 11th New York Battery and 12th New York Battery, Feb. 26, 1862, all Ser. 7, USSC Records, NYPL.

25. George L. Andrews return, 4th Vermont, Oct. 17, 1861; Bernard J. Bettelheim return, 57th Indiana, Mar. 17, 1863; and Bettelheim return, 22nd Indiana, Apr. 24–29, 1863, all Ser. 7, USSC Records, NYPL.

26. George L. Andrews return, 5th Wisconsin, Nov. 25, 1861, Ser. 7, USSC Records, NYPL.

27. T. B. Smith return, 7th New York Artillery, Dec. 30, 1862; Godfrey Aigner return, 27th Illinois, Dec. 24, 1861; Bernard J. Bettelheim return, 57th Indiana, Mar. 17, 1863; Edward A. Crane return, 2nd Vermont, Feb. 26, 1862; and Robert Collyer return, 19th Indiana, Aug. 20, 1861, all Ser. 7, USSC Records, NYPL.

28. George A. Blake return, 9th Connecticut, Feb. 13, 1862; Blake return, 26th Massachusetts, Feb. 13, 1862; Edward Meade return, 75th Ohio, Mar. 26, 1862; William M. Chamberlain return, 15th New York Engineers, Feb. 7, 1862; and Robert Ware return, 50th New York Engineers, Feb. 7, 1862, all Ser. 7, USSC Records, NYPL.

29. Marvin M. Marsh return, 1st Connecticut Battery, Mar. 14, 1862; Henry Oliver return, 8th Illinois Cavalry, Mar. 8, 1862; and William F. Swalm return, 26th Wisconsin, Mar. 17, 1863, all Ser. 7, USSC Records, NYPL.

30. Franklin B. Hough return, 3rd New York Cavalry, Apr. 10, 1862; John H. Douglas return, 12th Missouri, Dec. 24, 1861; Douglas return, 2nd Ohio Battery, Dec. 26, 1861; and Henry W. Warriner return, Battalion, 1st Nebraska Cavalry, Dec. 24, 1861, all Ser. 7, USSC Records, NYPL.

6. FOOD AND COOKING

1. O'Brien and Diefendorf, *General Orders of the War Department,* 1:95; *Revised Regulations,* 243.

2. Hammond, *Treatise on Hygiene,* 563; McClellan, *European Cavalry,* 127, 174–75; McClellan, *Armies of Europe,* 110–11.

3. De Fonblanque, *Treatise on the Administration and Organization of the British Army,* 356–57n, 363–65.

4. Hammond, *Treatise on Hygiene,* 497, 560–62.

5. Hammond, *Treatise on Hygiene,* 564; *Revised Regulations,* 36; Humphreys, *Intensely Human,* 129; Billings, *Hardtack and Coffee,* 112; "Dr. Aigner's Report on the Sanitary Conditions of the U.S. Forces in the District of Cairo during the months of December & January," Feb. 11, 1862, Ser. 1, Folder "Writings Re. Civil War, 1861–1865," Roll 12; and John H. Douglas to F. Law Olmsted, Aug. 15, 1861, Ser. 7, both USSC Records, NYPL; "Report of Lewis H. Steiner, Sanitary Inspector attached to the Division commanded by Maj. Genl. N. P. Banks, made Feb. 18, 1862, to the Sanitary Commission," 21, Lewis H. Steiner Papers, NLM.

6. Jackson and O'Donnell, *Back Home in Oneida,* 117; Bartow to wife, June 7, 1863, Sylvester Bartow Papers, Navarro College, Pearce Civil War Collection, Corsicana, TX; *OR,* 36(1):212; Sargent, "For Our Beloved Country," 50; Billings, *Hardtack and Coffee,* 116–17, 120–21; Albert S. Wright to unidentified recipient, [July] 10, 1863, Wright Family Papers, AU.

7. Knapp, "Major Dietary Changes," 188–91; Knapp, "Democratization of Meat and Protein," 541.

8. Billings, *Hardtack and Coffee,* 134; *Revised Regulations,* 241, 243; *OR,* 14:458; Lapham, *My Recollections,* 112.

9. *OR,* ser. 3, 4:482; *OR,* 30(3):247; Hess, "Meat-Eating in the Civil War," 154, 158–62.

10. Otto, *Memoirs of a Dutch Mudsill,* 73–74; Franklin B. Hough note in Baudens, *On Military and Camp Hospitals,* 35 (1st note).

11. Lapham, *My Recollections,* 112; Burt to wife, July 2, 1863, Richard W. Burt Papers, State Historical Society of Missouri, Research Center Columbia; Congdon, *Congdon's Cavalry Compendium,* 31; Ordronaux, *Hints on Health in Armies,* 118.

12. Billings, *Hardtack and Coffee,* 112; Lapham, *My Recollections,* 112–13.

13. "Remarks to accompany Report of Acting Med. Inspector of the 15th Army Corps, Dept. of the Tennessee, for the week ending April 12th 1863," Ser. 1, Folder 1; and "Remarks to accompany the weekly report of the Acting Medical Inspector of the 15th Army Corps, Dept. of the Tennessee, for the week ending April 19th 1863," Ser. 1, Folder 2, both Roll 1, USSC Records, NYPL.

14. "Remarks to accompany (Tabular) Report of Acting Med. Inspector of 15th Army Corps, Dept. of the Tennessee, for the week ending September 12th 1863," Ser. 1, Folder 4; and "Remarks to accompany the Tabular Report of Act. Med. Inspector E. O. F. Roler, 15th Army Corps, for the week ending Sept. 27th 1863, Camp near Black River, Miss.," Ser. 1, Folder 5, both Roll 1, USSC Records, NYPL.

15. John M. Woodworth to L. D. Huntington, June 21, 1865, Ser. 1, Folder 301, Roll 2, USSC Records, NYPL.

16. Henry Oliver return, Battery G, 1st New York Light Artillery, Jan. 14, 1862, Ser. 7, USSC Records, NYPL.

17. Godfrey Aigner return, 27th Illinois, Dec. 24, 1861, Ser. 7, USSC Records, NYPL.

18. M. P. Buel return, 1st Nebraska, Sept. 8, 1861; William M. Chamberlain return, 39th New York, Nov. 2, 1861; George A. Blake return, 1st Louisiana Native Guards, Dec. 12, 1862; Blake return, 12th Connecticut, June 16, 1862; Robert Jones return, 40th New York, July 15, 1861; and Jones return, 2nd Rhode Island, July 16, 1861, all Ser. 7, USSC Records, NYPL.

19. Bernard J. Bettelheim returns, 9th Kentucky, 79th Indiana, 19th Ohio, Mar. 26–27, 1863; and Edward A. Crane return, 7th Maine, Jan. 14, 1862, all Ser. 7, USSC Records, NYPL; [Olmsted], "Report of a Preliminary Survey of the Camps," 11.

20. Franklin B. Hough return, 6th Maine Battery, Apr. 10, 1862; and Bernard J. Bettelheim return, 6th Ohio, Mar. 31, 1863, both Ser. 7, USSC Records, NYPL.

21. Lewis H. Steiner return, 3rd Wisconsin, Jan. 31, 1862; George L. Andrews return, Brickel's 1st New York Artillery Battalion, Dec. 3, 1861; and Franklin B. Hough return, 19th Indiana, Feb. 10, 1862, all Ser. 7, USSC Records, NYPL; Newberry, "Report on the Condition of the Troops and the Operations of the Sanitary Commission," 25, 30.

22. Bernard J. Bettelheim return, 58th Indiana, Mar. 25, 1863, Ser. 7, USSC Records, NYPL.

23. Robert Collyer return, 5th Wisconsin, Aug. 19, 1861; Bernard J. Bettelheim return, 3rd Kentucky, Mar. 19, 1863; and Henry Oliver return, 4th New York Battery, Feb. 1, 1862, all Ser. 7, USSC Records, NYPL.

24. Franklin B. Hough return, 19th Indiana, Feb. 10, 1862; and Robert Jones return, 40th New York, July 15, 1861, both Ser. 7, USSC Records, NYPL.

25. "Dr. Aigner's Report on the Sanitary Conditions of the U.S. Forces in the District of Cairo during the months of December & January," Ser. 1, Folder "Writings Re. Civil War, 1861–1865," Roll 12; and Franklin B. Hough return, 2nd New Jersey, Feb. 12, 1862, both USSC Records, NYPL; Newberry, "Report on the Condition of the Troops and the Operations of the Sanitary Commission," 25, 30.

26. Godfrey Aigner return, 28th Illinois, Dec. 29, 1861; and Aigner return, 10th Iowa, Jan. 5, 1862, both Ser. 7, USSC Records, NYPL.

27. Bernard J. Bettelheim returns, 110th Illinois, 9th Indiana, Apr. 1, 3, 1863; and E. J. Dunning return, 20th New York, July 17, 1861, all Ser. 7, USSC Records, NYPL.

28. Edward Mead return, 75th Ohio, Mar. 26, 1862, Ser. 7; and Alex McDonald, "Notes on Sanitation in the Field," Ser. 1, Folder 1107, Roll 8, both USSC Records, NYPL.

29. Ordronaux, *Hints on Health in Armies,* 71, 73–74.

30. Kautz, *Customs of Service,* 269; Viele, *Hand-Book for Active Service,* 79–82; Grafton, *Treatise on the Camp and March,* 9; Butterfield, *Camp and Outpost Duty,* 104; De Fonblanque, *Treatise on the Administration and Organization of the British Army,* 362.

31. *Revised Regulations,* 23.

32. Howe, *Letters and Journals,* 490–92.

33. Bull, *Soldiering,* 95; Wild, *Memoirs and History of Capt. F. W. Alexander's Baltimore Battery,* 34.

34. "Report of Lewis H. Steiner, Sanitary Inspector attached to the Division commanded by Maj. Genl. N. P. Banks, made Feb. 18, 1862, to the Sanitary Commission," 19, Lewis H. Steiner Papers, NLM.

35. Wild, *Memoirs and History of Capt. F. W. Alexander's Baltimore Battery,* 24; Johnson, *Muskets and Medicine,* 46–47; Billings, *Hardtack and Coffee,* 135.

36. *OR,* 14:458–59; [Marsh], "Report on the Sanitary State of the Troops at Charleston," 80; Wilder, *Practicing Medicine,* 87; Hammond, *Treatise on Hygiene,* 512–14; *OR,* 11(3):350–51.

37. *OR*, 25(2):491–92, 46(2):562–63.

38. "Remarks to accompany Report of Acting Med. Inspector of the 15th Army Corps, Dept. of the Tennessee, for the week ending April 12th 1863," Ser. 1, Folder 1; and "Remarks to accompany the weekly report of the Acting Medical Inspector of the 15th Army Corps, Dept. of the Tennessee, for the week ending April 19th, 1863," Ser. 1, Folder 2, both Roll 1, USSC Records, NYPL.

39. "Remarks to accompany Tabular Report, Act. Med. Inspector E. O. F. Roler, 15th Army Corps 2nd Div. for the week ending Sept. 19th 1863"; and "Remarks to accompany the Tabular Report of Act. Med. Inspector E. O. F. Roler, 15th Army Corps, for the week ending Sept. 27th 1863, Camp near Black River, Miss.," both Ser. 1, Folder 5, Roll 1, USSC Records, NYPL.

40. "Remarks to accompany Report of Acting Medical Inspector 15th Army Corps, Dept. and Army of the Tennessee for the month of Feb. 1864," Ser. 1, Folders 302–5; and "Remarks to accompany Report of Act. Med. Inspector of the 15th Army Corps, Army and Dept. of the Tennessee, for the month of March 1864," Ser. 1, Folders 297–98, both Roll 2, USSC Records, NYPL.

41. "Remarks of Acting Med. Inspector Edward D. Kittoe, for the 15th Army Corps, Dept. of the Tennessee, for the week ending April 12th, 1863," Ser. 1, Folder 1; and "Report of Acting Med. Inspector E. O. F. Roler, for the 15th Army Corps, Dept. of the Tennessee, for the week ending Sept. 12th, 1863," Ser. 1, Folder 4, both Roll 1, USSC Records, NYPL.

42. W. S. Hough return, 1st and 2nd US Sharpshooters, Feb. 6, 1862; Robert Ware return, 71st Pennsylvania, Dec. 21, 1861; Edward A. Crane return, 3rd Vermont, Jan. 3, 1862; Franklin B. Hough return, 2nd New Jersey, Feb. 12, 1862; Franklin B. Hough return, 1st Connecticut Artillery, Feb. 5, 1862; Franklin B. Hough return, 19th Indiana, Feb. 10, 1862; and Bernard J. Bettelheim return, artillery of Van Cleve's division, Mar. 27, 1863, all Ser. 7, USSC Records, NYPL.

43. Bernard J. Bettelheim returns, 22nd Indiana and 59th Illinois, Apr. 24–29, 1863, Ser. 7, USSC Records, NYPL.

44. Bernard J. Bettelheim return, 58th Indiana, Mar. 25, 1863; and E. J. Dunning return, 1st Vermont, July 21, 1861, both Ser. 7, USSC Records, NYPL.

7. WATER, ALCOHOL, AND MORALE

1. McClellan, *European Cavalry*, 127; McClellan, *Armies of Europe*, 110.

2. Ordronaux, *Hints on Health in Armies*, 90–92; Craighill, *Army Officer's Pocket Companion*, 248.

3. Hammond, *Treatise on Hygiene*, 214–19.

4. Benjamin Woodward, "Notes on Water," Ser. 1, Folder 42, Roll 1, USSC Records, NYPL.

5. Woodward, "Notes on Water."

6. Woodward, "Notes on Water."

7. Congdon, *Congdon's Cavalry Compendium*, 32; "Civil War Letters of Brigadier General William Ward Orme," 283; Sargent, "For Our Beloved Country," 47; Mc-

Gregor, *Dearest Susie,* 30; Cooke, *Badger Boy in Blue,* 69; William P. Black to mother, June 22, 1863, John Charles Black Papers, ALPL; Pugh to wife. May 29. 1863, Isaac C. Pugh Papers, University of California, Special Collections and Archives, Riverside.

8. Taylor to Jane, June 18, 1863, William Taylor Letters, College of William and Mary, Special Collections Research Center, Williamsburg, VA; Tracey to sister, June 20, 1863, George Boardman Tracey Letters, Library of Virginia, Richmond; Shepherd, *To Rescue My Native Land,* 272.

9. "The Hospital Transport Service in the Western Medical Department," Ser. 1, Folder marked "Western Medical Dept. Hospital Transport," Roll 11, USSC Records, NYPL; Johnson, *Muskets and Medicine,* 69; Cooke, *Badger Boy in Blue,* 70–71; Benjamin F. Pease Memoir, 42, Syracuse University, Special Collections Research Center, Syracuse, NY; William P. Black to mother, June 17, 1863, John Charles Black Papers, ALPL.

10. Scherneckau, *Marching with the First Nebraska,* 181; Orpheus Everts, "Medical History of the 20th Ind Vol Infy July 1861 to August 1862," 3, Ser. 1, Folder 35, Roll 1; and John M. Woodworth to L. D. Huntington, June 21, 1865, Ser. 1, Folder 301, Roll 2, both USSC Records, NYPL; Sargent, "For Our Beloved Country," 94.

11. Perry, *Letters from a Surgeon,* 152; Congdon, *Congdon's Cavalry Compendium,* 32; Billings, *Hardtack and Coffee,* 273; Hammond, *Treatise on Hygiene,* 242, 244–45, 247–50; Post and Van Buren, *Report on Military Hygiene and Therapeutics,* 15; Muffly, *Story of Our Regiment,* 167.

12. *OR,* 25(2):491; Barton, *Autobiography,* 147; Buell, *"Cannoneer,"* 247.

13. Jesse W. Page return, 3rd Massachusetts, June 9, 1863; Robert Jones return, 2nd Rhode Island, July 16, 1861; Alfred L. Castleman return, 88th Indiana, Apr. 6, 1863, all Ser. 7; and Orpheus Everts, "Medical History of the 20th Ind Vol Infy July 1861 to August 1862," 5–6, 14, Ser. 1, Folder 35, Roll 1, all USSC Records, NYPL; Copp, *Reminiscences,* 94; *OR,* 36(1):254.

14. "Report of Acting Med. Inspector E. O. F. Roler for the 15th Army Corps, Dept. of the Tennessee, Camp near Black River, Miss., for the week ending Sept. 19th 1863," Ser. 1, Folder 5, Roll 1, USSC Records, NYPL.

15. John H. Douglas return, 1st Minnesota, Nov. 3, 1861; George L. Andrews return, 3rd Pennsylvania Cavalry, Nov. 3, 1861; and Lewis H. Steiner return, 3rd Wisconsin, Jan. 31, 1863, all Ser. 7, USSC Records, NYPL.

16. Rorabaugh, "Estimated U.S. Alcoholic Beverage Consumption," 357, 360–62; Bever, *At War with King Alcohol,* 3–5, 7.

17. Bever, *At War with King Alcohol,* 13–14, 36–37.

18. Warner, "Physiological Theory and Therapeutic Explanation," 235–39, 253–55; Ordronaux, *Hints on Health in Armies,* 97; Hammond, *Treatise on Hygiene,* 535–40, 542.

19. Dwight, "Feeding an Army," 102; Joseph H. Waite Diaries, June 24, 1863, IHS; *OR,* 42(1):192; Hawley to father and mother, July 12, 1863, Thomas S. Hawley Papers, Missouri History Museum, St. Louis; Hard, *Eighth Cavalry Regiment Illinois Volunteers,* 68–69.

20. Billings, *Hardtack and Coffee,* 139–41; De Forest, *Volunteer's Adventures,* 94; Johnson, *Muskets and Medicine,* 80; Jones, *Artilleryman's Diary,* 208; Remley and Remley, *Southern Sons,* 42; Williams, *From the Cannon's Mouth,* 38.

21. *Medical and Surgical History,* pt. 3, 1:171, 890–91.

22. Post and Van Buren, *Report on Military Hygiene and Therapeutics,* 15; "Soldier's Health," attached to Franklin B. Hough return, 2nd DC, Apr. 8, 1862, Ser. 7; D. F. Leavitt questionnaire, Ser. 1, Folder 1480, Roll 10; J. C. Batdorf questionnaire, Sept. 16, 1865, Ser. 1, Folder 487, Roll 3; Henry Manfred questionnaire, Ser. 1, Folder 779, Roll 6; and J. Wright questionnaire, Ser. 1, Folder 876, Roll 6, all USSC Records, NYPL.

23. Bernard J. Bettelheim returns, 74th Illinois and 75th Illinois, Apr. 24–25, 1863; George A. Blake return, 3rd Maine, Nov. 14, 1861; and Edward A. Crane return, 159th New York, Dec. 25, 1862, all Ser. 7, USSC Records, NYPL; Newberry, "Report on the Condition of the Troops and the Operations of the Sanitary Commission," 30.

24. Orpheus Everts, "Medical History of the 20th Ind Vol Infy July 1861 to August 1862," 7, Ser. 1, Folder 35, Roll 1; and William M. Chamberlain return, 39th New York, Nov. 2, 1861, Ser. 7, both USSC Records, NYPL; McClellan, *McClellan's Own Story,* 141–42; "Sketches of Field and Camp in a Series of Letters from a Sanitary Inspector to the Little Folks at Home, Vol. 1, Washington, Feb. 1862," Box 37, Folder 1, Franklin Benjamin Hough Papers, NYSL.

25. William M. Chamberlain return, 39th New York, Nov. 2, 1861; Edward A. Crane return, 5th Vermont, Jan. 6, 1862; Franklin B. Hough return, 1st Connecticut Artillery, Feb. 5, 1862; and T. B. Smith return, 2nd Pennsylvania Artillery, Jan. 7, 1863, all Ser. 7, USSC Records, NYPL.

26. W. S. Hough return, 1st and 2nd US Sharpshooters, Feb. 6, 1862; Robert Ware return, 2nd and 4th Battalions, 1st Wisconsin Artillery, Feb. 2, 1862; and Bernard J. Bettelheim returns, Battery A, 1st Ohio Light Artillery and 5th Indiana Battery, May 20–21, 1863, Ser. 7; and Elisha Harris to J. Foster Jenkins, Oct. 29, 1863, Ser. 1, Folder 480, Roll 3, all USSC Records, NYPL.

27. George L. Andrews return, Brickel's 1st New York Artillery Battalion, Dec. 3, 1861; Robert Ware return, 7th New York, Feb. 2, 1862; Alex McDonald return, 1st Maine Cavalry, Apr. 10, 1863; John H. Douglas return, 2nd Missouri, Dec. 26, 1861; and George A. Blake return, 3rd Maine, Nov. 14, 1861, all Ser. 7, USSC Records, NYPL.

28. Barber, *Army Memoirs,* 42–43; Jones, *Artilleryman's Diary,* 208. See also *Medical and Surgical History,* pt. 3, 1:691.

29. Martin, "American Civil War and the Course of Late Nineteenth-Century Temperance Reform," 193–96.

30. McClellan, *Armies of Europe,* 60, 62; De Fonblanque, *Treatise on the Administration and Organization of the British Army,* 113, 262n, 421.

31. Hammond et al., "Scurvy," 25; Van Buren, *Rules for Preserving the Health of the Soldier,* 8. William A. Hammond, who launched an all-out assault on masturbation in his *Treatise on Hygiene,* argued that officers should divert the men's attention to avoid this practice. Ironically, when John H. Douglas inspected the 2nd Ohio Battery in December 1861, someone told him that a member of the unit had died "from Masturbation." Since no one in the battery had died prior to that month, according to the state published roster, it apparently was said as a joke. See Hammond, *Treatise on Hygiene,* 142; and John H. Douglas return, 2nd Ohio Battery, Dec. 26, 1861, Ser. 7, USSC Records, NYPL.

32. *OR,* 41(2):181.

33. Perry, *Letters from a Surgeon,* 124.

34. Hard, *Eighth Cavalry Regiment Illinois Volunteers,* 69; Wild, *Memoirs and History of Capt. F. W. Alexander's Baltimore Battery,* 30.

35. Sargent, "For Our Beloved Country," 49; Gleason, "U.S. Mounted Bands and Cavalry Field Musicians," 113.

36. O'Brien and Diefendorf, *General Orders of the War Department,* 1:344–45; *OR,* ser. 3, 1:705, 728, 2:336.

37. General Orders No. 2, Headquarters, 1st Brigade, Grover's Division, Jan. 5, 1863, Box 3a, Simon G. Jerrard Papers, LSU.

38. Robert Jones return, 40th New York, July 15, 1861; Edward Mead return, 3rd West Virginia, Mar. 28, 1862; Bernard J. Bettelheim return, 21st Illinois, Apr. 29, 1863; and Bettelheim returns, 1st Kentucky and 2nd Kentucky, Apr. 3–4, 1863, all Ser. 7, USSC Records, NYPL. The 2nd Minnesota also used its company-level musicians to form a new regimental band after its first one was dissolved in the summer of 1862. See Bishop, *Story of a Regiment,* 178.

39. Robert Ware return, 2nd and 4th Battalions, 1st Wisconsin Artillery, Feb. 2, 1862; Franklin B. Hough return, 1st Connecticut Artillery, Feb. 5, 1862; Jesse W. Page return, 45th Massachusetts, Jan. 23, 1863; and John H. Douglas return, 1st Minnesota, Nov. 3, 1861, all Ser. 7, USSC Records, NYPL.

40. Newberry, "Report on the Condition of the Troops and the Operations of the Sanitary Commission," 30; Henry Oliver return, 1st Massachusetts, Dec. 13, 1861; Alex McDonald return, 119th Pennsylvania, Mar. 27, 1863; William M. Chamberlain return, 15th New York Engineers, Oct. 10, 1861; Robert Collyer return, 36th New York, Sept. 3, 1861; William M. Chamberlain return, 2nd Rhode Island, Nov. 28, 1861; George A. Blake return, Battery A, New Jersey Light Artillery, Dec. 11, 1861; Robert Ware return, 7th New York, Feb. 2, 1862; Ware return, 1st Minnesota, Feb. 20, 1862; and Bernard J. Bettelheim return, 1st Michigan Engineers and Mechanics, May 9, 1863, all Ser. 7, USSC Records, NYPL.

41. Franklin B. Hough return, 2nd New Jersey, Feb. 12, 1862; Franklin B. Hough return, 1st Connecticut Artillery, Feb. 5, 1862; and Bernard J. Bettelheim return, Pioneer Corps, [1863], all Ser. 7, USSC Records, NYPL.

42. John H. Douglas return, 48th Pennsylvania, Nov. 6, 1861; Edward A. Crane return, 2nd Vermont, Feb. 26, 1862; Franklin B. Hough return, 1st Connecticut Artillery, Feb. 5, 1862; John H. Douglas return, 36th Illinois, Dec. 28, 1861; W. S. Hough return, 1st and 2nd US Sharpshooters, Feb. 6, 1862; Godfrey Aigner return, 10th Iowa, Jan. 5, 1862; Alfred L. Castleman return, 36th Illinois, Apr. 22, 1863; and George A. Blake return, Battery A, Massachusetts Light Artillery, Dec. 12, 1861, all Ser. 7, USSC Records, NYPL.

43. Bernard J. Bettelheim return, 21st Illinois, Apr. 29, 1863; Alfred L. Castleman return, 36th Illinois, Apr. 22, 1863; Bernard J. Bettelheim returns, Battery A, 1st Ohio and 5th Indiana Battery, May 20–21, 1863; Marvin M. Marsh return, 1st Connecticut Battery, Mar. 14, 1863; Marsh return, 174th Pennsylvania, Mar. 11, 1863; and Godfrey Aigner return, 31st Illinois, Oct. 18, 1861, all Ser. 7, USSC Records, NYPL.

44. T. B. Smith return, 2nd Pennsylvania Artillery, Jan. 7, 1863; Robert Jones return, 3rd Maine, Aug. 31, 1861; Henry W. Warriner return, 2nd Iowa Battery, Jan. 3,

1862; F. U. Johnston return, 9th New Hampshire, Jan. 7–29, 1863; George G. Edgerly return, 1st Regiment Corps d'Afrique, Oct. 25, 1863; and Henry W. Warriner return, Battalion, 1st Nebraska Cavalry, Dec. 24, 1861, all Ser. 7, USSC Records, NYPL.

45. Gordon H. Winslow return, Battery A, 1st West Virginia, Feb. 1, 1862; and E. J. Dunning return, 20th New York, July 17, 1861, both Ser. 7, USSC Records, NYPL.

46. *Medical and Surgical History,* pt. 3, 1:884–86; O. W. Long to Elisha Harris, Nov. 29, 1865, Ser. 1, Folder 735, Roll 5, USSC Records, NYPL; Anderson, "Dying of Nostalgia," 264–70, 272; Clarke, "So Lonesome I Could Die," 253–54.

8. Recruit Examination and Vaccination

1. Marshall, *On the Enlisting,* 9–14, 16; Bartholow, *Manual of Instructions,* 151, 153–55, 157, 176, 200–201.

2. Bartholow, *Manual of Instructions,* 28, 35, 41–42; Coolidge, *Statistical Report,* 625–27; *OR,* ser. 3, 3:1057.

3. *Revised Regulations,* 130, 495; *OR,* ser. 3, 1:384, 4:966; O'Brien and Diefendorf, *General Orders of the War Department,* 1:102.

4. Newberry, "Report on the Condition of the Troops and the Operations of the Sanitary Commission," 25–26, 31–32; "Dr. Aigner's Report on the Sanitary Conditions of the U.S. Forces in the District of Cairo during the months of December & January," Feb. 11, 1862, Ser. 1, Folder "Writings Re. Civil War, 1861–1865," Roll 12, USSC Records, NYPL. Col. William B. Franklin of the 12th US Infantry inspected 4,500 New York volunteers in late May and concluded, "from the cursory examination I was able to make, that at least one-eighth ought to be rejected on account of physical disability, youth, disease, & c." *OR,* ser. 3, 1:237.

5. Hammond, *Treatise on Hygiene,* 19; Peters, "Remarks on the Evils of Youthful Enlistments and Nostalgia," 75.

6. Hard, *Eighth Cavalry Regiment Illinois Volunteers,* 36; Bartholow, *Manual of Instructions,* 168; Sargent, "For Our Beloved Country," 39.

7. *OR,* 5:713, 36(1):213; Bartholow, *Manual of Instructions,* 37–38.

8. Bartholow, *Manual of Instructions,* 38–40, 169–74, 189–90.

9. Hammond, *Treatise on Hygiene,* 19–21, 25–26, 30–33, 35–36, 50–52.

10. Hammond, *Treatise on Hygiene,* 79–88.

11. Grace, *Army Surgeon's Manual,* 18; *OR,* ser. 3, 5:679, 763–65.

12. Franklin B. Hough return, 3rd New York Cavalry, Apr. 10, 1862; T. B. Smith return, 2nd Pennsylvania Artillery, Jan. 7, 1863; and Edward A. Crane return, 2nd Louisiana, Dec. 29, 1862, all Ser. 7, USSC Records, NYPL.

13. [George L. Andrews] return, 8th Illinois Cavalry, Nov. 30, 1861; and Edward Mead return, 2nd Virginia (US), Mar. 27, 1862, both Ser. 7, USSC Records, NYPL.

14. Robert Ware return, 2nd and 4th Battalions, 1st Wisconsin Artillery, Feb. 2, 1862; Franklin B. Hough return, 11th New York Battery and 12th New York Battery, Feb. 26, 1862; and E. J. Dunning return, 20th New York, July 17, 1861, all Ser. 7, USSC Records, NYPL. Surgeon Sanford B. Hunt of the 109th New York performed a quick but surprisingly effective examination of the regiment's recruits. Each company

soldier stripped in whole or in part, and Hunt spent one minute per man "to cover all aspects possible." With the cooperation of regimental officers, he rejected 26 percent of the men. "Testimony of Medical Officers," 102.

15. George L. Andrews return, 19th Indiana, Oct. 9, 1861; and Bernard J. Bettelheim return, 100th Illinois, Mar. 13, 1863, both Ser. 7, USSC Records, NYPL; Franklin B. Hough return, 3rd Battalion, 2nd New York Light Artillery, Feb. 27, 1862, Box 37, Folder 2, Franklin Benjamin Hough Papers, NYSL. Although Col. Joshua W. Sill was a regular-army officer, he allowed Surgeon Alonzo J. Phelps to do only a minimal examination of recruits for the 33rd Ohio. That "consisted of but little more than opening and shutting the hands, bending the elbows and knees, and rotating the shoulder-joint, with a casual glance at the teeth and eyes, and a question as to age and previous general health. They were then, with few exceptions, mustered in to the service." Phelps, "Remarks on Various Circumstances," 45.

16. Franklin B. Hough return, 19th Indiana, Feb. 10, 1862; T. B. Smith return, 2nd Pennsylvania Artillery, Jan. 7, 1863; George G. Edgerly return, 11th Regiment Corps d'Afrique, Oct. 22, 1863; and James Gall return, 1st US Colored Troops, Sept. 24, 1863, all Ser. 7, USSC Records, NYPL.

17. Doyle and Smith, "'Very Best Soldiers in the World,'" 64–80; *OR*, ser. 3, 3:894, 1054, 1057.

18. Becker, "Smallpox in Washington's Army," 383, 386–90, 394–95; Cirillo, "Two Faces of Death," 126.

19. Becker, "Smallpox in Washington's Army," 385.

20. Kaufman, "American Anti-Vaccinationists," 463–64, 466–68, 471; Toner, "Propriety and Necessity of Compulsory Vaccination," 310, 313–14.

21. Gillett, *Army Medical Department*, 134–35; Humphreys, *Intensely Human*, 95–96; Toner, "Propriety and Necessity of Compulsory Vaccination," 315–16.

22. Humphreys, *Intensely Human*, 96–97; Hicks, "Scabrous Matters," 138–42.

23. Bell et al., "Protection from Smallpox," 274–75.

24. Gillett, *Army Medical Department*, 278; Ordronaux, *Hints on Health in Armies*, 18n; Smith and Stillé, "Report . . . on the Value of Vaccination in Armies," 3, 6–16, 18–19, 22–23, 26.

25. Wilcox and Peters, "Vaccination of the Twenty-First Regiment," 80–81; Bell et al., "Protection from Smallpox," 272.

26. Wilcox and Peters, "Vaccination of the Twenty-First Regiment," 81–82; Bell et al., "Protection from Smallpox," 272.

27. *Medical and Surgical History*, pt. 3, 1:625.

28. Claiborne J. Walton questionnaire, Ser. 1, Folder 990, Roll 7, USSC Records, NYPL.

29. Beecham, *As If It Were Glory*, 15–16.

30. Hard, *Eighth Cavalry Regiment Illinois Volunteers*, 46.

31. *OR*, 7:675, 44:79, 46(1):624, 47(1):695–96; Jones to parents, Dec. 20, 1862, John G. Jones Civil War Letters, WHS; C. M. Campbell questionnaire, Ser. 1, Folder 206, Roll 2, USSC Records, NYPL; Scherneckau, *Marching with the First Nebraska*, 173; Poak, *"Dear Sister Sadie,"* 49; Hicks, *Civil War Medicine*, 176–77.

32. Romeyn, "With Colored Troops," 56–58.

33. Gordon H. Winslow return, 5th New York, Jan. 22, 1862; George A. Blake return, 91st New York, Mar. 24, 1862; John H. Douglas return, 2nd Missouri, Dec. 26, 1861; and William M. Chamberlain return, 8th New York, Nov. 7, 1861, all Ser. 7, USSC Records, NYPL.

34. Henry Oliver return, 3rd Maine, Feb. 18, 1862; and William M. Chamberlain return, 50th New York Engineers, Feb. 7, 1862, both Ser. 7, Records, NYPL.

35. Henry Oliver return, 8th Illinois Cavalry, Jan. 9, 1862, Ser. 7; Henry Manfred questionnaire, 22nd Kentucky, Ser. 1, Folder 779, Roll 6; and R. G. Bogue questionnaire, 19th Illinois, Ser. 1, Folder 52, Roll 1, all USSC Records, NYPL.

36. Robert Ware return, 1st Minnesota, Feb. 20, 1862; Edward Mead return, 2nd West Virginia, Mar. 27, 1862; Bernard J. Bettelheim returns, 9th Kentucky, 79th Indiana, 19th Ohio, Mar. 26–27, 1863; Bettelheim returns, 74th Illinois, 75th Illinois, Apr. 24–25, 1863, Ser. 7; D. F. Leavitt questionnaire, 3rd Massachusetts Cavalry, Ser. 1, Folder 1480, Roll 10; Claiborne J. Walton questionnaire, 22nd Kentucky, Ser. 1, Folder 990, Roll 7; and R. G. Bogue questionnaire, 19th Illinois, Ser. 1, Folder 52, Roll 1, all USSC Records, NYPL.

37. *Medical and Surgical History,* pt. 3, 1:626, 634, 648, 690.

38. *Medical and Surgical History,* pt. 3, 1:625.

9. REGIMENTAL HOSPITALS AND OFFICER SUPERVISION

1. McClellan, *McClellan's Own Story,* 126; "Report of Lewis H. Steiner, Sanitary Inspector attached to the Division commanded by Maj. Genl. N. P. Banks, made Feb. 18, 1862, to the Sanitary Commission," 26, Lewis H. Steiner Papers, NLM; Ira Russell, "Hygienic & Hospital Records of the 11th Regt. Mass. Vols.," Ser. 1, Folder 678, Roll 5, USSC Records, NYPL.

2. Billings, *Hardtack and Coffee,* 50, 300, 302; *OR,* 23(1):418.

3. Billings, *Hardtack and Coffee,* 302–3, 315; Phelps, "Remarks on Various Circumstances," 59.

4. "Dr. Aigner's Report on the Sanitary Condition of the U.S. Forces in the District of Cairo during the months of December & January," Feb. 11, 1862, Ser. 1, Folder "Writings Re. Civil War, 1861–1865," Roll 12, USSC Records, NYPL.

5. Phelps, "Remarks on Various Circumstances," 62; "Remarks to accompany Report of Acting Med. Inspector of the 15th Army Corps, Dept. of the Tennessee, for the week ending April 12th 1863," Ser. 1, Folder 1, Roll 1; "Remarks to accompany the Tabular Report of Act. Med. Inspector E. O. F. Roler, 15th Army Corps, for the week ending Sept. 27th 1863, Camp near Black River, Miss.," Ser. 1, Folder 5, Roll 1; "Remarks to accompany Report of Act. Med. Inspector of the 15th Army Corps, Dept. and Army of the Tennessee, for the month of Feb. 1864," Ser. 1, Folder 305, Roll 2; and "Remarks to accompany Report of Act. Med. Inspector of the 15th Army Corps, Army and Dept. of the Tennessee, for the month of March 1864," Ser. 1, Folder 297, Roll 2, all USSC Records, NYPL.

6. Henry Oliver return, Battery B, 1st New York, Jan. 17, 1862; and Edward A. Crane return, 3rd New York Battery, Jan. 22, 1862, both Ser. 7, USSC Records, NYPL.

7. George A. Blake return, 12th Connecticut, June 16, 1862; E. J. Dunning return, 1st Vermont, July 16, 1861; and F. U. Johnston return, 26th New Jersey, Feb. 9, 1863, all Ser. 7, USSC Records, NYPL.

8. Robert Ware return, 50th New York Engineers, Feb. 7, 1862; T. B. Smith return, 2nd Pennsylvania Artillery, Jan. 7, 1863; Godfrey Aigner return, 28th Illinois, Dec. 29, 1861; John H. Douglas return, 12th Missouri, Dec. 24, 1861; Edward A. Crane return, 52nd Massachusetts, Dec. 24, 1862; Bernard J. Bettelheim returns, 30th Indiana and 90th Ohio, Apr. 5, 20, 1863; Bettelheim return, Harker's Brigade, Mar. 20, 1863; and William W. Estabrook return, 39th Ohio, Apr. 15, 1863, all Ser. 7, USSC Records, NYPL.

9. George L. Andrews returns, 1st Massachusetts Cavalry, Feb. 25, Apr. 4, 1862; John H. Douglas return, 1st Missouri Cavalry, Dec. 25, 1861; Henry W. Warriner return, 55th Illinois, Jan. 2, 1862; and F. U. Johnston return, 9th New Hampshire, Jan. 7–29, 1863, all Ser. 7, USSC Records, NYPL.

10. George L. Andrews return, 5th Vermont, Oct. 16, 1861; Godfrey Aigner return, 10th Iowa, Jan. 5, 1862, USSC Records, NYPL.

11. Franklin B. Hough return, 1st Connecticut Artillery, Feb. 5, 1862; and Godfrey Aigner return, 27th Illinois, Dec. 24, 1861, both Ser. 7, USSC Records, NYPL.

12. William M. Chamberlain return, 8th New York, Dec. 29, 1861, Ser. 7, USSC Records, NYPL.

13. William M. Chamberlain return, 2nd Rhode Island, Jan. 20, 1862; Henry Oliver return, 8th Illinois Cavalry, Jan. 9, 1862; William M. Chamberlain return, 15th New York Engineers, Feb. 7, 1862; John H. Douglas return, 15th Missouri, Dec. 26, 1861; Henry W. Warriner return, 55th Illinois, Jan. 2, 1862; and John H. Douglas return, 17th Missouri, Dec. 24, 1861, all Ser. 7, USSC Records, NYPL.

14. William M. Chamberlain return, Battery A, 1st New York Light Artillery, Nov. 9, 1861; Henry W. Warriner return, 2nd Iowa Battery, Jan. 3, 1862; and George A. Blake return, 15th Maine, June 14, 1862, all Ser. 7, USSC Records, NYPL.

15. William M. Chamberlain return, 2nd Rhode Island, Jan. 20, 1862; Bernard J. Bettelheim return, 57th Indiana, Mar. 17, 1863; and Edward A. Crane return, 161st New York, Dec. 25, 1862, all Ser. 7, USSC Records, NYPL.

16. Ordronaux, *Hints on Health in Armies,* 58–59; Viele, *Hand-Book for Active Service,* 32–33, 35; McClellan, *Armies of Europe,* 108; Ira Russell, "Hygienic & Hospital Records of the 11th Regt. Mass. Vols.," Ser. 1, Folder 678, Roll 5, USSC Records, NYPL.

17. Newberry, "Report on the Condition of the Troops and the Operations of the Sanitary Commission," 25–26, 32, 36; "Dr. Aigner's Report on the Sanitary Condition of the U.S. Forces in the District of Cairo during the months of December & January," Feb. 11, 1862, Ser. 1, Folder "Writings Re. Civil War, 1861–1865," Roll 12, USSC Records, NYPL.

18. Grace, *Army Surgeon's Manual,* 76–77; *OR,* 11(1):192–94, 196; McClellan, *McClellan's Own Story,* 126.

19. *OR,* 11(2):153; Franklin B. Hough return, 102nd New York, Apr. 5, 1862, Box 37, Folder 2, Franklin Benjamin Hough Papers, NYSL; Castleman, *Army of the Potomac,* 7, 9, 18–19,44, 48, 50–51, 56–57, 60, 75.

20. "Remarks to accompany Report of Acting Med. Inspector of the 15th Army Corps, Dept. of the Tennessee, for the week ending April 12th 1863," Ser. 1, Folder 1, Roll 1; "Remarks to accompany (Tabular) Report of Acting Med. Inspector of 15th Army Corps, Dept. of the Tennessee, for the week ending September 12th 1863," Ser. 1, Folder 4, Roll 1; and "Remarks to accompany Report of Acting Medical Inspector 15th Army Corps, Dept. and Army of the Tennessee for the month of Feb. 1864," Ser. 1, Folders 302, 304, Roll 2, all USSC Records, NYPL.

21. "Remarks to accompany the Tabular Report of Act. Med. Inspector E. O. F. Roler, 15th Army Corps, for the week ending Sept. 27th 1863, Camp near Black River, Miss.," Ser. 1, Folder 5, Roll 1; "Remarks to accompany Report of Acting Medical Inspector of the 15th Army Corps, Dept. and Army of the Tennessee, for the month of Feb. 1864," Ser. 1, Folder 304, Roll 2; and "Remarks to accompany Report of Act. Med. Inspector of the 15th Army Corps, Army and Dept. of the Tennessee, for the month of March 1864," Ser. 1, Folder 297, Roll 2, all USSC Records, NYPL.

22. Opdycke, *To Battle for God and the Right,* 66, 232–33; Williams, *From the Cannon's Mouth,* 23; Ripley, *Vermont General,* 279; Sargent, "For Our Beloved Country," 49–50; Welch, "Port Hudson."

23. *Harvard Memorial Biographies,* 1:264, 2:342.

24. William M. Chamberlain return, 36th New York, Oct. 9, 1861; George L. Andrews return, 5th Wisconsin, Oct. 21, 1861; and William M. Chamberlain return, 8th New York, Nov. 7, 1861, all Ser. 7, USSC Records, NYPL.

25. George A. Blake returns, 4th Wisconsin and 1st Louisiana Colored Heavy Artillery, Mar. 4, Nov. 7, 1863, Ser. 7, USSC Records, NYPL.

26. James Gall return, 1st US Colored Troops, Sept. 24, 1863, Ser. 7, USSC Records, NYPL.

27. Robert Collyer return, 19th Indiana, Aug. 21, 1861; William M. Chamberlain return, 15th New York Engineers, Oct. 10, 1861; Gordon H. Winslow return, 5th New York, Jan. 22, 1862; T. B. Smith return, 2nd Pennsylvania Artillery, Jan. 7, 1863; and Robert Jones return, 3rd Maine, Aug. 31, 1861, all Ser. 7, USSC Records, NYPL.

28. William W. Estabrook return, 39th Ohio, Apr. 15, 1863, Ser. 7, USSC Records, NYPL.

29. E. J. Dunning return, 1st Vermont, July 21, 1861; Alfred L. Castleman return, 17th Indiana Mounted Infantry, May 21, 1863; and George A. Blake return, 37th New York, Nov. 21, 1861, all Ser. 7, USSC Records, NYPL.

30. Henry W. Warriner return, Battalion, 1st Nebraska Cavalry, Dec. 24, 1861, Ser. 7, USSC Records, NYPL.

31. Robert Collyer return, 5th Wisconsin, Aug. 20, 1861; George L. Andrews return, 5th Wisconsin, Nov. 25, 1861; and Alfred L. Castleman return, 79th Pennsylvania, Mar. 19, 1863, all Ser. 7, USSC Records, NYPL.

32. George L. Andrews return, 9th Maine, Jan. 1, 1862; F. U. Johnston return, 9th New Hampshire, Jan. 7–29, 1863; Bernard J. Bettelheim return, 75th Illinois, Apr. 24–25, 1863; and John H. Douglas return, 1st Missouri Flying Battery, Dec. 27, 1861, all Ser. 7, USSC Records, NYPL.

10. CONFEDERATE SANITATION

1. *Atlanta Constitution,* Aug. 3, 1892; Kaufman, "John Stainback Wilson," 395–99; Wilson, *Southern Soldier's Health Guide,* 6–7.

2. *OR,* ser. 4, 1:692–93.

3. *OR,* ser. 4, 1:794.

4. *OR,* ser. 4, 1:890.

5. Davis, *Papers,* 8:55.

6. Balicki, "'Masterly Inactivity,'" 97, 119, 122, 125, 127; Reeves and Geier, "Under the Forest Floor," 194, 196, 199, 203; Balicki, "Confederate Cantonment at Evansport," 255, 269.

7. *Regulations for the Army of the Confederate States,* 54; T. F. Sevier to Leonidas Polk, Dec. 20, 1862; and Joseph Vaulx Jr. to T. F. Sevier, Mar. 28, 1863, Reel 18, M935, Inspection Reports, NARA.

8. Vaulx to Sevier, Mar. 28, 1863.

9. *OR,* 24(3):924, 29(2):820–21, 42(3):1202–3; Callaway, *Civil War Letters,* 27.

10. For an example of a Confederate inspection report that skirted many aspects of camp sanitation, see "Inspection Report of Anderson's Brigade, Withers' Division," Mar. 24, 1863, Reel 18, M935, Inspection Reports, NARA.

11. Wainwright, *Diary of Battle,* 23; Buckman to Smith, May 11, 1862, George Buckman Civil War Papers, Minnesota Historical Society, St. Paul; Grosh to mother, Feb. 1, 1863, John N. Grosh Letters, HL; Barnhart, "Hoosier Invades the Confederacy," 174; Wills, *Army Life,* 254; Bull, *Soldiering,* 169.

12. Nugent and Nugent, *My Dear Nellie,* 185; Ellison Capers to wife, Sept. 9, 1864, Ellison Capers Papers, The Citadel, Archives and Museum, Charleston, SC.

13. Redfield, "Characteristics of the Armies," 361–62.

14. Lee, *Memoirs of William Nelson Pendleton,* 144, 164; Mott, "War Journal," 237–38; P. L. Prudhomme to mother, Dec. 14, 1862, Prudhomme Family Papers, LSU; Dame, *From the Rapidan to Richmond,* 17–19.

15. Callaway, *Civil War Letters,* 29; Cumming, *Kate,* 118; Goodloe, *Confederate Echoes,* 196–98; Moore, *Story of a Cannoneer,* 169–70; George C. Porter and H. L. Douglas report, May 2, 1862; "Inspection Report of Anderson's Brigade, Withers' Division," Mar. 24, 1863; and Joseph Vaulx Jr. to T. F. Sevier, Mar. 28, 1863, Reel 18, M935, Inspection Reports, NARA.

16. Stanley, *Sir Henry Morton Stanley,* 112.

17. Callaway, *Civil War Letters,* 15, 29; William Dixon diary, July 21, 1863, William Y. Dixon Papers, LSU; Williams, "Company C," 546; Lee, *Memoirs of William Nelson Pendleton,* 163.

18. *Regulations for the Army of the Confederate States,* 11; Vaulx to Sevier, Mar. 28, 1863; "Inspection Report of Anderson's Brigade," Mar. 24, 1863; "Semimonthly report of Clayton's Brigade, Stewart's Division Camp on Missionary Ridge," Oct. 12, 1863, Reel 18, M935, Inspection Reports, NARA.

19. *Regulations for the Army of the Confederate States,* 12; Callaway, *Civil War Letters,* 15, 28.

20. Wise, *End of an Era,* 347.

21. Goodloe, *Confederate Echoes,* 224; Nugent and Nugent, *My Dear Nellie,* 185.

22. Green, *Johnny Green of the Orphan Brigade,* 120; Davis to Bettie, Jan. 11, 1862 [1863], Newton N. Davis Papers, ADAH; John W. Caldwell to Sarah, Jan. 7, 1863, 9th Kentucky Infantry (CS) Regimental File, Stones River National Battlefield, Murfreesboro, TN; Ely and Ely, *Just and Holy Cause?,* 122; Andrew White to Margaret, May 22, 1864, Andrew J. White Letters, Duke University, Rubenstein Rare Book and Manuscript Library, Durham, NC; Goodloe, *Confederate Echoes,* 220, 223.

23. *Regulations for the Army of the Confederate States,* 9–10; Alfred Roman to George W. Brent, Jan. 22, 1865, Alfred Roman Papers, LC.

24. *OR,* ser. 2, 6:577–78, 645, 743.

25. [Steiner], *Report of Lewis H. Steiner,* 8–9, 26.

26. *Regulations for the Army of the Confederate States,* 54; General Orders No. 69, Headquarters, Western Department, June 12, 1862, "General Orders from January 6th 1862 to August 24th 1862," Bragg-Beauregard Order Book, Bound Volumes, Louisiana Research Collection, TU; T. F. Sevier to Leonidas Polk, Dec. 20, 1862, Reel 18, M935, Inspection Reports, NARA; *OR,* 42(3):1203.

27. Sevier to Polk, Dec. 20, 1862; Davis, *Papers,* 9:361.

28. Owsley et al., "Man in the Iron Coffin," 93; Kuttruff, "Confederate Forward Line," 309; *Memphis Daily Appeal,* June 29, 1864; Cashin, "Hungry People in the Wartime South," 160–75.

29. Simeon R. Martin, "Facts About Co. 'I' of the 46th Mississippi Infantry," 77, 46th Mississippi Folder, VNMP; *OR,* 26(1):241–42, 244.

30. *Regulations for the Army of the Confederate States,* 11, 196.

31. *OR,* ser. 4, 1:887, 889.

32. Stanley, *Sir Henry Morton Stanley,* 110–11; Callaway, *Civil War Letters,* 19.

33. Callaway, *Civil War Letters,* 15, 28.

34. George C. Porter and H. L. Douglas report, May 2, 1862; T. F. Sevier to Leonidas Polk, Dec. 20, 1862; Joseph Vaulx Jr. to T. F. Sevier, Mar. 28, 1863; and "Inspection Report of Anderson's Brigade, Withers' Division," Mar. 24, 1863, all Reel 18, M935, Inspection Reports, NARA.

35. William Mattison to Elvira, May 5, Aug. 25, 1862, William N. Mattison Civil War Correspondence, AHC; Williams, *From That Terrible Field,* 99; John Crittenden to Bettie, Jan. 20, 1863, John Crittenden Collection, AU; W. B. Lance to Delia and children, May 31, 1863, Samuel J. Lance Papers, LSU.

36. Moore, *Story of a Cannoneer,* 170; *OR,* ser. 4, 2:1021.

37. *Regulations for the Army of the Confederate States,* 193; *OR,* ser. 4, 1:834–35; *OR,* 20(2):404.

38. T. J. Walker Reminiscences, University of Tennessee, Special Collections, Knoxville; Ingham, "Captain Valentine Merriwether M'Gehee," 142; Jones, "Recollections," 341; Charles Jacob Armstrong Diary, Dec. 30, 1862, ADAH; O'Brien, *Things Grew Beautifully Worse,* 4; Yeary, *Reminiscences of the Boys in Gray,* 404; Hampton, *Eyewitness to the Dark Days of 1861–65,* 24; Charles Barney Dennis Memoirs, 22, Rutherford B. Hayes Presidential Library & Museum, Fremont, OH; Bird, "Stone River."

39. Goodloe, *Confederate Echoes,* 191; Moore, *Story of a Cannoneer,* 172; Davis, *Papers,* 8:45.

40. *OR*, ser. 4, 2:2, 51, 408–9.

41. Hicks, "Scabrous Matters," 131.

42. *Medical and Surgical History*, pt. 3, 1:638, 645; Jones, *Researches upon "Spurious Vaccination,"* 3–4.

43. William Sykes to wife, Dec. 18, 1862, William E. Sykes Papers, Mississippi State University, Special Collections, Starkville; "Diary of Dr. Thomas J. Blackwell," 122; West, "Thirteenth Tennessee," 187; "William J. Rogers' Memorandum Book," 76–77; Newberry, "Civil War Letters," 54; Thompson, "Gallant Old Forty-Fourth Mississippi," 406; Maxwell, *Autobiography*, 159.

44. McGarity, "Letters of a Confederate Surgeon," pt. 1, 98; McGarity, "Letters of a Confederate Surgeon," pt. 3, 229; Owen, "Letters of a Confederate Surgeon in the Army of Tennessee," 79.

45. Williams, *From That Terrible Field*, 59.

46. Taylor and Taylor, *This Cruel War*, 25; Joseph Vaulx Jr. to T. F. Sevier, Mar. 28, 1863, Reel 18, M935, Inspection Reports, NARA; Ely and Ely, *Just and Holy Cause?*, 126.

47. *Regulations for the Army of the Confederate States*, 11, 29, 193; Order No. 1, Mar. 11, 1862, Order Book, 5th Company, Box 12, Folder 1, Louisiana Research Collection, Battalion of Washington Artillery Collection, TU.

48. Roman to George W. Brent, Jan. 22, 1865, Alfred Roman Papers, LC.

49. Jones, "Observations upon the Losses of the Confederate Armies," 349; *Medical and Surgical History*, pt. 3, 1:33.

11. AFTER THE CIVIL WAR

1. *Medical and Surgical History*, pt. 3, 1:7–10.

2. *OR*, ser. 3, 5:668.

3. Cirillo, "'Winged Sponges,'" 54.

4. Cirillo, "'Patriotic Odor,'" 18. For health-care progress in the British Army establishment during the last half of the nineteenth century, see Bricknell and Ross, "Fit to Fight," 2–3.

5. Cirillo, "'Winged Sponges,'" 53–54, 56, 58.

6. Cirillo, "'Patriotic Odor,'" 18–21.

7. Cirillo, "'Winged Sponges,'" 53, 60.

8. Traub, "Military Hygiene," 1, 4–8.

9. Woodhull, *Military Hygiene*, iii, 1, 3–4, 337.

10. Woodhull, *Military Hygiene*, 32–39, 46–153, 178–94, 202, 204–5, 212, 215, 261–88, 325, 341, 345.

11. Woodhull, *Military Hygiene*, 217, 220, 345.

12. Woodhull, "Teaching of Military Hygiene," 531.

13. Sternberg, *Sanitary Lessons of the War*, 1, 4–5, 8–14.

14. Sternberg, *Sanitary Lessons of the War*, 14–15, 17.

15. Coffman, *War to End All Wars*, 13–15.

16. Coffman, *War to End All Wars*, 29.

17. Hauser, "'Violent Desire for the Amusements,'" 885, 887, 892.

18. Cirillio, "Two Faces of Death," 123.
19. Harrison, *Medicine and Victory,* 2, 85, 87, 278.
20. Harrison, *Medicine and Victory,* 276–78.
21. Landers, "Destructiveness of Pre-Industrial Warfare," 457.
22. Cirillo, "Two Faces of Death," 122, 127.
23. Cirillo, "Two Faces of Death," 123–24, 128–29.
24. Hess, *Union Soldier in Battle,* 158–64; Young, *Camping Grounds,* chap. 1.

CONCLUSION

1. Bowditch, *Public Hygiene in America,* 36.
2. Derby, "Lessons of the War," 218, 223–25.
3. Derby, "Lessons of the War," 224.
4. Humphreys, *Marrow of Tragedy,* 271–72; Meier, "U.S. Sanitary Commission Physicians," 19; Hoy, *Chasing Dirt,* 59–60.
5. Howe, *Letters and Journals,* 495.
6. Howe, *Letters and Journals,* 496–97.
7. A. N. Read and M. C. Read, "General Hygienic conditions in the Armies of the Cumberland & Tennessee during the War," Ser. 1, Folder 930, Roll 7, USSC Records, NYPL; Newberry, "Report on the Condition of the Troops and the Operations of the Sanitary Commission," 18, 21.
8. Henry W. Warriner return, 3rd Michigan Cavalry, Dec. 25, 1861, Ser. 7, USSC Records, NYPL.
9. Alex McDonald, "Notes on Sanitation in the Field," Feb. 20, 1866, Ser. 1, Folder 1107, Roll 8; and John H. Douglas to F. Law Olmsted, Aug. 15, 1861, Ser. 7, both USSC Records, NYPL; Meier, "U.S. Sanitary Commission Physicians," 33.
10. *OR,* ser. 2, 4:106, 166, 5:588–89, 686–87.
11. *OR,* ser. 2, 6:575–79.
12. *OR,* ser. 2, 6:644–45, 742–45.
13. *OR,* ser. 2, 6:705–6, 763.
14. "Faults and Failures of the Army Medical System," Ser. 1, Folder "Writings: Faults and Failures of the Army Medical System," Roll 12; William F. Swalm return, Battery I, 1st New York Light Artillery, Mar. 5, 1863, Ser. 7; and James P. Prince, "The Peninsula Campaign 1862," Ser. 1, Folder 511, Roll 4, all USSC Records, NYPL.
15. Phelps, "Remarks on Various Circumstances," 43.
16. Boynton, *History of West Point,* 362–90; McClellan, *Armies of Europe,* 60, 62; Mordecai, *Military Commission to Europe,* 31, 49–50, 134; De Fonblanque, *Treatise on the Administration and Organization of the British Army,* 91, 174, 190–92.
17. Phelps, "Remarks on Various Circumstances," 43–44. For a discussion of the regular army's role in the Civil War generally, see Hsieh, *West Pointers and the Civil War.*
18. "Dr. Aigner's Report on the Sanitary Conditions of the U.S. Forces in the District of Cairo during the months of December & January," Feb. 11, 1862, Ser. 1, Folder "Writings Re. Civil War, 1861–1865," Roll 12; and Marvin M. Marsh return, Battery E, 3rd US Light Artillery, Mar. 18, 1863, Ser. 7, both USSC Records, NYPL.

19. Julius Nichols return, 1st German New York Rifles, Feb. 9, 1863, Ser. 7, USSC Records, NYPL; Higginson, *Life and Letters,* 159; *OR,* 5:720; Hyde, *Following the Greek Cross,* 239–40.

20. F. U. Johnston return, 148th Pennsylvania, Mar. 5, 1863; and Alfred L. Castleman return, 36th Illinois, Apr. 22, 1863, Ser. 7, both USSC Records, NYPL. As a regimental surgeon before he became interested in commission work, Castleman came to understand "that the great mortality of camp life is owing much more to neglect of the proper means within our reach of preserving health, than to any exposures to which the soldier is peculiarly liable." Castleman, *Army of the Potomac,* 39–40.

21. *OR,* ser. 3, 2:235–36.

22. *OR,* ser. 3, 2:237–38.

23. *OR,* ser. 3, 1:115, 225; *OR,* 5:599; Franklin B. Hough comment in Baudens, *On Military and Camp Hospitals,* 189n.

24. *OR,* ser. 3, 3:790–91, 966.

25. *OR,* ser. 3, 3:894, 1054, 1057.

26. *OR,* ser. 3, 5:664.

27. *OR,* ser. 3, 2:564; McDonald, "Notes on Sanitation in the Field," Feb. 20, 1866, Ser. 1, Folder 1107, Roll 8, USSC Records, NYPL.

28. Stanley, *Sir Henry Morton Stanley,* 110–11.

29. Smith, "'Cleanse or Die,'" 178–79.

30. Roberts, *Now for the Contest,* 76–77; *ORN,* 24:324–25.

31. For the latest study of officer effectiveness in the Civil War, see Bledsoe, *Citizen-Officers.*

32. Hammond, *Treatise on Hygiene,* 461.

33. Stillé, *United States Sanitary Commission,* 98–99.

34. *Medical and Surgical History,* pt. 2, vol. 1, 29.

35. Ryan, *Samuel Stouffer and the GI Survey,* 8, 37–40, 71–72, 107–8.

Bibliography

ARCHIVES

Abraham Lincoln Presidential Library, Springfield, Illinois
John Charles Black Papers
George Ditto Diary
Alabama Department of Archives and History, Montgomery
Charles Jacob Armstrong Diary
Newton N. Davis Papers
James Innes Davidson Papers
Atlanta History Center, Atlanta, Georgia
William N. Mattison Civil War Correspondence
James Neuman and Tripp Family Civil War Correspondence
Auburn University, Special Collections and Archives, Auburn, Alabama
John Crittenden Collection
Wright Family Papers
The Citadel, Archives and Museum, Charleston, South Carolina
Ellison Capers Papers
College of William and Mary, Special Collections Research Center, Williamsburg, Virginia
William Taylor Letters
Duke University, Rubenstein Rare Book and Manuscript Library, Durham, North Carolina
Andrew J. White Letters
Eastern Washington University, Archives and Special Collections, Cheney
Thomas Evans Letters and Diary
Harvard University, Center for the History of Medicine, Boston, Massachusetts
Robert Ware Scrapbook

Huntington Library, San Marino, California
John N. Grosh Letters
Lovel Newton Parker Diary
Indiana Historical Society, Indianapolis
Joseph Wright Chamberlain Papers
Joseph H. Waite Diaries
Library of Congress, Manuscripts Division, Washington, DC
Alfred Roman Papers
William Frank Wilder Collection
Library of Virginia, Richmond
George Boardman Tracey Letters
Louisiana State University, Louisiana and Lower Mississippi Valley Collection, Baton Rouge
William Y. Dixon Papers
Simon G. Jerrard Papers
Samuel J. Lance Papers
Prudhomme Family Papers
Massachusetts Historical Society, Boston
Wolcott Family Civil War Carte de Visite Album
Miami University, Special Collections, Oxford, Ohio
Edwin Witherby Brown, "Under a Poncho with Grant and Sherman"
Minnesota Historical Society, St. Paul
George R. Buckman Civil War Papers
Mississippi State University, Special Collections, Starkville
William E. Sykes Papers
Missouri History Museum, St. Louis
Thomas S. Hawley Papers
National Archives and Records Administration, Washington, DC
Inspection Reports and Related Records Received by the Inspection Branch in the Confederate Adjutant and Inspector General's Office, M935, RG 109
National Library of Medicine, Bethesda, Maryland
Lewis H. Steiner Papers
Navarro College, Pearce Civil War Collection, Corsicana, Texas
Sylvester Bartow Papers
New York Public Library, Manuscripts and Archives Division, Astor, Lenox, and Tilden Foundations, New York City
United States Sanitary Commission Records
New York State Library, Albany
Franklin Benjamin Hough Papers
Rutherford B. Hayes Presidential Library & Museums, Fremont, Ohio
Charles Barney Dennis Memoirs
State Historical Society of Missouri, Research Center Columbia
Richard W. Burt Papers
Stones River National Battlefield, Murfreesboro, Tennessee
Ninth Kentucky Infantry (CS) Regimental File

Syracuse University, Special Collections Research Center, Syracuse, New York
Benjamin F. Pease Memoir
Tulane University, Special Collections, New Orleans, Louisiana
"General Orders from January 6th 1862 to August 24th 1862," Bragg-Beauregard Order Book, Louisiana Research Collection
Order Book, 5th Company, Battalion of Washington Artillery, Louisiana Research Collection, Battalion of Washington Artillery Collection
University of California, Special Collections and Archives, Riverside
Isaac C. Pugh Papers
University of Michigan, William L. Clements Library, Ann Arbor
Clement Abner Boughton Papers
John S. Hedges Report
University of Tennessee, Special Collections, Knoxville
T. J. Walker Reminiscences
University of Washington, Special Collections, Seattle
M. F. Force Papers
Vicksburg National Military Park, Vicksburg, Mississippi
Eighth Indiana Folder
Seventeenth Iowa Folder
Forty-Sixth Mississippi Folder
Fifty-Sixth Ohio Folder
Western Reserve Historical Society, Cleveland, Ohio
Wells A. Bushnell Memoirs
Wisconsin Historical Society, Madison
John G. Jones Civil War Letters
Sylvester and Albert Strong Civil War Letters

NEWSPAPERS

Atlanta Constitution
Memphis Daily Appeal
The Morning Call (Paterson, NJ)
New York Times
Springfield (MA) Union
Tuscarawas Advocate (New Philadelphia, OH)

WEBSITES

"Bernard Jean Bettelheim." *Wikipedia.* http://en.wikipedia.org/wiki/Bernard_Jean_Bettelheim.
Estilow, Betsy. "Clara Barton's Network." National Museum of Civil War Medicine, Dec. 5, 2018. https://www.civilwarmed.org/surgeons-call/barton-network/.

"Gordon H. Winslow (1805–1864)." WikiTree. https://www.wikitree.com/wiki/winslow-1751.
"John Ordronaux (doctor)." *Wikipedia*. https://en.wikipedia.org/wiki/John_Ordronaux_(doctor).
"Lewis Henry Steiner." *Wikipedia*. https://en.wikipedia.org/wiki/Lewis_Henry_Steiner.
"Muster-In Roll of Field, Staff and Non-Commissioned Staff in the 84th Regt., N.Y.S.V." New York Division of Military and Naval Affairs. https://dmna.ny.gov/historic/reghist/civil/MusterRolls/Infantry/84thInf_NYSV_MusterRoll.pdf.
"Robert Ware—Union Surgeon." National Museum of Civil War Medicine, https://civilwarmed.org/robert-ware/.
William F. Swalm. Memorial ID 153103427. Find a Grave. Added Oct. 1, 2015. https://www.findagrave.com/memorial/153103427/william-f-swalm.

ARTICLES AND BOOKS

Anderson, David. "Dying of Nostalgia: Homesickness in the Union Army during the Civil War." *Civil War History* 56, no. 3 (Sept. 2010): 247–82.
Babcock, Willoughby M., Jr. *Selections from the Letters and Diaries of Brevet Brigadier General Willoughby Babcock of the Seventy-Fifth New York Volunteers*. Univ. of the State of New York, 1922.
Baker, Levi W. *History of the Ninth Mass. Battery*. J. C. Clark, 1888.
Balicki, Joseph F. "The Confederate Cantonment at Evansport, Virginia." In *Fields of Conflict: Battlefield Archaeology from the Roman Empire to the Korean War*, edited by Douglas Scott, Lawrence Babits, and Charles Haecker, 255–77. Potomac Books, 2009.
Balicki, Joseph F. "The Fall 1863 Bivouac of the 14th Connecticut Infantry." In *From These Honored Dead: Historical Archaeology of the American Civil War*, edited by Clarence R. Geier, Douglas D. Scott, and Lawrence E. Babits, 159–76. Univ. Press of Florida, 2014.
Balicki, Joseph F. "'Masterly Inactivity': The Confederate Cantonment Supporting the 1861–1862 Blockade of the Potomac River, Evansport, Virginia." In *Huts and History: The Historical Archaeology of Military Encampment During the American Civil War*, edited by Clarence R. Geier, David G. Orr, and Matthew B. Reeves, 97–135. Univ. Press of Florida, 2006.
Barber, Lucius W. *Army Memoirs of Lucius W. Barber, Company "D," 15th Illinois Volunteer Infantry, May 24, 1861, to Sept. 30, 1865*. J. M. W. Jones, 1894.
Barnhart, John D., ed. "A Hoosier Invades the Confederacy: Letters and Diaries of Leroy S. Mayfield." Contributed by Ura Sanders. *Indiana Magazine of History* 39, no. 2 (June 1943): 144–91.
Bartholow, Roberts. *A Manual of Instructions for Enlisting and Discharging Soldiers*. J. B. Lippincott, 1864.
Barton, T. H. *Autobiography of Dr. Thomas H. Barton, the Self-Made Physician of Syracuse, Ohio*. West Virginia Printing, 1890.

Baudens, Jean-Baptiste Louis. *On Military and Camp Hospitals, and the Health of Troops in the Field.* Translated and edited by Franklin B. Hough. Bailliere Brothers, 1862.

Beatty, John. *Memoirs of a Volunteer, 1861–1863.* W. W. Norton, 1946.

Becker, Ann M. "Smallpox in Washington's Army: Strategic Implications of the Disease During the American Revolutionary War." *Journal of Military History* 68, no. 2 (April 2004): 381–430.

Beecham, R. K. *As If It Were Glory: Robert Beecham's Civil War from the Iron Brigade to the Black Regiments.* Edited by Michael E. Stevens. Madison House, 1998.

Belknap, William W. "The Obedience and Courage of the Private Soldier." In *War Sketches and Incidents as Related by Companions of the Iowa Commandery, Military Order of the Loyal Legion of the United States,* 1:157–71. Broadfoot, 1994.

Bell, A. N., J. P. Loines, H. D. Bulkley, A. Nebinger, and James F. Hibberd. "Protection from Smallpox by Means of Vaccination and Revaccination for the Eradication of Smallpox." *Transactions of the American Medical Association* 16 (1866): 265–75.

Bellows, H. W. "Notes of a Preliminary Sanitary Survey of the Forces of the United States, in the Ohio and Mississippi Valleys, near Midsummer, 1861." In *Documents of the U.S. Sanitary Commission,* vol. 1, *Numbers 1 to 60,* no. 26. N.p., 1866.

Bentz, Brandon G., Elliot W. Strong, Gayle E. Woodson, and Jatin P. Shah. "The Magnanimous Professional Life and Tragic Demise of J. H. Douglas, MD." *Laryngoscope* 115, no. 8 (Aug. 2005): 1499–1504.

Bentz, Charles, and Yong W. Kim, eds. *The Sevierville Hill Site: A Civil War Union Encampment on the Southern Heights of Knoxville, Tennessee.* Tennessee Anthropological Association Miscellaneous Papers, no. 17. Univ. of Tennessee, 1993.

Bever, Megan L. *At War with King Alcohol: Debating Drinking and Masculinity in the Civil War.* Univ. of North Carolina Press, 2022.

Bies, Brandon S. "Guarding the Junction: The Encampment of the 14th New Jersey Volunteer Infantry." In *Huts and History: The Historical Archaeology of Military Encampment During the American Civil War,* edited by Clarence R. Geier, David G. Orr, and Matthew B. Reeves, 74–91. Univ. Press of Florida, 2006.

Billings, John D. *Hardtack and Coffee, or, The Unwritten Story of Army Life.* George M. Smith, 1887.

Bird, S. W. "Stone River: Comrade Bird Says the Rebels Drank Whisky and Gunpowder." *National Tribune,* July 22, 1886.

Bishop, Judson W. *The Story of a Regiment: Being a Narrative of the Service of the Second Regiment, Minnesota Veteran Volunteer Infantry, in the Civil War of 1861–1865.* N.p., 1890.

Bledsoe, Andrew S. *Citizen-Officers: The Union and Confederate Volunteer Junior Officer Corps in the American Civil War.* Baton Rouge: Louisiana State Univ. Press, 2015.

Bowditch, Henry I. *Public Hygiene in America: Being the Centennial Discourse Delivered Before the International Medical Congress, Philadelphia, September, 1876.* Little, Brown, 1877.

Bowen, J. R. *Regimental History of the First New York Dragoons (Originally the 130th N. Y. Vols. Infantry) During Three Years of Active Service in the Great Civil War.* N.p., 1900.

Boyd, Cyrus F. *The Civil War Diary of Cyrus F. Boyd, Fifteenth Iowa Infantry, 1861–1863.* Edited by Mildred Throne. Louisiana State Univ. Press, 1998.

Boynton, Edward C. *History of West Point, and Its Military Importance During the American Revolution; and the Origin and Progress of the United States Military Academy.* D. Van Nostrand, 1864.

Bricknell, Marin C. M., and David A. Ross. "Fit to Fight: From Military Hygiene to Wellbeing in the British Army." *Military Medical Research* 7, no. 18 (2020): 1–7.

Brown, Kathleen M. *Foul Bodies: Cleanliness in Early America.* Yale Univ. Press, 2009.

Browning, Judkin, and Timothy Silver. *An Environmental History of the Civil War.* Univ. of North Carolina Press, 2020.

Buell, Augustus. *"The Cannoneer": Recollections of Service in the Army of the Potomac.* National Tribune, 1890.

Bull, Rice C. *Soldiering: The Civil War Diary of Rice C. Bull, 123rd New York Volunteer Infantry.* Edited by K. Jack Bauer. Presidio, 1977.

Bushman, Richard L., and Claudia L. Bushman. "The Early History of Cleanliness in America." *Journal of American History* 74, no. 4 (Mar. 1988): 1213–38.

Butterfield, Daniel. *Camp and Outpost Duty for Infantry.* Harper and Brothers, 1862.

Callaway, Joshua K. *The Civil War Letters of Joshua K. Callaway.* Edited by Judith Lee Hallock. Univ. of Georgia Press, 1997.

Cashin, Joan E. "Hungry People in the Wartime South: Civilians, Armies, and the Food Supply." In *Weirding the War: Stories from the Civil War's Ragged Edges,* edited by Stephen Berry, 160–75. Univ. of Georgia Press, 2011.

Castleman, Alfred L. *The Army of the Potomac: Behind the Scenes, a Diary of Unwritten History.* Strickland, 1863.

Cirillo, Vincent J. "'The Patriotic Odor': Sanitation and Typhoid Fever in the National Encampments During the Spanish-American War." *Army History* 49 (Spring 2000): 17–23.

Cirillo, Vincent J. "Two Faces of Death: Fatalities from Disease and Combat in America's Principal Wars, 1775 to the Present." *Perspectives in Biology and Medicine* 51 (2008): 121–33.

Cirillo, Vincent J. "'Winged Sponges': Houseflies as Carriers of Typhoid Fever in 19th- and Early 20th Century Military Camps." *Perspectives in Biology and Medicine* 49, no. 1 (Winter 2006): 52–63.

"Civil War Letters of Brigadier General William Ward Orme—1862–1866." *Journal of the Illinois State Historical Society* 23, no. 2 (July 1930): 246–315.

Clarke, Frances. "So Lonesome I Could Die: Nostalgia and Debates over Emotional Control in the Civil War North." *Journal of Social History* 41, no. 2 (Winter 2007): 253–82.

Coffman, Edward M. *The War to End All Wars: The American Military Experience in World War I.* Univ. Press of Kentucky, 1986.

Coolidge, Richard H. *Statistical Report on the Sickness and Mortality of the Army of the United States, Compiled from the Records of the Surgeon General's Office, Embracing a Period of Sixteen Years, from January, 1839, to January, 1855.* A. O. P. Nicholson, 1856.

Congdon, James A. *Congdon's Cavalry Compendium: Containing Instructions for Non-Commissioned Officers and Privates in the Cavalry Service.* J. B. Lippincott, 1864.

Cooke, Chauncey H. *A Badger Boy in Blue: The Civil War Letters of Chauncey H. Cooke.* Introduction and appendix by William H. Mulligan Jr. Wayne State Univ. Press, 2007.

Copp, Elbridge J. *Reminiscences of the War of the Rebellion, 1861–1865.* Telegraph, 1911.

Craighill, William P. *The Army Officer's Pocket Companion: Principally Designed for Staff Officers in the Field.* D. Van Nostrand, 1862.

Cumming, Kate. *Kate: The Journal of a Confederate Nurse.* Edited by Richard Barksdale Harwell. Louisiana State Univ. Press, 1959.

Dame, William Meade. *From the Rapidan to Richmond and the Spottsylvania Campaign: A Sketch and Personal Narrative of the Scenes a Soldier Saw.* Green-Lucas, 1920.

Davis, Jefferson. *The Papers of Jefferson Davis.* 17 vols. Edited by Lynda Lasswell Crist. Louisiana State Univ. Press, 1971–2008.

De Fonblanque, Edward Barrington. *Treatise on the Administration and Organization of the British Army, with Especial Reference to Finance and Supply.* Longman, Brown, Green, Longmans, and Roberts, 1858.

De Forest, John William. *A Volunteer's Adventures: A Union Captain's Record of the Civil War.* Edited by James H. Croushore. Yale Univ. Press, 1946.

Delafield, Richard. *Report of the Art of War in Europe, 1854, 1855, and 1856.* George W. Bowman, 1860.

Derby, George. "The Lessons of the War to the Medical Profession." *Publications of the Massachusetts Medical Society* 2 (1868): 215–27.

"Diary of Dr. Thomas J. Blackwell, Co. C, 31st Miss. Vol. Inf., CSA, August 15, 1862–December 25, 1861." *Yalobusha Pioneer* 21, no. 3 (Fall 1996): 89–123.

Doyle, Julie A., and John David Smith. "'The Very Best Soldiers in the World': Two Surgeons Examine California's Civil War Recruits." *Military History of the West* 27, no. 1 (Spring 1997): 59–82.

"Dr. Robert Collyer Dead Following Illness of Month." *Chicago Sunday Tribune,* Dec. 1, 1912.

Dwight, Henry C. "Feeding an Army: Startling Quantities of Food Consumed." In *Camp and Field: Sketches of Army Life Written by Those Who Followed the Flag,* compiled by W. F. Hinman, 99–103. N. G. Hamilton, 1892.

Ely, Marcus Bethune, and Martha Frances Ely. *A Just and Holy Cause?: The Civil War Letters of Marcus Bethune and Martha Frances Ely, 1862–1865.* Edited by Linda S. McCardle. Mercer Univ. Press, 2016.

Farr, [William]. "The Health of the British Army, and the Efforts of Recent Sanitary Measures on its Mortality and Sickness." *Journal of the Statistical Society of London* 24, no. 4 (Dec. 1861): 472–84.

Ferguson, John Hill. *On to Atlanta: The Civil War Diaries of John Hill Ferguson, Illinois Tenth Regiment of Volunteers.* Edited by Janet Correll Ellison. Univ. of Nebraska Press, 2001.

Floyd, Fred C. *History of the Fortieth (Mozart) Regiment New York Volunteers.* F. H. Gilson, 1909.

"General Instructions to Sanitary Inspectors." In *Documents of the U.S. Sanitary Commission,* vol. 1, *Numbers 1 to 60,* no. 24. N.p., 1866.

Gillett, Mary C. *The Army Medical Department, 1818–1865.* Center of Military History, 1987.

Gleason, Bruce P. "U.S. Mounted Bands and Cavalry Field Musicians in the Union Army during the Civil War—Background, Duties, and Training." *Journal of Historical Research in Music Education* 27, no. 2 (Apr. 2006): 102–19.

Goodloe, Albert Theodore. *Confederate Echoes: A Voice from the South in the Days of Secession and of the Southern Confederacy.* M. E. Church, South, 1907.

Grace, William. *The Army Surgeon's Manual, for the Use of Medical Officers, Cadets, Chaplains, and Hospital Stewards.* Bailliere Brothers, 1864.

Grafton, Henry D. *A Treatise on the Camp and March, with Which Is Connected the Construction of Field Works and Military Bridges, with an Appendix of Artillery Ranges, &C., for Use of Volunteers and Militia in the United States.* Fetridge, 1854.

Grant, Ulysses S. *The Papers of Ulysses S. Grant.* 28 vols. Edited by John Y. Simon. Southern Illinois Univ. Press, 1967–2005.

Green, Johnny. *Johnny Green of the Orphan Brigade: The Journal of a Confederate Soldier.* Edited by A. D. Kirwan. Univ. Press of Kentucky, 2002.

[Haines, Zenas T.]. *Letters from the Forty-Fourth Regiment M.V.M.: A Record of the Experiences of a Nine Months' Regiment in the Department of North Carolina in 1862–3.* Herald, 1863.

Hall, Isaac. *History of the Ninety-Seventh Regiment New York Volunteers, ('Conkling Rifles'), in the War for the Union.* L. C. Childs and Son, 1890.

Hammond, William A. *A Treatise on Hygiene with Special Reference to the Military Service.* J. B. Lippincott, 1863.

Hammond, William A., Joseph Carson, Edward Hartshorne, Walter F. Atlee, and S. Weir Mitchell. "Scurvy." In *Military Medical and Surgical Essays Prepared for the United States Sanitary Commission, 1862–1864*, 3–29. N.p., 1865.

Hampton, N. J. *An Eyewitness to the Dark Days of 1861–65; or, A Private Soldier's Adventures and Hardships During the War.* By the author, 1898.

Hard, Abner. *History of the Eighth Cavalry Regiment Illinois Volunteers, During the Great Rebellion.* N.p., 1868.

Harrison, Carol E., and Thomas J. Brown. *Zouave Theaters: Transnational Military Fashion and Performance.* Louisiana State Univ. Press, 2024.

Harrison, Mark. *Medicine and Victory: British Military Medicine in the Second World War.* Oxford Univ. Press, 2004.

Harvard Memorial Biographies. 2 vols. Sever and Francis, 1866.

Hauser, Mark T. "'A Violent Desire for the Amusements': Boxing, Libraries, and the Distribution and Management of Welfare During the First World War." *Journal of Military History* 86, no. 4 (Oct. 2022): 883–913.

Hess, Earl J. "Meat-Eating in the Civil War: A Vegetarian Perspective." In *Animal Histories of the Civil War Era*, edited by Earl J. Hess, 149–66. Louisiana State Univ. Press, 2022.

Hess, Earl J. *The Union Soldier in Battle: Enduring the Ordeal of Combat.* Univ. Press of Kansas, 1997.

Hess, Earl J. "Wildlife and the Civil War." In *Animal Histories of the Civil War Era*, edited by Earl J. Hess, 101–20. Louisiana State Univ. Press, 2022.

Hicks, Robert D., ed. *Civil War Medicine: A Surgeon's Diary.* Indiana Univ. Press, 2019.

Hicks, Robert D. "Scabrous Matters: Spurious Vaccinations in the Confederacy."

In *War Matters: Material Culture in the Civil War Era,* edited by Joan E. Cashin, 123–50. Univ. of North Carolina Press, 2018.

Higginson, Henry Lee. *Life and Letters of Henry Lee Higginson.* Edited by Bliss Perry. Atlantic Monthly, 1921.

History of the Fifteenth Regiment, Iowa Veteran Volunteer Infantry, from October, 1861, to August, 1865. R. B. Ogden and Son, 1887.

History of the Seventy-Third Indiana Volunteers in the War of 1861–65. Carnahan, 1909.

Hodge, William Barwick. "On the Mortality Arising from Military Operations." *Journal of the Statistical Society of London* 19, no. 3 (Sept. 1856): 219–71.

Holmes, John Haynes. *The Life and Letters of Robert Collyer, 1823–1912.* 2 vols. Dodd Mead, 1917.

Hough, Franklin B. *History of Duryée's Brigade, During the Campaign in Virginia Under Gen. Pope, and in Maryland Under Gen. McClellan, in the Summer and Autumn of 1862.* J. Munsell, 1864.

Howe, Daniel Wait. *Civil War Times, 1861–1865.* Bowen-Merrill, 1902.

Howe, S. G. *A Letter on the Sanitary Condition of the Troops in the Neighborhood of Boston, Addressed to His Excellency the Governor of Massachusetts.* US Government Printing Office, 1861.

Howe, S. G. *Letters and Journals of Samuel Gridley Howe.* Edited by Laura E. Richards. Dana, Estes, 1909.

Hoy, Suellen. *Chasing Dirt: The American Pursuit of Cleanliness.* Oxford Univ. Press, 1996.

Hsieh, Wayne Wei-siang. *West Pointers and the Civil War: The Old Army in War and Peace.* Univ. of North Carolina Press, 2009.

Humphreys, Margaret. *Intensely Human: The Health of the Black Soldiers in the American Civil War.* Johns Hopkins Univ. Press, 2008.

Humphreys, Margaret. *Marrow of Tragedy: The Health Crisis of the American Civil War.* Johns Hopkins Univ. Press, 2013.

Humphreys, Margaret. "A Stranger to Our Camps: Typhus in American History." *Bulletin of the History of Medicine* 80, no. 2 (Summer 2006): 269–90.

Humphreys, Margaret. "'This Place of Death': Environment as Weapon in the American Civil War." *Southern Quarterly* 53, nos. 3–4 (Spring–Summer 2016): 12–36.

Hyde, Thomas W. *Following the Greek Cross; or, Memoirs of the Sixth Army Corps.* Univ. of South Carolina Press, 2005.

Ingham, Howard M. "Captain Valentine Merriwether M'Gehee." *Publications of the Arkansas Historical Association* 4 (1917): 140–51.

Jackson, Harry F., and Thomas F. O'Donnell. *Back Home in Oneida: Hermon Clarke and His Letters.* Syracuse Univ. Press, 1965.

Jackson, Robert. *A View of the Formation, Discipline, and Economy of Armies.* 3rd ed. Parker, Furnivall, and Parker, 1845.

Jacobsen, Edna L. "Franklin B. Hough, a Pioneer in Scientific Forestry in America." *New York History* 15, no. 3 (July 1934): 311–25.

Johnson, Charles Beneulyn. *Muskets and Medicine; or, Army Life in the Sixties.* F. A. Davis, 1917.

Jones, Jenkin Lloyd. *An Artilleryman's Diary.* Democrat Printing, 1914.

Jones, Joe B. "'Our Brigade Has Never Been in Winter Quarters, but Always in Tents & Moving About . . . ': Lessons Learned from the Archaeological Evaluations of Camp Mason, an Early Confederate Winter Encampment Near Winchester, Virginia." *Quarterly Bulletin of the Archeological Society of Virginia* 54, no. 1 (Mar. 1999): 20–35.

Jones, Joseph. "Observations upon the Losses of the Confederate Armies from Battle, Wounds and Disease During the American Civil War of 1861–1865, with Investigations upon the Number and Character of the Diseases Supervening upon Gun-Shot Wounds." Part 1. *Richmond and Louisville Medical Journal* 8, no. 4 (Oct. 1869): 339–58.

Jones, Joseph. *Researches upon "Spurious Vaccination"; or, The Abnormal Phenomena Accompanying and Following Vaccination in the Confederate Army During the Recent American Civil War, 1861–1865.* Univ. Medical Press, 1867.

Jones, P. R. "Recollections of the Battle of Murfreesboro." *Confederate Veteran* 31 (1923): 341–42.

Kaufman, Martin. "The American Anti-Vaccinationists and Their Arguments." *Bulletin of the History of Medicine* 41, no. 5 (Sept.–Oct. 1967): 463–78.

Kaufman, Martin. "John Stainback Wilson and Female Medical Education." *Journal of the History of Medicine and Allied Sciences* 28, no. 4 (Oct. 1973): 396–99.

Kautz, August V. *Customs of Service for Non-Commissioned Offices and Soldiers.* J. B. Lippincott, 1864.

Knapp, Vincent J. "The Democratization of Meat and Protein in Late Eighteenth- and Nineteenth-Century Europe." *Historian* 59, no. 3 (Spring 1997): 541–51.

Knapp, Vincent J. "Major Dietary Changes in Nineteenth-Century Europe." *Perspectives in Biology and Medicine* 31, no. 2 (Winter 1988): 188–93.

Kuttruff, Carl. "The Confederate Forward Line, Battle of Nashville, Tennessee." In *Fields of Conflict: Battlefield Archaeology from the Roman Empire to the Korean War,* edited by Douglas Scott, Lawrence Babits, and Charles Haecker, 294–313. Potomac Books, 2009.

Lapham, William B. *My Recollections of the War of the Rebellion.* Burleigh and Flynt, 1892.

Landers, John. "The Destructiveness of Pre-Industrial Warfare: Political and Technological Determinants." *Journal of Peace Research* 42, no. 4 (2005): 455–70.

Lee, Susan P. *Memoirs of William Nelson Pendleton, D. D.* J. B. Lippincott, 1893.

Luscombe, Edward Thornhill. *Practical Observations on the Means of Preserving the Health of Soldiers in Camp and in Quarters.* Archibald Constable, 1820.

Macleod, George H. B. *Notes on the Surgery of the War in the Crimea, with Remarks on the Treatment of Gunshot Wounds.* John Churchill, 1858.

[Marsh, M. M.]. "Report on the Sanitary State of the Troops at Charleston." *United States Sanitary Commission Bulletin* 1 (1866): 78–84.

Marshall, Henry. *On the Enlisting, Discharging and Pensioning of Soldiers with the Official Documents on These Branches of Military Duty.* 2nd British ed. A. Waldie, 1840.

Martin, Scott C. "The American Civil War and the Course of Late Nineteenth-Century Temperance Reform." *Social History of Alcohol and Drugs* 33, no. 2 (Fall 2019): 186–205.

Maxwell, James Robert. *Autobiography of James Robert Maxwell of Tuskaloosa, Alabama.* Greenberg, 1926.

Maxwell, William Quentin. *Lincoln's Fifth Wheel: The Political History of the United States Sanitary Commission.* Longman's, Green, 1956.

McClellan, George B. *The Armies of Europe: Comprising Descriptions in Detail of the Military Systems of England, France, Russia, Prussia, Austria, and Sardinia.* J. B. Lippincott, 1862.

McClellan, George B. *European Cavalry: Including Details of the Organization of the Cavalry Service Among the Principal Nations of Europe.* J. B. Lippincott, 1861.

McClellan, George B. *McClellan's Own Story: The War for the Union, the Soldiers Who Fought It, the Civilians Who Directed It, and His Relations to It and to Them.* Charles L. Webster, 1887.

McClellan, George B. *Regulations and Instructions for the Field Service of the U.S. Cavalry in Time of War.* J. B. Lippincott, 1862.

McGarity, Abner Embry. "Letters of a Confederate Surgeon: Dr. Abner Embry McGarity, 1862–1865. Part I." Edited by Edmund Cody Burnett. *Georgia Historical Quarterly* 29, no. 2 (June 1945): 76–114.

McGarity, Abner Embry. "Letters of a Confederate Surgeon: Dr. Abner Embry McGarity, 1862–1865. Part III." Edited by Edmund Cody Burnett. *Georgia Historical Quarterly* 29, no. 4 (Dec. 1945): 222–53.

McGregor, Frank Ross. *Dearest Susie: A Civil War Infantryman's Letters to His Sweetheart.* Edited by Carl E. Hatch. Exposition, 1971.

McNeil, Donald R. "Dr. Alfred L. Castleman, Agitator and Critic." *Wisconsin Medical Journal* 51, no. 3 (Mar. 1952): 291–96.

The Medical and Surgical History of the War of the Rebellion, 1861–65. 3 parts in 6 vols. US Government Printing Office, 1870–88.

Meier, Kathryn Shively. *Nature's Civil War: Common Soldiers and the Environment in 1862 Virginia.* Univ. of North Carolina Press, 2013.

Meier, Kathryn Shively. "Organic Armies: Military Engagement with Nature in the American Civil War." *South Central Review* 33, no. 1 (Spring 2016): 37–52.

Meier, Kathryn Shively. "U.S. Sanitary Commission Physicians and the Transformation of American Health Care." In *So Conceived and So Dedicated: Intellectual Life in the Civil War–Era North,* edited by Lorien Foote and Kanisorn Wongsrichanalai, 19–40. Fordham Univ. Press, 2015.

Moore, Edward A. *The Story of a Cannoneer Under Stonewall Jackson.* J. P. Bell, 1910.

Mordecai, Alfred. *Military Commission to Europe, in 1855 and 1856.* George W. Bowman, 1860.

Morhous, Henry C. *Reminiscences of the 123d Regiment, N.Y.S.V., Giving a Complete History of Its Three Years Service in the War.* Peoples' Journal, 1870.

Mott, Charles R., Jr., ed. "War Journal of a Confederate Officer [William H. Mott]." *Tennessee Historical Quarterly* 5, no. 3 (Sept. 1946): 234–48.

Muffly, Joseph Wendel, ed. *The Story of Our Regiment: A History of the 148th Pennsylvania Vols.* Kenyon, 1904.

Murray, Williamson. *War, Strategy, and Military Effectiveness.* Cambridge Univ. Press, 2011.

Nelson, Dean E. "'Right Nice Little House[s]': Winter Camp Architecture of the American Civil War." In *Huts and History: The Historical Archaeology of Military Encampment During the American Civil War,* edited by Clarence R. Geier, David G. Orr, Matthew B. Reeves, 177–93. Univ. Press of Florida, 2006.

Newberry, J. S. "Report on the Condition of the Troops and the Operations of the Sanitary Commission in the Valley of the Mississippi, for the Three Months Ending Nov. 30, 1861." In *Documents of the U.S. Sanitary Commission,* vol. 1, *Numbers 1 to 60,* no. 36. N.p., 1866.

Newberry, Thomas Jefferson. "The Civil War Letters of Thomas Jefferson Newberry." Edited by Enoch L. Mitchell. *Journal of Mississippi History* 19, no. 1 (Jan. 1948): 44–80.

Nightingale, Florence. *Notes on Hospitals.* 3rd ed. Longman, Green, Longman, Roberts, & Green, 1863.

Nolan, L. E. *Cavalry: Its History and Tactics.* 3rd ed. Bosworth and Harrison, 1860.

Nugent, William L., and Eleanor Smith Nugent. *My Dear Nellie: The Civil War Letters of William L. Nugent to Eleanor Smith Nugent.* Edited by William M. Cash and Lucy Somerville Howorth. Univ. Press of Mississippi, 1977.

O'Brien, John. *Things Grew Beautifully Worse: The Wartime Experiences of Captain John O'Brien, 30th Arkansas Infantry, C.S.A.* Edited by Brian K. Robertson. Butler Center of Arkansas Studies, 2001.

O'Brien, Thomas M., and Oliver Diefendorf, [eds.]. *General Orders of the War Department, Embracing the Years 1861, 1862, & 1863.* 2 vols. Derby and Miller, 1864.

Official Records of the Union and Confederate Navies in the War of the Rebellion. 30 vols. US Government Printing Office, 1894–1922.

[Olmsted, Frederick Law]. "Report of a Preliminary Survey of the Camps of a Portion of the Volunteer Forces Near Washington." In *Documents of the U.S. Sanitary Commission,* Vol. 1, *Numbers 1 to 60,* no. 17. N.p., 1866.

Opdycke, Emerson. *To Battle for God and the Right: The Civil War Letterbooks of Emerson Opdycke.* Edited by Glenn V. Longacre and John E. Haas. Univ. of Illinois Press, 2003.

Ordronaux, John. *Hints on Health in Armies, for the Use of Volunteer Officers.* 2nd ed. D. Van Nostrand, 1863.

Osborn, Thomas Ward. *No Middle Ground: Thomas Ward Osborn's Letters from the Field (1862–1864).* Edited by Herb S. Crumb and Katherine Dhalle. Edmonston, 1993.

Otto, John Henry. *Memoirs of a Dutch Mudsill: The "War Memories" of John Henry Otto, Captain, Company D, 21st Regiment Wisconsin Volunteer Infantry.* Edited by David Gould and James B. Kennedy. Kent State Univ. Press, 2004.

Owen, U. G. "Letters of a Confederate Surgeon in the Army of Tennessee to His Wife." [Part 2]. Edited by Enoch L. Mitchell. *Tennessee Historical Quarterly* 5, no. 1 (Mar. 1946): 60–81.

Owsley, Douglas W., Karin S. Bruevelheide, Larry W. Cartmell Sr., Laurie E. Burgess, Shelly J. Foote, Skye M. Chang, and Nick Fielder. "The Man in the Iron Coffin: An Interdisciplinary Effort to Name the Past." *Historical Archaeology* 40, no. 3 (2006): 89–108.

Perry, John Gardner. *Letters from a Surgeon of the Civil War.* Compiled by Martha Derby Perry. Little, Brown, 1906.

Peters, DeWitt C. "Remarks on the Evils of Youthful Enlistments and Nostalgia." *American Medical Times* 6, no. 7 (Feb. 14, 1863): 75–76.

Peterson, Robert K. D. "Insects, Disease, and Military History: The Napoleonic Campaigns and Historical Perception." *American Entomologist* 41, no. 3 (Fall 1995): 147–60.

Phelps, A. J. "Remarks on Various Circumstances Relating to the Causation of Disease, Especially Among Volunteer Troops, Based on Personal Observations in the Field, During the Years 1861–65." In *Contributions, Relating to the Causation and Prevention of Disease, and to Camp Diseases: Together with a Report of the Diseases, Etc., Among the Prisoners at Andersonville, GA,* edited by Austin Flint, 42–63. Hurd and Houghton, 1867.

Phisterer, Frederick, comp. *New York in the War of the Rebellion, 1861 to 1865.* 6 vols. 3rd ed. J. B. Lyon, 1912.

Poak, David W. *"Dear Sister Sadie": The Letters of David W. Poak, 30th Illinois Infantry During the Civil War: Also the Diary of Edward Grow and Letters of Henry M. McLain.* Edited by Matthew Anderson. Create Space, 2013.

Post, Alfred C., and W. H. Van Buren. *Report on Military Hygiene and Therapeutics.* 4th ed. US Sanitary Commission, 1865.

Pringle, John. *Observations on the Diseases of the Army.* Fry and Kammerer, 1812.

Raoult, Didier, Olivier Dutour, Linda Houhamdi, Rimantas Jankauskas, Pierre-Edouard Fournier, Yann Ardagna, Michel Drancourt, Michel Signoli, Vu Dang La, Yves Macia, and Gérard Aboudharam. "Evidence for Louse-Transmitted Diseases in Soldiers of Napoleon's Grand Army in Vilnius." *Journal of Infectious Diseases* 193, no. 1 (Jan. 2006): 112–20.

Record of the Service of the Forty-Fourth Massachusetts Volunteer Militia in North Carolina, August 1862 to May 1863. Privately printed, 1887.

Redfield, H. V. "Characteristics of the Armies." In *Annals of the War Written by Leading Participants North and South Originally Published in the Philadelphia Weekly Times,* 357–71. Blue & Grey, 1996.

Reeves, Matthew B., and Clarence R. Geier. "Under the Forest Floor: Excavations at a Confederate Winter Encampment, Orange, Virginia." In *Huts and History: The Historical Archaeology of Military Encampment During the American Civil War,* edited by Clarence R. Geier, David G. Orr, Matthew B. Reeves, 194–215. Univ. Press of Florida, 2006.

Regulations for the Army of the Confederate States, 1864. J. W. Randolph, 1864.

Remley, George A., and Lycurgus Remley. *Southern Sons, Northern Soldiers: The Civil War Letters of the Remley Brothers, 22nd Iowa Infantry.* Edited by Julie Holcomb. Northern Illinois Univ. Press, 2004.

Revised Regulations for the Army of the United States, 1861. J. G. L. Brown, 1861.

Rhodes, John H. *The History of Battery B, First Regiment Rhode Island Light Artillery in the War to Preserve the Union, 1861–1865.* Snow and Farnham, 1894.

Ripley, Edward Hastings. *Vermont General: The Unusual War Experiences of Edward Hastings Ripley, 1862–1865.* Edited by Otto Eisenschiml. Devin-Adair, 1960.

Roberts, William H. *Now for the Contest: Coastal and Oceanic Naval Operations in the Civil War.* Univ. of Nebraska Press, 2004.

Roemer, J. *Cavalry: Its History, Management, and Uses in War.* D. Van Nostrand, 1863.

Roemer, Jacob. *Reminiscences of the War of the Rebellion, 1861–1865, by Bvt. Maj. Jacob Roemer.* Edited by L. A. Furney. Flushing Journal, 1897.

Romeyn, Henry. "With Colored Troops in the Army of the Cumberland." In *War Papers: Being Papers Read Before the Commandery of the District of Columbia, Military Order of the Loyal Legion of the United States,* 3: 49–72. Broadfoot, 1993.

Rorabaugh, W. J. "Estimated U.S. Alcoholic Beverage Consumption, 1790–1860." *Journal of Studies on Alcohol* 37, no. 3 (Mar. 1976): 357–64.

Roster of All Regimental Surgeons and Assistant Surgeons in the Late War, with Their Service, and Last-Known Post-Office Address. N. A. Strait, 1882.

Ryan, Joseph W. *Samuel Stouffer and the GI Survey: Sociologists and Soldiers during the Second World War.* Univ. of Tennessee Press, 2013.

Sargent, George. "For Our Beloved Country: The Diary of a Bugler." Edited by Morgan Speer. *Missouri Review* 12, no. 3 (1989): 35–142.

Scherneckau, August. *Marching with the First Nebraska: A Civil War Diary.* Edited by James E. Potter and Edith Robbins. Univ. of Oklahoma Press, 2007.

[Shattuck, Lemuel]. *Report of a General Plan for the Promotion of Public and Personal Health.* Dutton and Wentworth, 1850.

Sheldon, Winthrop D. *"The Twenty-Seventh": A Regimental History.* Morris and Benham, 1866.

Shepherd, William T. *To Rescue My Native Land: The Civil War Letters of William T. Shepherd, First Illinois Light Artillery.* Edited by Kurt H. Hackemer. Univ. of Tennessee Press, 2005.

Sherman, William T. *Sherman's Civil War: Selected Correspondence of William T. Sherman, 1860–1865.* Edited by Brooks D. Simpson and Jean V. Berlin. Univ. of North Carolina Press, 1999.

Simmons, L. A. *The History of the 84th Reg't Ill. Vols.* Hampton Brothers, 1866.

Small, Abner Ralph. *The Road to Richmond: The Civil War Memoirs of Major Abner R. Small of the Sixteenth Maine Volunteers.* Edited by Harold Adams Small. Univ. of California Press, 1939.

Smith, Elise Juzda. "'Cleanse or Die': British Naval Hygiene in the Age of Steam, 1840–1900." *Medical History* 62, no. 2 (Apr. 2018): 177–98.

Smith, F. G., and Alfred Stillé. "Report of a Committee Appointed by the Sanitary Commission to Prepare a Paper on the Value of Vaccination in Armies." In *Military, Medical, and Surgical Essays.* Collins, 1861.

Stanley, David Sloane. *Personal Memoirs of Major-General D. S. Stanley, U.S.A.* Harvard Univ. Press, 1917.

Stanley, Henry M. *Sir Henry Morton Stanley: Confederate.* Edited by Nathaniel Cheairs Hughes Jr. Louisiana State Univ. Press, 2000.

[Steiner, Lewis H.]. *Report of Lewis H. Steiner, M.D., Inspector of the Sanitary Commission, Containing a Diary Kept During the Rebel Occupation of Frederick, MD. and an Account of the Operations of the U.S. Sanitary Commission During the Campaign in Maryland, September 1862.* Anson D. F. Randolph, 1862.

Sternberg, George M. *Sanitary Lessons of the War and Other Papers.* Byron S. Adams, 1912.

Stevenson, Thomas M. *History of the 78th Regiment O.V.V.I., from Its "Muster-In" to Its "Muster-Out."* Hugh Dunne, 1865.

Stewart, Robert B. "The Battle of Stone River, as Seen by One Who Was There." *Blue and Gray* 5 (1895): 10–14.

Stillé, Charles J. *History of the United States Sanitary Commission, Being the General Report of Its Work During the War of the Rebellion.* J. B. Lippincott, 1866.

Stormont, Gilbert R., comp. *History of the Fifty-Eighth Regiment of Indiana Volunteer Infantry.* Clarion, 1895.

Supplement to the Official Records of the Union and Confederate Armies. 100 vols. Broadfoot, 1993–2000.

Taylor, Grant, and Malinda J. Slaughter Taylor. *This Cruel War: The Civil War Letters of Grant and Malinda Taylor, 1862–1865.* Edited by Ann K. Blomquist and Robert A. Taylor. Mercer Univ. Press, 2000.

"Testimony of Medical Officers Respecting the Relations of Physical Endurance and the Power of Resisting Disease to Age, Period of Service, Season, Climate, and Locality; Residence in City or Country Prior to Enlistment; and the Influence of Previous Habits of Life, Remarks on the Physical Characteristics of Different Classes of Recruits and the Influence of Previous Habits, by Dr. S. B. Hunt, Remarks by Dr. Hunt on the Effects of Altitude, Opinions and Facts Pertaining to Alimentation, the Use of Tea and Coffee, and the Whisky Ration." In *Contributions, Relating to the Causation and Prevention of Disease, and to Camp Diseases: Together with a Report of the Diseases, Etc., Among the Prisoners at Andersonville, GA,* edited by Austin Flint, 95–117. Hurd and Houghton, 1867.

Thompson, J. N. "The Gallant Old Forty-Fourth Mississippi." *Confederate Veteran* 28 (1920): 406–7.

Thompson, S. Millett. *Thirteenth Regiment of New Hampshire Volunteer Infantry in the War of the Rebellion, 1861–1865.* Houghton Mifflin, 1888.

Toner, J. M. "A Paper on the Propriety and Necessity of Compulsory Vaccination." *Transactions of the American Medical Association* 16 (1866): 305–30.

Traub, Peter E. "Military Hygiene: How Best to Enforce Its Study in Our Military and Naval Schools and Promote Its Intelligent Practice in Our Army." *Journal of the Military Service Institution of the United States* 36 (Jan.–Feb. 1905): 1–38.

Tuttle, Russell M. *The Civil War Journal of Lt. Russell M. Tuttle, New York Volunteer Infantry.* Edited by George H. Tappan. McFarland, 2006.

Valenčius, Conevery Bolton. *The Health of the Country: How American Settlers Understood Themselves and Their Land.* Basic, 2002.

Van Buren, W. H. *Rules for Preserving the Health of the Soldier.* 5th ed. N.p., originally 1861.

Vance, J. W., ed. *Report of the Adjutant General of the State of Illinois.* 8 vols. H. W. Rokker, 1886.

Viele, Egbert L. *Hand-Book for Active Service: Containing Practical Instructions in Campaign Duties for the Use of Volunteers.* D. Van Nostrand, 1861.

Wainwright, Charles S. *A Diary of Battle: The Personal Journals of Colonel Charles S. Wainwright, 1861–1865.* Edited by Allan Nevins. Harcourt, Brace and World, 1962.

The War of the Rebellion: A Compilation of the Official Records of the Union and Confederate Armies. 70 vols. in 128 pts. US Government Printing Office, 1880–1901.

Warner, John Harley. "Physiological Theory and Therapeutic Explanation in the 1860s: The British Debate on the Medical Use of Alcohol." *Bulletin of the History of Medicine* 54, no. 2 (Summer 1980): 235–57.

Warren, John C. *The Preservation of Health, with Remarks on Constipation, Old Age, Use of Alcohol in the Preparation of Medicines.* Ticknor, Reed, and Fields, 1854.

Webster, Dan, and Don C. Cameron. *History of the First Wisconsin Battery Light Artillery.* N.p., 1907.

Welch, Robert. "Port Hudson: Terrible Days When the Besieging Ranks Were Thinned by Disease and Hostile Bullets." *National Tribune,* Jan. 1, 1903.

West, James Durham. "The Thirteenth Tennessee Regiment—Confederate States of America." *Tennessee Historical Magazine* 7, no. 3 (Oct. 1921): 180–89.

Whitehorne, Joseph W. A. "Blueprint for Nineteenth-Century Camps: Castramentation, 1778–1865." In *Huts and History: The Historical Archaeology of Military Encampment During the American Civil War,* edited by Clarence R. Geier, David G. Orr, Matthew B. Reeves, 28–50. Univ. Press of Florida, 2006.

Whitman, George Washington. *Civil War Letters of George Washington Whitman.* Edited by Jerome M. Loving. Duke Univ. Press, 1975.

Whittaker, Frederick. *Volunteer Cavalry: The Lessons of the Decade by a Volunteer Cavalryman.* By the author, 1871.

Widney, Lyman S. *Campaigning with "Uncle Billy": The Civil War Memoirs of Sgt. Lyman S. Widney, 34th Illinois Volunteer Infantry.* Edited by Robert I. Girardi. Trafford, 2008.

Wilcox, Charles H., and Joseph A. Peters. "Report on Vaccination of the Twenty-First Regiment, New York State Volunteers." *Buffalo Medical and Surgical Journal and Reporter* 1, no. 3 (Oct. 1861): 80–82.

Wild, Frederick W. *Memoirs and History of Capt. F. W. Alexander's Baltimore Battery of Light Artillery, U.S.V.* Maryland School for Boys, 1912.

Wilder, Burt G. *Practicing Medicine in a Black Regiment: The Civil War Diary of Burt G. Wilder, 55th Massachusetts.* Edited by Richard M. Reid. Univ. of Massachusetts Press, 2010.

Wiley, Bell Irvin. *The Life of Billy Yank: The Common Soldier of the Union.* Louisiana State Univ. Press, 1983.

"William J. Rogers' Memorandum Book." *West Tennessee Historical Society Papers* 9 (1955): 59–92.

Williams, A. B. "Company C—Light Battery." In *Histories of the Several Regiments and Battalions from North Carolina in the Great War, 1861–'65,* edited by Walter Clark, 1: 537–50. E. M. Uzzell, 1901.

Williams, Alpheus S. *From the Cannon's Mouth: The Civil War Letters of General Alpheus S. Williams.* Edited by Milo M. Quaife. Wayne State Univ. Press, 1959.

Williams, James M. *From That Terrible Field: Civil War Letters of James M. Williams, Twenty-First Alabama Infantry Volunteers.* Edited by John Kent Folmar. Univ. of Alabama Press, 1981.

Williams, Reub. *General Reub Williams's Memories of Civil War Times.* Edited by Sally Coplen Hogan. Heritage Books, 2004.

Wills, Charles W. *Army Life of an Illinois Soldier.* Globe, 1906.

Wilson, John Stainback. *The Southern Soldier's Health Guide.* N.p., 1861.

Wilson, John Stainback. *Woman's Home Book of Health, Embracing Her Physical Life, Hygiene, and Peculiar Diseases: Being a Brief Description of the Structure and Functions of the Human Body.* J. B. Lippincott, 1860.

Wilson, Mark R. "The Extensive Side of Nineteenth-Century Military Economy: The Tent Industry in the Northern United States during the Civil War." *Enterprise and Society* 2 (June 2001): 297–337.

Winter, Susan E. "Civil War Fortifications and Campgrounds on Maryland Heights: The Citadel of Harpers Ferry." In *Look to the Earth: Historical Archaeology and the American Civil War,* edited by Clarence R. Geier Jr. and Susan E. Winter, 101–29. Univ. of Tennessee Press, 1994.

Wise, John S. *The End of an Era.* Houghton, Mifflin, 1902.

Woodhull, Alfred A. *Military Hygiene for Officers of the Line.* John Wiley and Sons, 1909.

Woodhull, Alfred A. "The Teaching of Military Hygiene." *Journal of the Military Service Institution of the United States* 36 (May–June 1905): 531–34.

Wright, T. J. *History of the Eighth Regiment Kentucky Vol. Inf.* St. Joseph Steam Printing, 1880.

Wyeth, John J. *Leaves from a Diary Written While Serving in Co. E, 44 Mass. Dep't of No. Carolina, from September, 1862 to June, 1863.* L. F. Lawrence, 1878.

Yeary, Mamie, comp. *Reminiscences of the Boys in Gray, 1861–1865.* Smith-Lamar, 1912.

Young, Phoebe S. K. *Camping Grounds: Public Nature in American Life from the Civil War to the Occupy Movement.* Oxford Univ. Press, 2021.

Index

www.ingramcontent.com/pod-product-compliance
Lightning Source LLC
Chambersburg PA
CBHW030800030526
44270CB00031BA/739
9781606355053